Titles of related interest

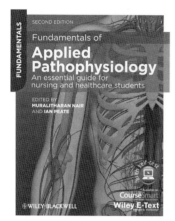

SECOND EDITION

FUNDAMENTALS

Fundamentals of
**Applied
Pathophysiology**
An essential guide for
nursing and healthcare students

EDITED BY
**MURALITHARAN NAIR
AND IAN PEATE**

WILEY-BLACKWELL

Wiley E-Text

ISBN: 978-0-4706-7062-0
Review of the first edition:
"Totally suitable for my module,
covers all the topics in the
module specification. Especially
impressed with diagrams,
MCQs, learning outlines and
test your knowledge" (Senior
Lecturer, Huddersfield
University)

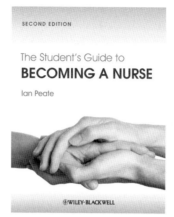

SECOND EDITION

The Student's Guide to
BECOMING A NURSE

Ian Peate

WILEY-BLACKWELL

ISBN: 978-0-470-67270-9
"This comprehensive book will
be indispensable throughout a
student's education." (Nursing
Standard by Sarah Lovie, nursing
student, Royal Cornhill Hospital)

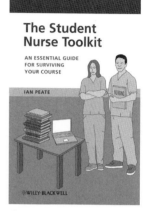

**The Student
Nurse Toolkit**

AN ESSENTIAL GUIDE
FOR SURVIVING
YOUR COURSE

IAN PEATE

WILEY-BLACKWELL

ISBN: 978-1-1183-9378-9
"I instantly felt like I could
relate to the book and to
the ideas of the author in a
way that really built trust
between me as the reader
and what the book was
teaching me." (Second year
adult nursing student,
University of Nottingham)

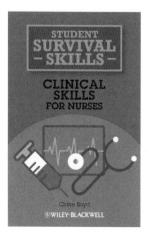

STUDENT
**SURVIVAL
-SKILLS-**

**CLINICAL
SKILLS
FOR NURSES**

Claire Boyd
WILEY-BLACKWELL

ISBN: 978-1-1184-4877-9

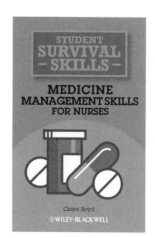

STUDENT
**SURVIVAL
-SKILLS-**

**MEDICINE
MANAGEMENT SKILLS
FOR NURSES**

Claire Boyd
WILEY-BLACKWELL

ISBN: 978-1-1184-4885-4

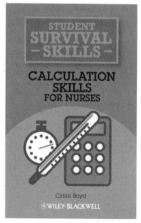

STUDENT
**SURVIVAL
-SKILLS-**

**CALCULATION
SKILLS
FOR NURSES**

Claire Boyd
WILEY-BLACKWELL

ISBN: 978-1-1184-4889-2

"I love this series. . . . I am truly looking forward to them being published as I can't wait to get my hands on them."
(Second year nursing student, University of Abertay, Dundee)

This title is also available as an e-book.
For more details, please see
www.wiley.com/buy/9781118306659 or scan this QR code:

SECOND EDITION

Fundamentals of

Infection Prevention and Control

Theory and practice

DEBBIE WESTON

Deputy Lead Nurse and Operational Lead for Infection Prevention and Control at
East Kent Hospitals University NHS Foundation Trust, Kent, UK

WILEY Blackwell

Library of Congress Cataloging-in-Publication Data

Weston, Debbie.
   Fundamentals of infection prevention and control : theory and practice / Debbie Weston. – 2nd ed.
      p. ; cm.
   Rev. ed. of: Infection prevention and control / Debbie Weston. c2008.
   Includes bibliographical references and index.
   ISBN 978-1-118-30665-9 (pbk. : alk. paper) – ISBN 978-1-118-30769-4 – ISBN 978-1-118-30770-0 (ePub) –
ISBN 978-1-118-30771-7 – ISBN 978-1-118-67383-6 – ISBN 978-1-118-67388-1
   I. Weston, Debbie. Infection prevention and control.   II. Title.
   [DNLM: 1. Cross Infection–prevention & control.   2. Hospitals.   3. Infection Control–methods. WX 167]
   RA761
   362.196'9–dc23

                                        2013012753

A catalogue record for this book is available from the British Library.

Cover image: iStockphoto File #22313218 © Mark Bowden
Cover design by Fortiori Design

Set in 10/12 pt Calibri by Toppan Best-set Premedia Limited
Printed and bound in Singapore by Markono Print Media Pte Ltd

1   2013

Contents

Contents

About the series

Wiley's *Fundamentals* series are a wide-ranging selection of textbooks written to support pre-registration nursing and other healthcare students throughout their course. Packed full of useful features such as learning objectives, activities to test knowledge and understanding and clinical scenarios, the titles are also highly illustrated and fully supported by interactive MCQs, and each one includes access to a Wiley E-Text powered by VitalSource – an interactive digital version of the book including downloadable text and images and highlighting and note-taking facilities. Accessible on your laptop, mobile phone or tablet device, the *Fundamentals* series is *the* most flexible, supportive textbook series available for nursing and healthcare students today.

Preface

Since I wrote the first edition in 2007, which was published in February 2008, much has changed. The threat of an influenza pandemic became a reality in 2009 with the H1N1 'swine flu' pandemic, antibiotic resistance remains an ever-increasing concern, particularly with the emergence of carbapenemase resistance and NDM-1, and although the overall prevalence of healthcare-associated infections (HCAIs) has decreased (and infections caused by meticillin-resistant *Staphylococcus aureus*, or MRSA, and *Clostridium difficile* have decreased significantly), the prevalence of some specific HCAIs has increased. The NHS is experiencing a period of turmoil with the NHS reforms and there are huge concerns in the media not so much around HCAIs but around patient care.

Infection prevention and control are integral parts of patient care and they are everyone's responsibility. HCAIs are harm events, and the principles of infection prevention and control have to be embedded into everyday clinical practice and not be viewed as something separate. The focus now is very much on preventing avoidable HCAIs, with a culture of zero tolerance for avoidable infections and poor practice, and holding staff to account, and it is becoming even more essential that healthcare professionals have a firm grasp of both the principles of infection control that they can relate to clinical practice, and the current issues.

'Infection control' as a speciality is fascinating, complex (although the basic principles are simple), challenging, sometimes very frustrating and extremely diverse, and it is my passion. I hope that this revised and updated second edition will provide the reader with an insight into the work of the Infection Prevention and Control Team and that it will be a valuable resource, not only enhancing their knowledge and understanding of infection control but also encouraging them to look at their own clinical practice and that of others. I also hope that it fosters a real interest in, and enthusiasm for, the subject.

Debbie Weston
Deputy Lead Nurse / Operational Lead, Infection Prevention and Control
East Kent Hospitals University NHS Foundation Trust, Kent, UK

How to get the best out of your textbook

Welcome to the new edition of *Fundamentals of Infection Prevention and Control*. Over the next few pages you will be shown how to make the most of the learning features included in the textbook.

Features contained within your textbook

Every chapter begins with a contents list, an introduction to the topic, and the learning outcomes you should have achieved by the end of the chapter.

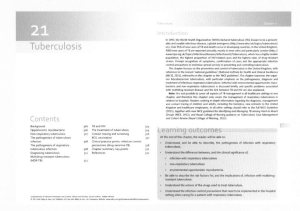

Fact boxes highlight need-to-know information.

Fact Box 5.4   Biofilm activity

Biofilm have been defined as 'a community of micro-organisms irreversibly attached to a surface' (Lindsay and von Holy, 2006) and 'a complex, highly multi-cultural community with a level of activity within the biofilm that resembles a city' (Watnick and Koiter, 2000).

Reflection boxes help you consider the wider implications of the topic or how it relates to your practice.

Reflection point

What other examples can you think of where failure to demonstrate compliance with infection control practice may be viewed as negligent or as a breach of duty of care?

The glossary at the back of the book explains the meaning of the words in bold coloured text.

re based on antigenic differences and
ility, epidemiology and clinical f
ans, also circulate among   y mamm
ies barrier that makes t   serotype the
a viruses with pandemic potential, as
ch originated in Mexico and spread glo
th Organization in 2010). While influen
nza C causes mild disease throughout th
vious pandemics, although that does n

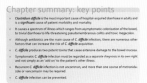

Global outbreak of infection or disease.

Every chapter ends with a summary listing the key points of the topic.

Chapter summary: key points

- *Clostridium difficile* is the most important cause of hospital-acquired diarrhoea in adults and is a significant cause of patient morbidity and mortality.
- It causes a spectrum of illness which ranges from asymptomatic colonisation of the bowel, to trivial diarrhoea to life-threatening pseudomembranous colitis and toxic megacolon.
- Although antibiotics are the main cause of *C. difficile* infection, there are numerous other factors that can increase the risk of *C. difficile* acquisition.
- *C. difficile* produces two potent toxins that cause extensive damage to the bowel mucosa.
- Symptomatic *C. difficile* infection must be regarded as a separate diagnosis in its own right and not simply as an 'add on' to the patient's other illness.
- Recurrent *C. difficile* infection is not uncommon, and more than one course of metronidazole or vancomycin may be required.
- *C. difficile* infection can be prevented.

How to get the best out of your textbook

The anytime, anywhere textbook

Wiley E-Text

For the first time, your textbook comes with free access to a Wiley E-Text Edition – a digital, interactive version of this textbook which you own as soon as you download it.

Your Wiley E-Text Edition allows you to:

Search: Save time by finding terms and topics instantly in your book, your notes, even your whole library (once you've downloaded more textbooks)

Note and Highlight: Colour code, highlight and make digital notes right in the text so you can find them quickly and easily

Organize: Keep books, notes and class materials organized in folders inside the application

Share: Exchange notes and highlights with friends, classmates and study groups

Upgrade: Your textbook can be transferred when you need to change or upgrade computers

Link: Link directly from the page of your interactive textbook to all of the material contained on the companion website

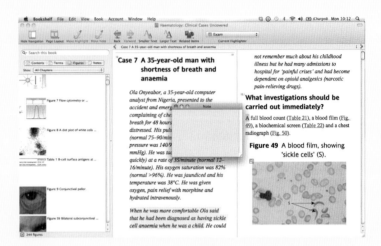

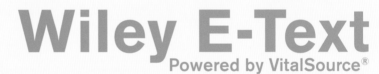

To access your Wiley E-Text Edition:

- Find the redemption code on the inside front cover of this book and carefully scratch away the top coating of the label. Visit www.vitalsource.com/software/bookshelf/downloads to download the Bookshelf application to your computer, laptop or mobile device.
- If you have purchased this title as an e-book, access to your Wiley E-Text Edition is available with proof of purchase within 90 days. Visit http://support.wiley.com to request a redemption code via the 'Live Chat' or 'Ask A Question' tabs.
- Open the Bookshelf application on your computer and register for an account.
- Follow the registration process and enter your redemption code to download your digital book.
- For full access instructions, visit www.wiley.com/go/fundamentalsofinfectionprevention

The VitalSource Bookshelf can now be used to view your Wiley E-Text on iOS, Android and Kindle Fire!

- **For iOS:** Visit the app store to download the VitalSource Bookshelf: http://bit.ly/17ib3XS
- **For Android:** Visit the Google Play Market to download the VitalSource Bookshelf: http://bit.ly/ZMEGvo
- **For Kindle Fire, Kindle Fire 2 or Kindle Fire HD:** Simply install the VitalSource Bookshelf onto your Fire (see how at http://bit.ly/11BVFn9). You can now sign in with the email address and password you used when you created your VitalSource Bookshelf Account.

Full E-Text support for mobile devices is available at: http://support.vitalsource.com

CourseSmart

CourseSmart gives you instant access (via computer or mobile device) to this Wiley eTextbook and its extra electronic functionality, at 40% off the recommended retail print price. See all the benefits at www.coursesmart.com/students.

Instructors . . . receive your own digital desk copies!
It also offers instructors an immediate, efficient, and environmentally-friendly way to review this textbook for your course.

For more information visit www.coursesmart.com/instructors.

With CourseSmart, you can create lecture notes quickly with copy and paste, and share pages and notes with your students. Access your Wiley CourseSmart digital textbook from your computer or mobile device instantly for evaluation, class preparation, and as a teaching tool in the classroom.

Simply sign in at http://instructors.coursesmart.com/bookshelf to download your Bookshelf and get started.

To request your desk copy, hit 'Request Online Copy' on your search results or book product page.

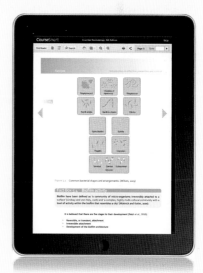

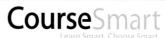

We hope you enjoy your new textbook. Good luck with your studies!

How to use the companion website

Don't forget to visit the companion website for this book:

www.wiley.com/go/fundamentalsofinfectionprevention

There you will find valuable instructor and student material designed to enhance your learning, including:

- interactive multiple choice questions
- scenarios
- fact sheets
- website content glossary
- instructions on how to access your free Wiley e-Text

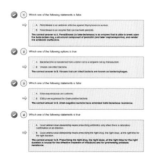

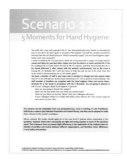

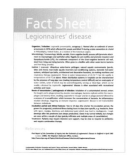

The website contains a number of clinical practice scenarios to work through that are relevant to Chapters 2–5, 9–14 and 20–24.

They can be undertaken from any perspective (e.g. that of a nurse in training, infection control (IC) link practitioner, staff nurse or new-in-post infection prevention and control nurse) and they can be adapted to make them relevant to the reader's workplace.

The reader should apply his or her own local IC policies when responding to the questions where relevant. However, there aren't necessarily any right and wrong answers to some of the questions posed. This is because there are always slight differences in the application of the evidence base for infection prevention and control between different organisations, and therefore minor differences in local policy and practice.

Acknowledgements

I would like to thank:

My family and friends for their patience with me over the last 12 months or so.

The Infection Prevention and Control Specialist Nursing Team at East Kent Hospitals University NHS Foundation Trust for being so supportive – Sue Roberts, Alison Burgess, Zoe Nixon, Kathrin Penticost-Turnbull, Esther Taborn and Catherine Maskell.

I would particularly like to thank Zoe for her assistance with the Scenarios for Chapters 12 and 13 on the companion website.

Dr Angela Kearns at the Staphylococcus Reference Laboratory, HPA Colindale, London for the information regarding the evolution of MRSA and clones.

My very grateful thanks to those at Wiley in particular Magenta Styles, Executive Editor; Madeleine Hurd, Associate Commissioning Editor; Catriona Cooper, Project Editor; Angela Cohen, Production Manager; Cheryl Adam, Copy Editor and Kathy Syplywczak, Project Manager.

Introduction

This book is written with the intention of providing healthcare staff working within acute and primary care with a valuable and comprehensive text that will enable them to understand the theory behind the practice of infection prevention and control, and apply the principles in their day-to-day work. It is envisaged that this book will be a particularly useful resource for student nurses, nurses undertaking postgraduate education, staff nurses, ward or department managers, infection prevention and control link practitioners, and new-in-post infection prevention and control nurses. I hope that it will also be a resource for medical students and foundation year 1 junior doctors.

The book is in four parts. **Part** 1 consists of Chapters 1–10. **Chapter 1** introduces the reader to the problem of healthcare-associated infections (HCAIs), looking at the national and global burden of HCAIs, the risk factors for their development and the threat that infectious diseases pose to public health. It also briefly discusses the challenges of infection prevention and control in acute trust and primary care settings. **Chapter 2** describes the role of the infection prevention and control team and discusses the responsibility, accountability and duty of care that healthcare staff have regarding the prevention and control of infection. **Chapter 3** introduces audit and surveillance, and explains their value in HCAI prevention and reduction, and **Chapter 4** describes aspects of the investigation and management of clusters and outbreaks of infection. In **Chapter 5**, the reader is introduced to the classification, structure and properties of bacteria and viruses, and is also introduced to some of the medically important viruses. **Chapters 6 and 7** aim to give the reader an insight into the importance of obtaining good-quality clinical specimens and the workings of the clinical microbiology laboratory, so that they will understand some of the processes that occur in order to identify the cause of the patient's infection, which in turn influences the patient's treatment. **Chapter 8** describes the basic components and functions of the immune system and how an immune response is generated in patients with an infection, giving rise to systemic signs and symptoms of illness. **Chapter 9** looks at sepsis and neutropenia. Part 1 concludes with **Chapter 10**, which examines the problem of antimicrobial resistance and the implications for patient care and public health, and discusses specific antibiotic-resistant bacteria and associated infections.

In **Part** 2, **Chapters 11–15** focus on the basic principles of infection prevention and control and the underpinning evidence base for hand hygiene, the principles of isolation and cohort nursing, the use of personal protective equipment, the safe use and disposal of sharps, and cleaning.

In **Part** 3, **Chapters 16–19** focus on clinical practice in relation to the management of vascular devices and the prevention of bloodstream infections caused by them, the prevention and management of catheter-associated urinary tract infections, the prevention and management of surgical site infections, and the prevention and management of hospital and community-acquired

Fundamentals of Infection Prevention and Control: Theory and Practice, Second Edition. Debbie Weston.
© 2013 John Wiley & Sons, Ltd. Published 2013 by John Wiley & Sons, Ltd. Companion Website: www.wiley.com/go/fundamentalsofinfectionprevention

pneumonia. In **Part** 4, **Chapters 20–24** are concerned with specific organisms and examine in detail *Staphylococcus aureus* (particularly meticillin-resistant *S. aureus*, or MRSA), tuberculosis, *Clostridium difficile*, norovirus and blood-borne viruses (HIV, hepatitis B and hepatitis C). Each organism is described along with the pathogenesis of infection, the clinical features of infection, laboratory testing and diagnosis, and the infection control management of infected or colonised patients, along with clinical practice points.

The book can be read as a whole from cover to cover, or dipped in and out of. All chapters are cross-referenced and contain learning outcomes, fact boxes, and reflection and clinical practice points. Throughout the book, reference is made to the evidence base arising from national and international guidance and Department of Health policies, drives and initiatives, and there is an emphasis on best practice.

The glossary at the back of the book explains words and terms used (in bold coloured print) in the text. It also directs the reader to the **companion website** at www.wiley.com/go/ fundamentalsofinfectionprevention, where there are numerous fact sheets relating to specific organisms and infections (e.g. *Neisseria meningitidis*, the causative agent of meningococcal disease, and invasive group A streptococcal disease) and clinical practice points (such as aseptic non-touch technique), which are referred to within the chapters but not covered within the text in detail. The website also contains multiple choice questions (MCQs) and clinical practice scenarios for each chapter.

Note: Readers should always refer to the policies in the 'Infection Prevention and Control Manual' within their own place of work. There are often slightly different approaches and variations in local policies, although the basic principles are the same.

Part One

Introduction to infection prevention and control

1

The burden of healthcare-associated infections, and disease threats old and new

Contents

Fundamentals of Infection Prevention and Control: Theory and Practice, Second Edition. Debbie Weston.
© 2013 John Wiley & Sons, Ltd. Published 2013 by John Wiley & Sons, Ltd. Companion Website: www.wiley.com/go/fundamentalsofinfectionprevention

Introduction

This introductory chapter is in two parts. The first part looks at the burden and impact of healthcare-associated infections on the NHS as an organisation and on patients, including risk factors for, and risk factors contributing to, the development of these infections, and the threats to public health posed by old and new infectious diseases. The second part briefly reflects on the changing face of healthcare and summarises some of the key differences and challenges regarding infection control in acute and community care settings.

Learning outcomes

After reading this chapter, the reader will be able to:

- Define healthcare-associated infections (HCAIs).

- List six patient risk factors for the development of HCAIs.

- List 10 general factors that can increase the risk of HCAIs.

- List six ways in which HCAIs can affect patients and healthcare providers.

- Understand the continuing threat to public health from old and new diseases.

Background

The problem of healthcare-associated infections (HCAIs) is not a new one. In 1941, seven years before the creation of the NHS, the British Medical Council recommended that 'control of infection officers' be appointed in hospitals to oversee the control of infection. This was followed in 1944 by the setting up of control of infection committees consisting of clinical and laboratory staff, nurses and administrators.

Fact Box 1.1   The first Infection Control Nurse

The first Infection Control Nurse was appointed in the United Kingdom in 1959 (Gardner *et al.*, 1962). The appointment of Miss E.M. Cottrell, formerly an Operating Theatre Superintendent, as Infection Control Sister at Torbay Hospital, Devon, was in response to a large outbreak of staphylococcal infections affecting both patients and staff. Staphylococci (see Chapters 5 and 20) had been causing problems in UK hospitals since 1955, and staphylococcal surveillance at Torbay Hospital revealed that the carriage rate amongst nursing staff on two of the major hospital wards was 100%, with high staff absentee levels due to staphylococcal skin sepsis, and evidence of post-operative wound infections and skin sepsis amongst the patients.

Miss Cottrell was appointed for an experimental period to assist in the collection of surveillance data and advise healthcare staff on the prevention of cross-infection through rigorous adherence to the principles of asepsis.

6

In 1961, a report on the development of the post of Infection Control Sister was submitted by Dr Brendan Moore, Director of the Public Laboratory in Exeter, to the Joint Advisory Committee on Research of the South West Region Hospital Board. Although the appointment of a nurse as a full-time member of the Infection Control Team was nationally opposed by consultants, Infection Control Sisters were subsequently appointed in many other hospitals.

During the 1960s, an increase in infections caused by Gram-negative bacteria such as *Escherichia*, *Klebsiella*, *Pseudomonas* (see Chapter 10) and *Proteus* started to overtake *Staphylococcus aureus* as agents of cross-infection (Selwyn, 1991). (There are Fact Sheets on all these organisms on the companion website.) *Pseudomonas* in particular established itself as a major opportunistic hospital pathogen in those with underlying illness. During the 1960s and 1970s antibiotic resistance was recognised as an increasing problem, and lurking just around the corner were major resistance problems with staphylococci against methicillin (known as meticillin since 2005), which gave rise to meticillin-resistant *S. aureus* (MRSA). MRSA really started to become problematic in the 1970s, and it exploded during the 1980s (see Chapter 20). Since then, antibiotic resistance has become increasingly common with most strains of bacteria now resistant to one or more antibiotics, and as discussed in Chapter 10, the emergence of pan-resistant strains currently represents a major threat to public health.

The problem of HCAIs

Fact Box 1.2   Definition of a healthcare-associated infection

A healthcare-associated infection can be defined as 'an infection occurring in a patient during the process of care in a hospital or other healthcare facility, which was not present or incubating at the time of admission. This includes infections acquired in the hospital but appearing after discharge and also occupational infections amongst staff of the facility' (World Health Organization [WHO], 2011). An infection occurring within 48–72 hours of admission is considered to be community acquired (unless there is a link with a previous hospital admission); an infection occurring more than 48–72 hours post admission is healthcare associated. HCAIs, especially those that are avoidable, are harm events.

HCAIs are a global concern affecting hundreds of millions of patients per year, with the highest prevalence in developing or low-income countries (WHO, 2011), where resources are limited and reporting and surveillance strategies are weak. In 2011, the publication of the *Report on the Burden of Endemic Healthcare Associated Infection Worldwide* by WHO identified that:

- The prevalence of HCAIs in low and middle-income countries varies between 5.7% and 19.1%.
- Infection rates in newborn babies are 3–20 times higher in low and middle-income countries than in developed or high-income countries; in the former, HCAIs are responsible for 4–56% of deaths in the neonatal period (and 75% of neonatal deaths in Southeast Asia and Sub-Saharan Africa).
- The proportion of patients with infections acquired in intensive care units in low- and middle-income countries ranges from 4.4% to 88.9%.
- The incidence of surgical site infections is up to nine times higher than in developed countries.

As far back as 1995, the Department of Health (DH) (Department of Health and Public Health Laboratory Service, 1995) estimated that:

- Hospital-acquired infections (as they were referred to then) were responsible for the deaths of 5000 patients in the United Kingdom each year.
- HCAIs were probably a contributing factor, but not the primary cause, in at least 15 000 other deaths.
- At any one time, one in 10 patients receiving care in acute hospitals had a hospital-acquired infection, and a significant but undetermined number of patients discharged from hospital into the community also had, or developed, infections related to their hospital stay.
- While it was not possible to prevent all infections, there were several recognised risk factors which increased the risk to patients.
- Between 15 to 30% of infections could be prevented through good clinical or infection control practice.

In 1999, a report by Plowman *et al.* arising from a project funded by the DH had identified that:

- Of hospital in-patients, 7.8% had one or more hospital-acquired infections, and 19.1% of patients reported symptoms of infection post discharge.
- Costs associated with treating patients with infections were 2.9% higher than the costs associated with uninfected patients, representing approximately £3154 per case.
- The average length of stay for patients with an infection was 2.9 times longer and equivalent to an additional 11 days.
- Patients who had an infection identified either in hospital or post discharge took longer to return to normal activities and had more days away from employment as a result.
- Patients with an infection were seven times more likely to die than uninfected patients.
- Hospital-acquired infections were estimated to cost the NHS in England £986.36 million annually.

Concerns regarding the burden of HCAIs and their management and control within the NHS have been highlighted by the National Audit Office (NAO) over the last decade with the publication of three NAO Reports in 2000, 2004 and 2009.

The first NAO Report (2000) stated that the prevention and control of HCAIs were not seen as priorities within the health service, and that the strategic management of hospital-acquired infections needed to be strengthened nationally and at NHS Trust level, as it was clear that the NHS did not have a grip on either the extent of the problem or the resulting financial burden. It also clearly, and significantly, stated that responsibility for the prevention and control of infection did not rest solely with Infection Prevention and Control Teams (IP&CTs). While factors compounding the problem of trying to control infections were acknowledged, the message was clear; the NHS as an organisation had to get its act together, and individual NHS bodies had to accept responsibility and start to take action.

The second NAO Report, published in 2004, went on to identify that a root and branch shift across all levels of the NHS was required if infections were to be kept under control and the burden of HCAIs reduced. The Report acknowledged that although the profile of infection control had undoubtedly increased and there had been 'notable progress at trust level in putting the systems and processes in place and strengthening infection control teams . . . wider factors continue to impede good infection control practices'. The Report stated that the implementation of recommendations had been 'patchy', and that it was imperative that engagement at all levels had to be sought and obtained in order to effect change.

8

In the intervening years between the publication of the second Report and of the third Report, in 2009, a large number of **DH-led drives and initiatives** were developed and implemented. Amongst them were:

- The introduction of national MRSA bacteraemia reduction targets, which had to be investigated as adverse clinical incidents using root cause analysis (RCA) (replaced as of the 1st April 2013 by Post Infection Reviews, or PIRs) (see Chapter 2)
- Mandatory surveillance (beginning in 2004) for *Clostridium difficile* in patients over the age of 65, which was extended in 2007 to include patients aged two and over (see Chapter 3)
- The introduction of a national *C. difficile* reduction target in 2007 (along with the setting of local reduction rates with hospitals by primary care trusts [PCTs] in their role as commissioners of healthcare services) (see Chapter 22)
- The launch in 2005 by the DH of Saving Lives, a delivery programme to reduce healthcare-associated infections including MRSA
- Implementation of new legislation regarding healthcare associated infections with the introduction of the Health Act 2006: *Code of Practice for the prevention and control of healthcare associated infections* (DH, 2006).

The third NAO Report (2009) concluded that although there had been significant changes, including a change of culture, there were still numerous areas for improvement, particularly around strengthening surveillance, reporting HCAIs that contribute to death, significant disability or injury, and improving compliance with practice.

Reflection point

Box 1.1 lists the recognised patient risk factors for the development of HCAIs. How many risk factors can you identify in your patients?

Box 1.1   Patient risk factors for HCAIs

Age > 65 years (see Chapter 8)
Emergency admission to an intensive care unit
Hospital in-patient stay of > 7 days
Insertion of an invasive indwelling device (e.g. vascular access device, urinary catheter or endotracheal tube) (see Chapters 16, 17 and 19)
Surgery (see Chapter 18)
Trauma-induced immunosuppression
Neutropenic (see Chapter 9)
Rapidly, or ultimately fatal, disease
Impaired functional status.

Source: Data from WHO, 2011.

HCAI point prevalence surveys

HCAI point prevalence surveys provide a snapshot of the numbers of cases of illness or disease (e.g. HCAIs) in a population at a given time. A number of HCAI point prevalence surveys have been undertaken in the United Kingdom since the 1980s, as summarised in Table 1.1; Table 1.2 compares the prevalence of specific HCAIs.

Table 1.1   Summary of HCAI point prevalence, United Kingdom, 1980–2012

Year and location	Number of patients included in surveys	HCAI point prevalence
1980, United Kingdom	18 163	9.2%
1996, United Kingdom and Republic of Ireland	37 111	9.0%
2006, England, Wales and Ireland	58 775	8.2% England – 8.2% Wales – 6.3% Northern Ireland – 5.5% Republic of Ireland – 4.9%
2011, Wales	—	4%
2011, England	52 443	6.4%
2011, Scotland	13 558	4.9%

Source: Data from Meers *et al.*, 1981; Emmerson *et al.*, 1996; Hospital Infection Society and Infection Control Nurses Association, 2007; Welsh Healthcare Associated Infection and Antimicrobial Resistance Programme, 2011; Health Protection Agency, 2012; Health Protection Scotland and NHS National Services Scotland, 2012.

Table 1.2   Prevalence of specific HCAIs, 2006 and 2012

HCAI	2006	2012
Urinary tract infections	19.7%	17.2%
Pneumonia and respiratory tract infections	13.9%	22.8%
Surgical site infections	13.8%	15.7%
Gastro-intestinal infections	22%	8.8%
Bloodstream infections	6.8%	7.3%
MRSA prevalence	1.28%	<0.1%
C. difficile prevalence	1.98%	0.4%

Source: Data from Hospital Infection Society and Infection Control Nurses Association, 2007; Health Protection Agency, 2012.

Boxes 1.2 and 1.3 list the factors that contribute to the increase in HCAIs and the impact that HCAIs have on patients and the NHS.

Box 1.2   General factors contributing to the increase in HCAIs

Increase in the number of patients undergoing major surgery and invasive diagnostic procedures

An increasing elderly population with weakened immunity and increased susceptibility to infection
- > 18% of the UK population over retirement age
- 1.3 million people in the United Kingdom aged 85 or over
- 65% of hospital beds occupied by patients over the age of 65

Hospitals no longer able to cope with the patient population – design, layout, condition and maintenance of buildings and environment

Increased bed occupancy rates

Increased patient turnaround times

Increased movement of patients

Lack of isolation facilities

Use of invasive indwelling devices

Lack of equipment

Contaminated equipment and devices

Length of stay

Antibiotic resistance

Poor antimicrobial prescribing (see Chapter 10)

Poor infection control practice

Poor clinical leadership

Poor staff-to-patient ratios

Poor staff morale.

Source: Data from DH, 2000, 2004, 2007; Cunningham *et al.*, 2005; Wigglesworth and Wilcox, 2006; Griffiths *et al.*, 2008; National Office for Statistics, 2009; Poteliakhoff and Thomson, 2011; Imison *et al.*, 2012.

The challenge of disease threats old and new

It is difficult to predict when a new disease with the potential to wreak havoc and destruction will emerge, but an increase in the emergence of new diseases and the re-emergence of old foes such as tuberculosis (see Chapter 21) is inevitable, due to the astounding abilities that microorganisms possess, which enable them to diversify and mutate. Centuries-old infectious diseases such as

Box 1.3   The impact of HCAIs

- Effects on patients and their relatives – fear and anxiety, psychological effects of isolation in a single room or isolation ward, loss of earnings, harm, disability or death
- Increased length of stay
- Delayed discharges – lost bed days and loss of revenue
- Expenditure on litigation, antibiotic prescribing, extra equipment, extra staff and additional cleaning resources (outbreak situations)
- Financial penalties for failing to meet DH HCAI reduction targets and loss of Commissioning for Quality Innovation (CQUIN) funding (no avoidable infections)
- Public confidence in the NHS as an organisation and in local services badly dented
- Adverse publicity
- Poor morale amongst staff.

plague, one of the oldest notifiable diseases known to humans, remain endemic in many parts of the world today; smallpox was eradicated in 1979, but it is recognised as posing a potential public health threat in the event of a deliberate release as an act of bioterrorism. Childhood diseases such as measles (see Chapter 5) and pertussis, both of which are preventable through vaccination, still cause outbreaks. Since the 1970s, more than 30 new infectious diseases have emerged worldwide, including Legionnaires' disease, new-variant Creutzfeldt–Jakob disease (CJD), HIV and hepatitis C (Chapter 24). As demonstrated with the severe acute respiratory syndrome (SARS) pandemic, and decades earlier with the 1918–1919 Spanish influenza pandemic, increases in the global population and global travel have led to an increasingly densely packed and mobile population, meaning that an infectious disease can spread anywhere in the world within a matter of hours. Fact Sheets on plague, smallpox, pertussis, Legionnaires' disease, CJD (along with new-variant CJD) and Spanish influenza are available on the companion website.

SARS

Somewhat prophetically in January 2002, a report by the Chief Medical Officer (DH, 2002) acknowledged that it was inevitable that new infectious diseases would emerge, as at least 30 new infectious diseases had emerged since the 1970s, and that it was therefore 'essential to expect the unexpected'. Ten months later, one such new disease emerged in Southeast Asia, leading to a global outbreak between March and July 2003.

The new disease caused widespread fear and panic, badly affected trade and the travel industry, overwhelmed the provision of healthcare services where the highest burden of cases was seen amongst healthcare workers, and took advantage of the fact that the world is now a highly mobile society by efficiently spreading across the globe. That new disease was SARS, and it was the first new viral disease threat of the twenty-first century. In July 2003, WHO issued a global statement declaring that the last human chain of transmission had been broken and the first global outbreak of SARS had been contained, and in May 2005 it declared that SARS had been eradicated, although whether it has gone forever remains to be seen.

Fact Box 1.3   SARS

SARS affected more than 4300 people in 32 countries, with an additional 8400 probable cases, and resulted in more than 800 deaths (WHO, 2003). The highest mortality rate was seen amongst healthcare workers.

Further information regarding the origin of the SARS virus can be found in Chapter 5.

Fact Box 1.4   The emergence of a novel coronavirus in 2012

In the late summer of 2012, reports emerged out of the Middle East of a novel coronavirus that was causing isolated cases of an acute, severe respiratory illness. The virus appears to be distantly related to, but different from, the SARS virus. Like SARS, the respiratory illness presents as pneumonia, but it does not appear to be (certainly at the moment) readily transmissible. As of the 12th May 2013, there have been 34 laboratory cases, including 18 deaths. Although much is yet to be learnt about this new virus (now officially known as Middle East respiratory syndrome coronavirus, or MERS-CoV), early indications are that, like the SARS virus, it is a zoonosis, and is linked to the bat coronavirus. Further information on this new disease can be found on the WHO and Health Protection Agency (HPA)/Public Health England websites (www.who.int and www.hpa.org.uk).

Pandemic influenza

Microorganisms previously unknown or unrecognised, or thought to cause disease only in animals, can and have evolved to produce more virulent strains which can also affect humans. Avian influenza is one such example (see Fact Sheet 1.1 on the companion website). The world has recently experienced an influenza pandemic, and although it was not as devastating as initially feared, there were a number of deaths globally.

Fact Box 1.5   H1N1 'swine flu' pandemic

The 2009 H1N1 'swine flu' pandemic was caused not by the emergence of a new strain of influenza, but from a triple re-assortment (genes derived from human, swine and avian influenza A viruses) North American swine influenza virus, which in turn had acquired genes from Eurasian strains of influenza.

The story of the H1N1 pandemic, and lessons learnt, can be found on the HPA/Public Health England website at http://www.hpa.org.uk/Topics/InfectiousDiseases/InfectionsAZ/Influenza (HPA, 2013). Information about the influenza virus can be found in Chapter 5.

Changes within the NHS and the provision of healthcare

The healthcare arena has changed significantly since the early days of the NHS, and the NHS itself has undergone immense re-organisation over the last 60 years. It now faces what is widely deemed to be its most radical shake-up yet, with the implementation of the Health and Social Care Act 2012 and the controversial NHS reforms. These are too complex and too numerous to mention here, but the 'story' of the NHS reforms can be read on the Kings Fund website (www.kingsfund.org.uk) in *Never Again? The Story of the Health and Social Care Act 2012: A Study in Coalition Government and Policy Making* (Timmins, 2012), and also at www.nuffieldtrust.org.uk. Further information and updates regarding these reforms and healthcare generally (including HCAIs) can also be found on the DH website (http://www.gov.uk/government/organisations/department-of-health) by using the Search tool. Quite what the implications of these reforms will be regarding the prevention and control of HCAIs within acute trusts and community settings remains to be seen. At the time of writing, all healthcare providers are under tremendous pressure to rein in spending; budgets have been slashed, resources reduced, jobs downgraded or lost, and wards closed. Most healthcare providers have been through some kind of internal re-organisation and re-structuring and yet the pressures on the NHS continue to grow and grow. Certainly the political climate within the last decade, with the introduction of government targets to reduce waiting times in accident and emergency departments and on elective surgery waiting lists (DH, 2000), had an adverse knock-on effect as far as infection prevention and control were concerned, generally giving rise to claims of a 'target culture' within the NHS. The pursuit of targets and the avoidance of associated financial penalties were widely viewed by many frontline staff, including IP&CTs, to be at the expense of infection control, with short cuts taken in clinical practice and procedures and practices not always followed to the letter, giving rise to increased infection rates and some high-profile outbreaks of HCAIs (Healthcare Commission, 2006, 2007).

Secondary versus primary care: infection control in acute trust and primary care settings

Care within the NHS is divided into primary and secondary care, and NHS Trusts are divided into Clinical Commissioning Groups (CCGs), Acute Trusts (including Foundation Trusts), Ambulance Trusts, Mental Health Trusts and Care Trusts.

Fact Box 1.6   Primary care

Eighty percent of patient contact with the NHS happens within primary care settings, which encompass GP surgeries, health centres, walk-in clinics, dental clinics, polyclinics (essentially 'super-surgeries' offering a range of specialist treatments on an out-patient basis), residential and nursing homes, patients' own homes, hospices, schools and nurseries, prisons, podiatry, physiotherapy, speech and language therapy, occupational therapy and community mental health care (National Clinical Guidelines Centre, 2012; National Health Service, 2013).

NHS acute trusts (secondary care)

Acute hospitals provide a range of in-patient and out-patient services and have patients with health-care needs of varying complexity, many of whom require specialist care and invasive interventions. Increasingly within hospitals, ambulatory care wards or units have become commonplace, whereby certain medical conditions are managed as day case attendees. Patients may be referred by their GP or directly from the Emergency Department, negating the need for an emergency hospital admission and reducing the pressure on acute beds. Hospital at Home Teams, working as an arm of an Acute Trust, can facilitate the early release of patients who require long-term intravenous therapy, and provide that care in the patient's own home. Virtual Wards aim to prevent emergency admissions to hospitals through the provision of multi-disciplinary care in the community which is provided along the lines of care within a hospital ward (see Nuffield Trust, 2013).

Much of the focus on the prevention and control of HCAIs generally has been within the acute hospital setting as this has historically been where the risk to patients has been perceived to be the greatest. This is because of the mixing of different patient populations, patients admitted as medical or surgical emergencies and often presenting with associated co-morbidities, rapid turnaround times, high bed occupancy, length of stay, invasive procedures (both diagnostic and surgical), the use of invasive indwelling devices and exposure to pathogens associated with HCAIs. However, care in this type of setting is more controlled, and facilities and resources are more likely to be conducive to best practice. Infection prevention and control within the primary care community present many challenges, some of which are summarised in Box 1.4.

Guidelines that are specific to the primary care setting are available in the DH document *Prevention and Control of Infection in Care Homes – an information resource* (DH/HPA, 2013); the National Institute for Health and Clinical Excellence (NICE) Clinical Guideline *Infection Control: Prevention of Healthcare-associated Infections in Primary and Community Care* (National Clinical Guideline Centre, 2012) and the 2009 publication by the Care Quality Commission, *Working Together to Prevent and Control Infections: A Study of the Arrangements for Infection Prevention and Control between Hospitals and Care Homes*. Also relevant is the *Code of Practice on the Prevention and Control of Infections and Related Guidance* (DH, 2010). In 2007, the DH published *Essential Steps to Safe, Clean Care*, a series of review tools, audits and self-assessment exercises designed to be used by staff providing patient care outside of acute hospital settings, in order to reduce or prevent HCAIs and implement evidence-based best practice in infection prevention and control. These can be accessed at: http://webarchive.nationalarchives.gov.uk/20120118164404/hcai.dh.gov.uk (National Archives, 2012). Infection control advice to care homes, health care centres, hospices and GP surgeries may be given by the local Health Protection Unit (Public Health England), or covered by the Community Infection Control Team. There may be some that do not have any formal infection control 'cover' from an IP&CT at all, hence the importance of the guidelines as described above.

Box 1.4 Infection prevention and control in primary care – challenges

- Patients' own homes – poor standard of living, poverty, neglect and poor standards of hygiene/cleanliness
- Clinics and health centres – older buildings may be cramped, over-crowded and not fit for purpose

- Nursing and residential homes – designed to be 'homely' for residents (e.g. soft furnishings, fixtures and fittings, carpets and shared facilities)
- Décor and estates issues – can impede effective cleaning
- Patients with complex healthcare needs and associated co-morbidities – wounds, intravenous (IV) access and drug-resistant organisms
- Resources and facilities: medical devices (equipment and instruments) – single use (disposable) and re-usable; facilities for the cleaning and decontamination of medical devices that conform to national best-practice standards; adequate levels of staff and appropriate skill mix; and storage of equipment and medical devices
- Environmental cleaning: walls, floors, surfaces, beds, examination couches, chairs and other furnishings and furniture
- Staff in residential care facilities may have dual roles, such as caring for residents plus cleaning duties, and this can pose challenges during outbreaks.
- Staff education and training regarding standard precautions (e.g. hand hygiene, personal protective equipment [PPE], sharps, linen, waste, cleaning and decontamination), the method of delivery of mandatory training and updates, and measuring and ensuring compliance with best practice
- Staff knowledge around the different types of infections that can affect patients, residents and their management; access to policies, protocols and guidance documents
- Compliance with legislation and regulations (e.g. Control of Substances Hazardous to Health Regulations [COSHH], Reporting of Injuries, Diseases and Dangerous Occurrences Regulations [RIDDOR] and waste regulations)
- Implementation of audit and surveillance.

Chapter summary: key points

- Healthcare-associated infections are not a new problem, but they have had an increasingly high profile over the last 10–15 years.

- Community-acquired infections are infections present on admission, or occurring less than 48–72 hours after admission (unless there is a link with a previous episode of healthcare); HCAIs are infections which develop more than 48–72 hours after admission.

- The prevalence of HCAIs has decreased from 8.2% to 6.4% over the last 5 years, and during this time, a number of initiatives and drives to reduce HCAIs have been implemented.

- An increasingly elderly population, changes in healthcare provision, the re-emergence of old infectious diseases, the emergence of new ones and the emergence of novel pathogens mean that the threat of infections and infectious diseases is ever present.

- Although there are many general patient risk factors that increase the risk of HCAIs developing, and many other factors that compound the risk, HCAIs must not be accepted as an inevitable consequence of healthcare intervention.

Further resources are available for this book, including interactive multiple choice questions. Visit the companion website at:

www.wiley.com/go/fundamentalsofinfectionprevention

References

Care Quality Commission (2009). *Working Together to Prevent and Control Infections: A Study of the Arrangements for Infection Prevention and Control between Hospitals and Care Homes*. Care Quality Commission, London.

Cunningham J.B., Kernohan W.G., Sowney, R. (2005). Bed occupancy and turnover interval as determinant factors in MRSA infections in acute settings in Northern Ireland. *Journal of Hospital Infection*. 61 (3), 189–193.

Department of Health (2006). *Code of Practice on the prevention and control of healthcare associated infections*. Department of Health, London.

Department of Health (DH) (2000). *The NHS Plan: A Plan for Investment, a Plan for Reform*. DH, London.

Department of Health (DH) (2002). *Getting Ahead of the Curve: A Strategy for Combating Infectious Diseases (Including Other Aspects of Health Protection)*. Report by the Chief Medical Officer. DH, London.

Department of Health (DH) (2004). *Towards Cleaner Hospitals and Lower Rates of Infection: A Summary of Action*. DH, London.

Department of Health (DH) (2006). *Infection Control Guidance for Care Homes*. DH, London.

Department of Health (DH) (2007). *Essential Steps to Safe Clean Care: Reducing Healthcare Associated Infections*. DH, London.

Department of Health (DH) and Health Protection Agency (HPA) (2013). *Prevention and Control of Infections in Care Homes – an information resource*. Department of Health and Health Protection Agency, London.

Department of Health and Public Health Laboratory Service (1995). *Hospital Infection Control: Guidance on the Control of Infection in Hospitals*. The Hospital Infection Working Group of the Department of Health and Public Health Laboratory Service, London.

Emmerson A.M., Enstone J.E., Griffin M., Kelsey M.C., Smyth E.M. (1996). The second national prevalence survey of infection in hospitals – overview of results. *Journal of Hospital Infection*. 32 (3), 175–190.

Gardner A.M.N., Stamp M., Bowgen J.A., Moore B. (1962). The infection control sister: a new member of the control of infection team in general hospitals. *The Lancet*. October 6, 710–711.

Griffiths P., Renz A., Rafferty A.M. (2008). *The Impact of Organisation and Management Factors on Infection Control in Hospitals: A Scoping Review*. Royal College of Nursing and Kings College, London.

Healthcare Commission (2006). *Investigation into Outbreaks of* Clostridium difficile *at Stoke Mandeville Hospital, Buckinghamshire Hospitals NHS Trust*. Commission for Healthcare Audit and Inspection, London.

Healthcare Commission (2007). *Investigation in Outbreaks of Clostridium difficile at Maidstone and Tunbridge Wells NHS Foundation Trust*. Commission for Healthcare Audit and Inspection, London.

Health Protection Agency (HPA) (2012). *English National Point Prevalence Survey on Healthcare Associated Infections and Antimicrobial Use, 2011. Preliminary Data*. Health Protection Agency, London.

Health Protection Agency (HPA) (2013). http://www.hpa.org.uk/Topics/InfectiousDiseases/InfectionsAZ/Influenza (accessed 1 March 2013)

Health Protection Scotland and NHS National Services Scotland (2012). *Scottish National Point Prevalence Survey of Healthcare Associated Infections and Antimicrobial Prescribing, 2012*. Health Protection Scotland and NHS National Services Scotland, Glasgow.

Hospital Infection Society and Infection Control Nurses Association (2007). *The Third Prevalence Survey of Healthcare-associated Infections in Acute Hospitals: Report for the Department of Health (England)*. Hospital Infection Society, London.

Imison C., Poteliakhoff E.M., Thomson J. (2012). *Older People and Emergency Bed Use: Exploring Variation*. The Kings Fund, London.

Meers P.D., Ayliffe G.A., Emmerson A.M., Leigh D.A., Mayon-White R.T. *et al.* (1981). Report on the national surveillance of infection in hospitals, 1980. *Journal of Hospital Infection*. 2 (Suppl.), 1–11.

National Archives (2012). http://webarchive.nationalarchives.gov.uk/20120118164404/hcai.dh.gov.uk (accessed 2 March 2012)

National Audit Office (NAO) (2000). *The Management and Control of Hospital-acquired Infection in Acute NHS Trusts in England*. Report by the Comptroller and Auditor General, HC 230 Session 1999–2000, 17 February 2000. National Audit Office, London.

National Audit Office (NAO) (2004). *Improving Patient Care by Reducing the Risks of Hospital Acquired Infection: A Progress Report*. HC 876 Session 2003–2004. National Audit Office, London.

National Audit Office (NAO) (2009). *Reducing Healthcare Associated Infections in Hospitals in England*. Report by the Comptroller and Auditor General, HC 560 Session 2008–2009, 12 June 2009. National Audit Office, London.

National Clinical Guidelines Centre (2012). *Infection: Prevention and Control of Healthcare Associated Infections in Primary and Secondary Care*. National Institute for Health and Clinical Excellence, London.

National Health Service (2013). *The NHS in England*. http://www.nhs.uk/NHSEngland/thenhs/about/Pages/authoritiesandtrusts.aspx (accessed 28 February 2013)

National Office for Statistics (2009). *Older People's Day*. http://globalag.igc.org/elderrights/world/2009/olderpersonsday.pdf (accessed 15 December 2012)

Nuffield Trust (2013). *Examining the effectiveness of Virtual Wards*. http://www.nuffieldtrust.org.uk/our-work/projects/examining-effectiveness-virtual-wards (accessed 1 March 2013)

Plowman R., Graves N., Griffin M., Roberts J.A., Swan A.V. *et al.* (1999). *The Socio-economic Burden of Hospital Acquired Infection*. Public Health Laboratory Service, London.

Poteliakhoff E., Thomson J. (2011). *Emergency Bed Use: What the Numbers Tell Us*. The Kings Fund, London.

Selwyn S. (1991). Hospital infection: the first 2500 years. *Journal of Hospital Infection*. 18 (Suppl. A), 5–64.

Timmins N. (2012). *Never Again? The Story of the Health and Social Care Act 2012: A Study in Coalition Government and Policy Making*. The King's Fund and the Institute of Government, London.

Welsh Healthcare Associated Infection and Antimicrobial Resistance Programme (2011). *Point Prevalence Survey of Healthcare Associated Infections, Medical Devices and Antimicrobial Prescribing, 2011 Report*. Welsh Healthcare Associated Infection and Antimicrobial Resistance Programme, Cardiff.

Wigglesworth N., Wilcox M.H. (2006). Prospective evaluation of hospital isolation room capacity. *Journal of Hospital Infection*. 63 (2), 156–161.

World Health Organization (WHO) (2003). SARS: lessons from a new disease. In: *The World Health Report 2003 – Shaping the Future*. WHO, Geneva.

World Health Organization (WHO) (2011). *Report on the Burden of Healthcare-Associated Infection Worldwide: Clean Care Is Safer Care*. WHO, Geneva.

2

The Infection Prevention and Control Team

Contents

Fundamentals of Infection Prevention and Control: Theory and Practice, Second Edition. Debbie Weston.
© 2013 John Wiley & Sons, Ltd. Published 2013 by John Wiley & Sons, Ltd. Companion Website: www.wiley.com/go/fundamentalsofinfectionprevention

Introduction

Responsibility for the prevention and control of healthcare-associated infections does not rest with the Infection Prevention and Control Team. It is an organisational responsibility, an integral component of patient-centred care, and it is the responsibility of all staff to ensure that it is embedded into every aspect of patient care all of the time. This chapter describes the role of the Infection Prevention and Control Team and provides examples of the Team's scope and remit. Responsibility, accountability and duty of care are briefly discussed, along with the importance of ensuring competence with regard to clinical practice. Mention is made of the role of the Infection Control Link Practitioner, followed by determining avoidable and unavoidable infections and the process of root cause analysis (RCA).

Learning outcomes

After reading this chapter, the reader will:

- Understand the remit and activities of the Infection Prevention and Control Team.

- Understand what is meant by responsibility, accountability and duty of care and how these apply to them individually with regard to infection prevention and control.

- Understand the implications of not complying with the *Code of Practice on the Prevention and Control of Infections and Related Guidance*.

- Understand the role of root cause analysis.

The role of the Infection Prevention and Control Team

The *Code of Practice on the Prevention and Control of Infections and Related Guidance* (Department of Health [DH], 2010), part of the Health and Social Care Act 2008, requires healthcare organisations to have, or have access to, 'an appropriate mix of both nursing and consultant medical expertise (with specialist training in infection prevention and control)'. The Infection Prevention and Control Team (IP&CT), whose size and structure vary depending on where they work and the size of the Trust, are the nursing and medical experts responsible for providing the organisation with evidence-based best-practice advice on all aspects of infection prevention and control, and are the only specialist nursing and medical team with responsibility for patients, staff, the public **and** the environment. The Consultant Medical Microbiologists primarily advise on the medical management of patients, dealing with laboratory reports, reviewing patients and advising medical teams on treatment, laboratory testing and diagnosis, and antimicrobial prescribing. Box 2.1 lists some of the activities undertaken by the IP&CT, the majority of which fall under the remit of the IP&CT Specialist Nurses. This list is not all inclusive but is intended to illustrate the scope of the Team's work.

Box 2.1 Remit and activities of the IP&CT

Clinical advice

- Undertake clinical reviews of patients – liaise with nursing and medical staff.
- Respond to ad hoc enquiries.
- Advise on patient placement and patient movement.
- Document laboratory results and advice given.
- Maintain patient records.
- Escalate concerns regarding medical management to the Consultant Medical Microbiologist.
- Hold staff to account for clinical practice.

Liaison

- Executive Team and Trust Board
- All Ward and Department Managers, Matrons and nursing and other departmental staff
- Heads of Nursing and Divisional Directors
- Patients, visitors and other members of the general public
- Risk Management Department or Legal Department
- Human Resources Department
- Bed Manager
- Emergency Planning Officer
- Occupational Health Department
- Medical staff – all grades
- Allied Health Professionals
- Facilities and Hotel Services staff (e.g. contract cleaners, porters, catering staff and transport staff)
- Estates staff and building contractors
- Sterile Services Department
- Supplies Department
- Laboratory staff
- Health Protection Agency/Public Health England Reference Laboratories
- Ambulance Service
- IP&CTs at other Trusts
- Local and other Health Protection Units
- Clinical Commissioning Groups (CCGs)
- Community Infection Control Team
- Community Care Teams – District Nurses, GPs, Nursing and Residential Home Managers, and staff in Community Hospitals
- Communications Department
- Local and national media
- Patient Experience Team
- Local Involvement Network

- Care Quality Commission
- Department of Health
- Health and Safety Executive.

Education and training

- Induction for new staff
- Medical staff induction – all grades
- Student nurse training (links with local university)
- Mandatory training
- Ad hoc training, and participation in study days and education sessions
- Infection Control Link Worker or Link Practitioner programme
- Preceptorship programme for newly qualified staff
- Speaking and presenting at local and national conferences – promoting and sharing best practice
- Writing for publication.

Audit and evaluate clinical practice

- Develop audit tools, Key Performance Indicators and Clinical Indicators.
- Undertake audits in accordance with the annual audit programme – ensure feedback, devise action plans or assist the Ward or Department Manager with action plan development and implementation, monitor progress and compliance, and escalate issues or concerns.
- Audit compliance with the *Code of Practice on the Prevention and Control of Infections and Related Guidance* (DH, 2010).
- Prepare a monthly Infection Control Divisional Performance Report for the Trust Board.
- Participate in local and national surveillance.
- Hold staff to account for clinical practice.

Risk management

- Advise on patient placement, transfer and discharge.
- Patient risk factors for developing healthcare-associated infections (HCAIs).
- Assess the need for ward closure during outbreaks.
- Assess and review the availability of isolation facilities.
- Assess and determine staff knowledge and competency.
- Identify environmental risk factors (e.g. poor fabric or repair, cleanliness).
- Advise on the use and availability of equipment and decontamination processes.
- Engage in preparedness planning (e.g. for pandemic influenza).
- Undertake risk assessments (of patients, the environment and equipment).

Continued

- Engage in ongoing alert organism and alert condition surveillance.
- Comply with NHS Litigation Authority (NHSLA) standards.
- Hold staff to account for clinical practice.

Investigation and management of outbreaks and incidents

- Undertake investigations.
- Organise and chair meetings.
- Write or contribute to the writing of reports and minutes of meetings.
- Chair RCA/PIR meetings.
- Hold staff to account for clinical practice.

Service improvement

- Improve practice and patient care through audit, education and training.
- Develop business cases to support the implementation of best-practice recommendations where there are resource implications.
- Advise on building and refurbishment works.
- Hold staff to account for clinical practice.
- Trial and evaluate products and equipment.
- Assist with research.

Policy development and implementation

- Develop policies, protocols and guidelines based on national evidence-based best-practice recommendations.
- Review the Infection Control Manual.
- Hold staff to account for clinical practice.

Administrative and clerical work

- Maintain patient records or infection control databases.
- Manage emails.
- Write or issue reports.
- Respond to complaints.

The challenges of working as an Infection Prevention and Control (IP&C) Specialist Nurse

IP&C Specialist Nurses have to be many things to many people, often at the same time. They are leaders, educators, facilitators, collaborators, innovators, negotiators, change agents and complex decision makers. Aspiring IP&C Nurses looking to specialise and join an established IP&CT need to demonstrate that they possess a natural sense of curiosity, patience, tact and diplomacy, empathy, a sense of humour, considerable organisational and time management skills, the ability to multi-task, prioritise and work under pressure, as well as a genuine interest in and commitment to HCAI prevention and control.

One of the many challenges that IP&C Specialist Nurses face almost on a daily basis is that of challenging poor practice or non-compliance and holding staff to account (a common theme in Box 2.1) whilst also engaging with staff and fostering excellent working relationships at all levels of the organisation. To do this, they need excellent communication, negotiating and teaching skills, and continually need to show that they are competent, knowledgeable and credible practitioners.

For the IP&C Specialist Nurses to be seen as credible, they need to demonstrate possession of a body of specialist expert knowledge on all aspects of infection prevention and control, including microbiology, immunology, epidemiology (the study of infectious diseases) and decontamination, and in-depth knowledge of the evidence base and national guidance, and their application in everyday clinical practice. An understanding of, and experience working in, different specialities is particularly helpful here as it helps the IP&C Specialist Nurses relate to the challenges that nursing and medical staff face in caring for patients with complex nursing and medical needs. Contrary to popular belief, the IP&CT do not always have the perfect answer or solution to every question or dilemma. A credible IP&C Specialist Nurse, however, will always be consistent with his or her advice and arrive at a response or solution that is fair, reasonable, practical and based on a sound risk assessment.

As healthcare has advanced over the years and the nature of infections and infectious diseases has changed, so too has the role of IP&C Specialist Nurses, and the level of knowledge, skills and competencies that they need has increased substantially. Competencies for IP&C Nurses and Practitioners were first developed by the Infection Control Nurses Association in 2000 and reviewed in 2004, before being extensively revised in 2011 (Burnett and the Infection Prevention Society and Competency Steering Group, 2011). These currently consist of 17 competencies which sit within the four advanced practitioner domains (clinical practice, education, research, and leadership and management) and are linked to the NHS knowledge and skills framework (DH, 2004).

The role of Infection Control Link Practitioners

Infection Control Link Nurses or Link Practitioners play a very valuable role in HCAI prevention and control, working within their designated clinical areas (e.g. as nurses, healthcare assistants or therapy staff) and acting as role models and champions for infection prevention and control within their workplace. They assist the IP&C Specialist Nurses with promoting best practice and educating staff, and are a link between the ward or department and the IP&CT. They are **not** solely responsible for ensuring compliance with clinical practice and policies, or for challenging and dealing with non-compliance and poor practice. They need to be supported and developed in the role, and provided with the necessary skills, competencies and clinical support to enable them not only to perform the role effectively but also to derive professional satisfaction from undertaking it. If the Link Practitioner does not have the support of his or her line manager, if the role, remit and boundaries are not clearly defined, and if the culture within the ward or department is not one of promoting infection prevention and control, Link Practitioners will flounder. To this end, the Royal College of Nursing is currently in the process of developing a Link Nurse framework, which includes core competencies (Royal College of Nursing, 2011).

Responsibility, accountability and duty of care

All staff are **responsible** for the care that they give, and are **accountable**, or answerable to someone, for their actions. They also have a **duty of care**, which is a legal obligation to ensure that patients in their care come to no harm as a consequence of any acts or omissions by the healthcare worker. As has been mentioned in this chapter, one aspect of the role of the IP&CT is to hold staff to account and to challenge poor infection control practice and non-compliance (**compliance** essentially means acting in accordance with agreed standards or guidelines). Therefore, it is essential that staff understand that they are responsible for their practice in relation to infection prevention and control, and for protecting their patients, as far as is practically and reasonably possible, from HCAIs, and that they answerable to someone (i.e. the IP&CT) if they are non-compliant. For example, failure to record the visual infusion phlebitis (VIP) scores for two days on a patient with a peripheral cannula in situ (see Chapter 16), who subsequently develops a cannula site infection leading to a bloodstream infection, could be viewed as **negligent**, meaning that harm has been caused to the patient through careless omission (as opposed to a deliberate act), and that the duty of care to the patient has been breached.

Reflection point

What other examples can you think of where failure to demonstrate compliance with infection control practice may be viewed as negligent or as a breach of duty of care?

Holding staff to account is **not** about apportioning blame. It **is** about encouraging responsibility, ownership and engagement with and for infection prevention and control, and the IP&CT and healthcare staff working together to reduce, prevent, control and manage HCAIs and the risks to patients. Infection control is an integral component of patient centred care. Aspects of infection prevention and control practice such as screening patients for MRSA, inspecting cannula sites, and completing IC documentation (for example), must not be viewed as 'add-ons', only to be completed if there is time. They are as important as all other aspects of patient care and interventions, not separate to it.

Competency

Staff must have the competency or ability to undertake tasks or clinical interventions, and part of this ability means possessing the necessary knowledge and skills. There are several areas of clinical practice in relation to infection prevention and control where clinical staff are formally required to demonstrate competency. For example:

- Peripheral cannula insertion
- Urinary catheter insertion
- Blood culture collection
- Endoscope decontamination.

Other areas of clinical practice where competency is required but may not be formally assessed are:

- Surgical hand antisepsis (surgical scrubbing)
- Hand washing and application of alcohol hand rub
- Insertion and management of bowel management systems (used for patients with faecal incontinence or intractable diarrhoea)
- Specimen collection (may result in an inappropriately sized specimen being obtained, or contamination of the specimen)
- Administration of the meticillin-resistant *Staphylococcus aureus* (MRSA) decolonisation protocol (the patient may be inadequately decolonised if the 'decol' is not administered correctly – see Chapter 20).

The Nursing and Midwifery Council (NMC) Code, *The Code: Standards of Conduct, Performance and Ethics for Nurses and Midwives* (NMC, 2008), states that nurses 'must recognise and work within the limits of . . . competence'. To undertake certain clinical interventions or practices without the appropriate knowledge, skills and training places patients at risk of HCAI, and also places the healthcare worker at risk.

Documentation

All care given to patients should be accurately documented. This includes any verbal advice that the IP&CT have conveyed to staff (e.g. requests for screening or isolation) and infection control risk assessments. Screening and specimen collections should be recorded, invasive device insertion and ongoing care records completed each shift, stool charts completed and infection control patient management plans and patient pathways completed. Where there are gaps and omissions in the patient's paperwork, the legal interpretation is that care was not given.

The IP&CT have to make many complex decisions regarding patients, and to do so without the full picture is very difficult. If the Team are investigating a cluster of infections, a period of increased incidence or a ward-acquired MRSA bacteraemia, incomplete documentation relating to the management and care of the patients concerned serves to illustrate that there has been non-compliance with infection control clinical practice standards.

Avoidable versus unavoidable infections

The NHS Operating Framework for 2012–2013 (DH, 2011) continues to emphasize the ongoing drive towards zero avoidable infections.

Fact Box 2.1   Avoidable and unavoidable infections

Chapters 1 and 8 identify the various risk factors that can increase the risk of patients developing HCAIs. Sometimes, in spite of all appropriate measures being taken, a patient will develop an infection. If full compliance with infection control practice and policies can be demonstrated or evidenced, then the infection will be deemed to be unavoidable. If, however, there is evidence of poor clinical practice and non-compliance, the infection will be deemed avoidable. Any successful reduction in HCAIs requires a zero-tolerance approach by all healthcare staff with regard to poor infection control practice and non-compliance with policies, protocols and evidence-based best-practice recommendations.

Reflection point

What examples of poor clinical practice or non-compliance with infection control policy can you think of that may result in an avoidable HCAI? What are the reasons for non-compliance?

The Health and Social Care Act 2008: *Code of Practice on the Prevention and Control of Infections and Related Guidance*

Under the Health and Social Care Act 2008, the *Code of Practice on the Prevention and Control of Infections and Related Guidance* (DH, 2010) sets out the responsibilities of all healthcare and adult social care providers in England in relation to the prevention and control of HCAIs. It is a legal requirement that all registered providers of healthcare register with the Care Quality Commission (CQC) (www.cqc.org.uk), which is the independent regulator of health and social care in England, ensuring that national standards of safety and quality are met, and it is a requirement of registration that providers comply with the *Code*. There are 10 compliance criteria (Box 2.2).

Box 2.2   Compliance criteria: *Code of Practice on the Prevention and Control of Infections and Related Guidance*

- Have systems to manage and monitor the prevention and control of infection.
- Provide and maintain a clean and appropriate environment in managed premises that facilitates the prevention and control of infections.
- Provide suitable accurate information on infections to visitors.
- Provide suitable accurate information on infections to any person concerned with providing further support or nursing or medical care in a timely fashion.
- Ensure that people who have or develop an infection are identified promptly and receive the appropriate treatment and care to reduce the risk of passing on the infection to other people.
- Ensure that all staff and those employed to provide care in all settings are fully involved in the process of preventing and controlling infection.
- Provide or secure adequate isolation facilities.
- Secure adequate access to laboratory support as appropriate.
- Have and adhere to policies designed for the individual's care and provider organisations that will help to prevent and control infections.
- Ensure, so far as is reasonable practicable, that care workers are free of and are protected from exposure to infections that can be caught at work, and that all staff are suitably educated in the prevention and control of infection associated with the provision of healthcare.

Source: Data from DH, 2010.

Each criterion consists of subcriteria and examples of application or evidence, such as policies on standard infection control precautions (including hand hygiene), aseptic non-touch technique, outbreaks, MRSA, *C. difficile*, respiratory tuberculosis, 'diarrhoeal outbreaks' (i.e Norovirus), the safe handling of sharps and the prevention of occupational exposure to blood borne viruses (BBVs), and the management of invasive devices. The full requirements in relation to the above, plus many other requirements, are laid out within the Code, particularly in criterion 9. Some (not all) are covered within the Chapters within this book. The reader should be aware that compliance with the Code is implict in *every* chapter and integral to *every* topic/aspect of infection prevention and control that is described/discussed. Where healthcare providers breach compliance with the *Code*, the CQC can:

- Remove, or impose, conditions of registration.
- Suspend registration with the CQC.
- Cancel registration.
- Issue a warning notice.
- Issue a fixed penalty notice.
- Issue a caution.
- Prosecute.

Root Cause Analysis (RCA)/Post Infection Review (PIR)

RCA has been widely used in the investigation of HCAIs since the introduction of the MRSA bacteraemia target (see Chapter 3), when it became a requirement that RCA was undertaken for all MRSA bacteraemias. Since then it has been used for the investigation of *Clostridium difficile* infection and other HCAIs, and as part of the investigation and management of clusters, periods of increased incidence and outbreaks of infection (see Chapter 4). Like audit (see Chapter 3), RCA now forms part of any HCAI reduction programme. It is also widely used for the investigation and management of patient care incidents that are not related to infection prevention and control. Box 2.3 identifies the healthcare staff who may need to be present at an RCA/PIR meeting.

Box 2.3   Who needs to be present at an RCA/PIR?

Infection Prevention and Control Team
Ward Manager
Matron
Head of Nursing
Staff nurses and IC Link Practitioners as appropriate
Consultant, Registrar and Foundation Year Doctors
Antimicrobial Pharmacist
Representative from the Clinical Commissioning Group
Facilities and Hotels Services Manager (if there are concerns regarding cleanliness standards)
Other healthcare professionals as appropriate, such as the Community Infection Control Team, District Nurses if the patient has had community or primary care involvement, or if the RCA is being held in a community or primary care setting
If the RCA/PIR is being held in a community or primary care setting, the patient's GP will be involved.

The purpose of RCA, or in the case of an MRSA bacteraemia, a PIR is to determine why an incident happened, identify the critical issues or problems (root causes) that led to the incident occurring and take steps to ensure that it does not happen again. To be of value, it needs to be undertaken robustly and involve collaborative working with the multi-disciplinary team, and a detailed preliminary investigation before the RCA/PIR takes place, incorporating a timeline of events, is essential in order to piece together the 'story' of what happened. Box 2.4 lists the areas of compliance with infection control practice and policy that need to be investigated with regard to an MRSA bacteraemia.

Box 2.4   Investigating an MRSA bacteraemia

- Date and time of admission

- Type of admission (elective or emergency)

- Place of residence (own home or care facility) or contact with other health care providers (i.e. hospice/respite care)

- Reason for admission and diagnosis

- Whether the patient was known to be MRSA-positive at the time of admission (i.e. previous history of MRSA colonisation)

- Date and time of blood culture collection

- Number of positive blood culture bottles or sets

- The patient's medical history (may identify risk factors), including any previous admissions within the last year, and the dates and results of past MRSA screens and other significant laboratory results

- Was the patient screened for MRSA on admission in accordance with Trust policy? Record the date, time and sites screened (were clinical specimens obtained from all appropriate sites?) and where the patient was screened (e.g. Emergency Department, Admissions Unit or ward).

- Did the patient have a vascular access device inserted on admission? Was it put in by the ambulance crew or inserted in the department or ward? Who inserted it, when and why? Is there an insertion and care record? How was the skin decontaminated prior to insertion? If it was inserted by the ambulance crew, was it removed and re-sited within 24 hours of admission to hospital?

- Was the patient pyrexial or septic on admission? Were bloods taken? What were the inflammatory markers (see Chapter 8)?

- What interventions were undertaken, and why?

- What ward was the patient admitted or transferred to, and when?

- What was the result of the MRSA admission screen, and when was it confirmed? If positive, was the patient decolonised appropriately (i.e. decolonisation was prescribed and administered correctly for the full five days)? Was the commencement of decolonisation delayed, and if so, why? Are there gaps on the prescription chart, MRSA Patient Management Plan or MRSA Patient Pathway indicating missed doses? Who administered the decol – was the patient self-administering, or was it done by the nursing staff? Were they competent to administer the decol?

- If the patient was MRSA-positive from the admission screen, was he or she isolated or cohort nursed?

- If the patient was MRSA-negative on admission, were there other MRSA positive patients on the ward? If so, where were they nursed in relation to this patient? Had there been an increase in the number of ward-acquired MRSA colonisations amongst patients on the ward?

- Was the patient screened appropriately during his or her admission?

- Is there documentary evidence that all device-related interventions were undertaken appropriately? Examples include recording the dates and times for all interventions, recording VIP scores twice daily and removing or re-siting cannulae at 96 hours if still required, using Instillagel on insertion of urinary catheter (see Chapter 17) and not interrupting the circuit.

- Did the patient have any wounds/areas of non-intact skin or poor skin integrity?

- What were the patient's vital signs? Did he or she develop a pyrexia? Were the inflammatory markers raised? If so, when and why? What actions were taken?

- Was the patient prescribed antibiotics at any point? If so, what were they, why were they prescribed and were they the correct antibiotics? Had the Team liaised with the Consultant Microbiologist?

- Was the patient's overall condition improving or deteriorating?

- When was the blood culture taken, why, from which site and by whom? Was the person taking the blood culture competent to do so (evidence of competency required)? How was the skin decontaminated?

- Was the bacteraemia clinically significant, or was the blood culture contaminated through poor collection technique? Was the bacteraemia avoidable or unavoidable?

The role of the IP&CT in RCA/PIR is to hold staff to account, challenge poor practice and work with staff in identifying the points for learning and developing and implementing the action plan. However, it is also important that the process highlights and promotes good practice and that this is shared amongst healthcare teams.

Reflection point

Three patients on a ward in the same bay develop *C. difficile* infection (see Chapter 22) over a period of three weeks. It is known that there were delays in isolating the first patient and that there have been some issues regarding clinical practice. An RCA is to be undertaken. What aspects of infection control clinical practice do you think will be relevant to the RCA (you may wish to look at Chapter 3)? What do you think the learning might be?

Chapter summary: key points

- The IP&CT are the nursing and medical experts responsible for providing evidence-based best-practice advice on all aspects of infection prevention and control.

- They are the only specialist nursing and medical team with responsibility for patients, staff, the public and the environment.

- The IP&CT hold staff to account and challenge poor practice and non-compliance.

- Infection Control Link Nurses and Link Practitioners act as role models and champions for infection prevention and control within their workplace.

- Staff have a professional responsibility and duty of care to protect their patients from HCAIs, and are accountable for their actions.

- It is a requirement of registration with the Care Quality Commission that registered health-care providers are compliant with the *Code of Practice on the Prevention and Control of Infections and Related Guidance*.

- Root Cause Analysis/Post Infection Review of infection incidents helps healthcare teams to determine why an incident happened, identify the critical issues and problems (root causes) that led to the incident occurring and take steps to ensure that it does not happen again.

 Further resources are available for this book, including interactive multiple choice questions. Visit the companion website at:

www.wiley.com/go/fundamentalsofinfectionprevention

References

Burnett E., the Infection Prevention Society and Competency Steering Group (2011). Outcome competencies for practitioners in infection prevention and control. *Journal of Infection Prevention*. 12 (2): 67–90. http://bji.sagepub.com/content/12/2/67 (accessed 1 March 2013)

Department of Health (DH) (2004). *The NHS Knowledge and Skills Framework (KSF)*. Department of Health, London.

Department of Health (DH) (2010). *Code of Practice on the Prevention and Control of Infections and Related Guidance*. Department of Health, London.

Department of Health (DH) (2011). *The Operating Framework for the NHS in England, 2012/13*. Department of Health, London.

Royal College of Nursing (2011). *The Role of the Link Nurse in Infection Prevention and Control (IPC): Developing a Link Nurse Framework.* Royal College of Nursing, London.

Nursing and Midwifery Council (NMC) (2008). *The Code: Standards of Conduct, Performance and Ethics for Nurses and Midwives*. Nursing and Midwifery Council, London.

3

Audit and surveillance

Contents

Fundamentals of Infection Prevention and Control: Theory and Practice, Second Edition. Debbie Weston.
© 2013 John Wiley & Sons, Ltd. Published 2013 by John Wiley & Sons, Ltd. Companion Website: www.wiley.com/go/fundamentalsofinfectionprevention

Introduction

All healthcare staff are involved in audit and surveillance in some form, and it is an integral part of the Infection Prevention and Control Team's work as they undertake activities in accordance with their annual audit and surveillance programme. This chapter explains what audit and surveillance are, their importance in the prevention and control of healthcare-associated infections and how they are undertaken, and gives examples of routine audit and surveillance activities.

Learning outcomes

After reading this chapter, the reader will:

- Be able to state the benefits of audit with regard to patient care and infection control practice.

- List the five main purposes of surveillance.

- Understand what is meant by alert organism, alert condition and notifiable diseases surveillance.

- List at least six alert organisms, six alert conditions and six notifiable diseases.

- List the organisms that form part of the national mandatory surveillance scheme.

Audit

In a nutshell, the purpose of audit, or clinical audit to give it its proper title, is to review patient care in order to ensure that best practice is being implemented. Best practice equates to quality care for patients, and as has previously been emphasised, the prevention and control of healthcare-associated infections (HCAIs) are fundamental components of patient care. Therefore, assurance that best practice with regard to infection prevention and control is in place *and* is being adhered to is crucial, and auditing compliance with infection control standards forms an integral part of any HCAI prevention programme.

Fact Box: 3.1   Saving Lives and *Essential Steps*

In 2007, the Department of Health (DH) introduced Saving Lives High Impact Interventions (HIIs), a series of care bundles and simple audit tools relating to key clinical procedures and/or core components of patient care which, if all elements are applied consistently and correctly, can reduce the risk of infection and therefore improve patient care and promote best practice. These were designed for implementation within Acute Trusts. For healthcare staff working in a variety of community settings, *Essential Steps to Safe, Clean Care* was published (DH, 2006), consisting of a number of best-practice guidance and simple audit and review tools. Both Saving Lives and *Essential Steps* have evolved over the years, with existing audit and review tools being revised and new ones being developed.

With regard to infection prevention and control, the majority of audits, which are designed to review certain aspects of patient care and compliance with clinical practice, involve the use of simple audit tools and, for the most part, can be undertaken by pretty much anyone at any time – as long as healthcare staff understand *what* it is they are being asked to audit, *why* and *how* to do it. This is important as the results are only as good as the information obtained and while this may be influenced by the design of the audit tool itself, it may also be down to the individual who is undertaking the audit and collating the information.

Box 3.1 lists examples of some infection control audits that staff may be required to undertake weekly or monthly.

Box 3.1   Examples of infection control audits that may be undertaken weekly or monthly

- Hand hygiene observational audits – compliance with the 5 Moments for Hand Hygiene approach and hand decontamination at the point of care (see Chapter 12)
- Observational audit of compliance with a Bare Below the Elbows policy (see Chapter 12)
- Commodes – cleanliness; decontaminated in between each episode of patient use and labelled
- Meticillin-resistant *Staphylococcus aureus* (MRSA) screening within 24 hours of admission to hospital (see Chapter 20)
- The number of patients on a ward on a given day of the week or month with a peripheral cannula or a urinary catheter in situ
- Completion of visual infusion phlebitis (VIP) scores (peripheral cannulae) (see Chapter 16)
- Base or static mattresses, zipped seat cushions and other items with a foam interior – integrity and cleanliness of inner and outer covers and foam core
- Antimicrobial prescribing – evidence of antimicrobial stewardship and compliance with antimicrobial prescribing guidelines (usually undertaken by an Antimicrobial Pharmacist or medical staff)
- Observational audits of compliance with standard precautions (personal protective equipment use and disposal; sharps handling and disposal; segregation of healthcare waste)
- Documentation – for example, completion of Infection Control Patient Management Plans or Pathways and completion of stool charts.

Reflection point

How many infection control-related audits take place within your clinical area? Who is responsible for undertaking the audits? How are the results fed back and acted upon?

More in-depth and complex audits, such as annual audits of Infection Control Environmental and Clinical Practice Standards, and audits of compliance with decontamination procedures in

Endoscopy Departments, are generally undertaken by the Infection Prevention and Control Specialist Nurses in conjunction with Ward and Department Managers; antimicrobial prescribing audits may be undertaken by junior medical staff or the Antimicrobial Pharmacist. In some Infection Prevention and Control Teams (IP&CTs), the majority of audit and surveillance work may be undertaken by Audit and Surveillance Nurses. The Clinical Audit Department will also be involved, and may be asked by the IP&CT to undertake a Trust-wide audit across all clinical areas on a given day; for example, an audit of all patients with a vascular access device (VAD) in situ. Box 3.2 lists examples of some of the larger infection control audits.

Box 3.2   Some examples of larger infection control audits that may be undertaken annually or more frequently

- Audit of hand hygiene facilities – for example, number and location of sinks; availability of liquid soap, paper towels and moisturiser; availability of alcohol hand rub; hand hygiene posters displayed; sinks compliant with the standards for clinical wash hand basins; and sinks and splash backs intact
- Hospital-wide audit of commodes (undertaken on a particular day) – for example, the number of commodes available in each ward or department; cleanliness or evidence of soiling; labelled with date and time cleaned; whether frame or parts are intact or require replacement
- Compliance with MRSA screening – for example, admission and long-stay screens, including whether staff are obtaining the correct clinical specimens as part of the screening process, and screening within the correct time frame
- Management of VADs – for example, number of patients on all wards with a VAD in situ, indication for and date of insertion, completion of all components of device insertion and ongoing care records
- Annual audit of compliance with Infection Control Environmental and Clinical Practice Standards
- Hospital-wide annual audit of compliance with the safe handling and disposal of sharps
- Annual audit of the management of healthcare staff presenting in Occupational Health or the Emergency Department following a needlestick injury
- Isolation rooms – for example, the number of rooms available on site; the number that are en-suite; whether the rooms are used appropriately; if in use – is appropriate signage displayed? Is the door closed? Are the room and equipment within it clean?
- Availability of Patient Information Leaflets – for example, are the 'mandatory' Infection Control Patient Information Leaflets displayed and available, and are they given to patients when required?
- Audit of compliance with endoscope decontamination standards – within Endoscopy Departments and other departments where a variety of scopes may be used and processed (i.e. Outpatients, Theatres, Intensive Care Unit and Day Surgery).

Staff can feel overwhelmed with audit, as it can be applied to virtually any aspect of patient care, and subsequently it may actually be viewed by hard-pressed healthcare staff as a hindrance and an added burden in terms of paperwork. This may mean that it is poorly completed or not undertaken at all, and it may be viewed simply as another paper exercise, in which case it will lose its value. Equally, if audit results are not acted upon (some actions may be beyond the scope of Ward and Department Managers or Matrons to implement, particularly if they require expenditure), or if staff do not receive feedback, then it is easy to become disillusioned and see no real value or purpose in the audit process.

The IP&CT have to engage with staff regarding infection prevention and control audits; they can be a powerful tool for change, and should be viewed positively, either as an indicator of the effectiveness of clinical practice, or as a benchmark to raise standards and improve patient care. Poor audit findings indicate poor clinical practice and poor compliance with infection control policies, and while this can be demoralising for staff, it indicates that there are risks for patients.

As mentioned in Chapter 4, the IP&CT will usually undertake some spot audits of compliance with clinical practice and compliance with infection control policies, for example:

- MRSA admission and long-stay screening, including clinical specimen collection
- The prescribing and administration of the MRSA decolonisation protocol
- Isolation or cohort nursing
- Commode cleanliness
- Use of, and cleanliness of, isolation side rooms
- VIP score recording.

For audit to be effective, the results should be fed back to staff promptly; depending on the particular audit undertaken, immediate feedback is generally possible, followed by a written report. Audit results should also be fed back at staff meetings, form part of the agenda at clinical governance meetings, and be included in monthly and quarterly infection control reports to Divisions, Directorates and the Trust Board. Taking ownership of the results, good or bad, is all part of the process. This may mean developing an action plan, which may be undertaken by the IP&CT depending on the nature of the audit and then disseminated to the appropriate managers for implementation locally, or devised by Ward or Department Managers or Matrons, implemented and fed back to the IP&CT. The Action Plan itself will have to be audited to ensure effective implementation and sustained improvement.

Surveillance

Surveillance essentially means supervision or close observation and has several purposes:

- It enables the early identification of illnesses, infectious diseases and infections that can lead to outbreaks.
- It enables trends to be identified.
- It assists in the identification of risk factors for the development of infection.
- It allows control measures to be evaluated.
- It leads to improvements in practice and patient care, both locally and nationally.

Alert organism surveillance, alert condition surveillance, notifiable disease surveillance and mandatory or voluntary surveillance take place continuously. All healthcare staff are involved in surveillance activities on a daily basis, even if they are not directly aware that what they are doing forms part of surveillance.

Alert organism surveillance

Alert organisms (see Box 3.3) are those that can cause cross-infection and outbreaks in healthcare settings, and alert organism surveillance is routinely undertaken by the IP&CT and the Microbiology Laboratory. When these organisms are identified, the IP&CT will instruct the healthcare team to implement control measures to contain them and prevent their spread (i.e. standard precautions in conjunction with specific infection control policies).

Box 3.3   Alert organisms

- MRSA (see Chapter 20)
- 'Atypical' resistant MRSA (i.e. mupirocin-resistant)
- Panton–Valentine leukocidin-producing strains of *Staphylococcus aureus* and MRSA
- *Clostridium difficile* (antigen only or antigen and toxin) (see Chapter 22)
- *Streptococcus pyogenes* (group A streptococcus) (see Fact Sheet 3.9 on the companion website)
- *Legionella* species (see Fact Sheet 1.3 on the companion website)
- Extended-spectrum β-lactamases (ESBLs) and carbapenem-resistant organisms (see Chapter 10)
- Glycopeptide-resistant enterococci (GRE) (see Fact Sheet 3.2 on the companion website)
- Group B haemolytic streptococci (group B strep) in pregnant women or neonates
- Resistant Gram-negative bacilli – *Acinetobacter*, *Pseudomonas aeruginosa* and *Stenotrophomonas maltophilia* (see Chapter 10)
- *Campylobacter* species (see Fact Sheet 3.1 on the companion website)
- *Salmonella* species (see Fact Sheets 3.5 and 3.7 on the companion website)
- *Escherichia coli* 0157 (see Chapter 10).

Alert conditions

These are conditions that may have wider public health implications which become apparent on investigation, and may require escalation to the local Health Protection Unit (see Box 3.4). Alert condition surveillance is also undertaken by the IP&CT as part of their daily work, and alert conditions may be identified through routine visits to wards and departments. Some of these conditions may also be noticed or suspected by other healthcare staff and reported by telephone, or mentioned during a chance meeting in a corridor.

Box 3.4   Examples of alert conditions

- Infectious diarrhoea (see Chapters 22 and 23)
- Food poisoning
- Scabies and infestations (see Fact Sheet 3.6 on the companion website)
- Tuberculosis (see Chapter 21)
- Chickenpox and shingles (see Fact Sheet 3.11 on the companion website)
- Meningococcal disease (see Fact Sheet 3.4 on the companion website)
- Typhoid and paratyphoid fever (see Fact Sheet 3.10 on the companion website)
- Viral hepatitis
- Patients admitted with infections
- Post-operative surgical site infection and surgical sepsis (see Chapter 18)
- Creutzfeldt–Jakob disease (CJD) (see Fact Sheet 1.2 on the companion website).

Surveillance of notifiable diseases

Certain diseases (see Box 3.5), labelled notifiable diseases, can pose a serious threat to public health, with the potential to cause outbreaks and epidemics unless they are promptly investigated and control measures implemented. Notification, which has to be made to the proper officer (the Consultant in Communicable Disease Control at the local Health Protection Unit) by the doctor looking after the patient, is a statutory duty (legal requirement) and must not be delayed until positive laboratory confirmation has been received; it must be made as soon as a single case is suspected.

Fact Box 3.2   The origins of notifiable diseases

Diseases such as diphtheria, typhus, scarlet fever, cholera and smallpox, which regularly caused epidemics and carried a high mortality rate, first became notifiable in London in 1881 (McCormick 1993). Then, the head of the household, or landlord, and the doctor attending the patient were responsible for following the process for notification. Over the last 110 years or so, more diseases have been made notifiable, and under the Health Protection (Notification) Regulations (2010), there are also 60 notifiable bacteria and viruses (Health Protection Authority [HPA], 2010).

Box 3.5   List of notifiable diseases (England and Wales)

Note: All HPA citations in this box refer to web pages containing basic disease information and links for further reading.

- Acute encephalitis
- Acute infectious hepatitis
- Acute meningitis (see Fact Sheet 3.4 on the companion website)
- Acute poliomyelitis (see HPA, 2013h)
- Anthrax
- Botulism (see HPA, 2013a)
- Brucellosis (see HPA, 2013d)
- Cholera (see HPA, 2013b)
- Diphtheria (see HPA, 2013c)
- Enteric fever (typhoid and paratyphoid)
- Food poisoning
- Haemolytic uraemic syndrome
- Infectious bloody diarrhoea
- Invasive group A streptococcal disease (see Fact Sheets 3.3, 3.8 and 3.9 the companion website)
- Legionnaires' disease
- Leprosy (see HPA, 2013e)
- Malaria (see HPA, 2013f)
- Measles (see Chapter 5)
- Meningococcal septicaemia (see Fact Sheet 3.4 on the companion website)
- Mumps (see Chapter 5)
- Plague (see Fact Sheet 1.5 on the companion website)
- Rabies (see HPA, 2013i; World Health Organization [WHO], 2013b)
- Rubella (see Chapter 5)
- SARS (see Chapter 1 and Chapter 5)
- Scarlet fever
- Smallpox (see Fact Sheet 1.7 on the companion website)
- Tetanus (see HPA, 2013j)
- Tuberculosis (see Chapter 21)
- Typhus
- Viral haemorrhagic fever (see Fact Sheet 3.12 on the companion website; and see WHO, 2013a)
- Whooping cough (pertussis) (see Fact Sheet 1.4 on the companion website)
- Yellow fever (see HPA, 2013k).

Source: Health Protection Agency (http://www.hpa.org.uk/Topics/InfectiousDiseases/InfectionsAZ/NotificationsofInfectiousDiseases/ListofNotifiableDiseases).

Mandatory and voluntary surveillance

MRSA bacteraemia

Attributable mortality due to MRSA may be difficult to ascertain, but there is evidence to suggest that MRSA bacteraemia carries twice the attributable mortality of meticillin-sensitive *Staphylococcus aureus* (MSSA) bacteraemia (Gould, 2005), and colonisation with MRSA is a recognised risk factor for the development of an MRSA bloodstream infection. In April 2001, the Department of Health introduced mandatory surveillance and reporting of MRSA bacteraemias, which are largely avoidable HCAIs, potentially life-threatening and difficult to treat. Results from the fourth year of the surveillance scheme (2004–2005) showed that while there had been a slight decrease (7247 bacteraemias in 2001–2002, increases in 2002–2003 and 2003–2004, and then a decrease to 7212 in 2004–2005), it wasn't sufficient and something radical had to be done. In November 2004 the Health Secretary, John Reid, announced that the DH was setting each NHS Acute Trust in England the target of reducing its MRSA bacteraemia rate by 50% based on its 2004 baseline, to be achieved by March 2008. Each Trust was given a target which set out the number of MRSA bacteraemias 'allowed' each year, demonstrating a year-on-year reduction in order to reach the target. It was the setting of the bacteraemia reduction target, which came about through mandatory surveillance, which pushed infection control right to the top of every Trust's agenda, requiring engagement from senior managers and the appointment of nominated Infection Control Leads among nursing and medical staff in every service area and clinical directorate or division.

Fact Box 3.3   MRSA reduction target

In order to achieve their reduction targets, Trusts were required to examine a number of infection control interventions such as the screening of high-risk patients for MRSA colonisation, the isolation of colonised patients (often compounded by a lack of isolation facilities and by infections caused by other organisms, which place an added demand on isolation facilities), the effectiveness of hand hygiene programmes, the prevention of contaminated blood cultures (which accounted for a significant number of bacteraemias reported), the decontamination of equipment, environmental cleanliness and the use and management of invasive indwelling devices. Central to a successful reduction was the requirement to undertake a root cause analysis (RCA) (see Chapter 2) each time a bacteraemia was confirmed to assist in identifying where poor practice had occurred.

Mandatory surveillance of MRSA bacteraemia continues (and now also includes MSSA, although no reduction target has been set for MSSA), and each Trust has found that its target has become more challenging. As of April 2013, there are no set reduction targets. Instead, the new guidance from the NHS Commissioning Board states that there must be 'zero tolerance' for bacteraemias, and that 'the Government considers it unacceptable for a patient to acquire an MRSA bloodstream infection (MRSA BSI) while receiving care in a healthcare setting (NHS Commissioning Board, 2013).

Clostridium difficile

Voluntary reporting of laboratory-confirmed *C. difficile* isolates was introduced in 1990 and became mandatory in 2004, with Acute Trusts in England required to report all cases of *C. difficile* infection in patients over the age of 65 to the DH. The purpose of *C. difficile* surveillance was (and still is) to detect and interpret trends in the incidence, distribution and severity of *C. difficile*, by the collation of robust date which reports individual cases, outbreaks and periods of increased incidence (see Chapter 4). As discussed in Chapter 23, Trusts were set a 30% reduction target in 2008, based on their 2007–2008 baseline, to be achieved by 2010–2011, and targets have continued to be set.

E. coli and glycopeptide-resistant enterococci (GRE)

Voluntary reporting of *E. coli* bloodstream infections has indicated a year-on-year increase in bacteraemias caused by Gram-negative bacteria and *E. coli* in particular, leading to reporting becoming mandatory in 2011. This will enable the identification of risk factors for *E. coli* bacteraemia and interventions for the prevention of avoidable infections. Although no national reduction target has been set as yet, Trusts should examine their data in order to identify any local risk factors and implement prevention measures. The data collection form can be viewed on the HPA/Public Health England website (HPA, 2013g).

Mandatory reporting of bloodstream infections due to GRE was introduced in September 2003. See Fact Sheet 3.2 of the companion website for information on the clinical significance of GRE.

Surveillance of surgical site infections

The Nosocomial Infection National Surveillance Scheme (NINSS) was established by the DH and the Public Health Laboratory Service in 1996 with the aim of gathering information that would not only identify HCAIs but also lead to their reduction through identifying areas for improvement in care (e.g. conducting surgical site infection surveillance and identifying and reducing patient risk factors), and helping to guide national best practice to prevent avoidable infections (see Chapter 18). Up until 2004, participation was voluntary, but this was the year in which HCAIs were pushed right to the top of the political agenda and HCAI reduction was in the throes of rapidly becoming a national priority for action. It was in 2004 that it became mandatory for Trusts undertaking orthopaedic surgery (where the consequences of SSI can be severe) to annually submit three months of data regarding orthopaedic SSIs in relation to at least one of the four categories of orthopaedic surgery depicted in **Box 3.6**.

SSI surveillance is also undertaken in relation to other surgical procedures, which are sub-categorised (see **Box 3.7**) and which have been selected for surveillance because historically higher rates of infection have been detected for them (HPA, 2011).

Box 3.6   SSIs – orthopaedic surgery

Total hip replacement
Total knee replacement
Hip hemiarthroplasty
Open reduction of long bone fracture.

Surveillance involves completion of a data spreadsheet (simple tick boxes and short responses), which is commenced on admission and then completed throughout the patient's hospital stay until discharge. It can be completed by nursing and/or medical staff (who often complete it poorly) but is often overseen by Audit and Surveillance Nurses or dedicated Surveillance Clerks. The data are entered onto the SSI website, where they are checked for completeness and errors, and any queries are referred back to the hospital reporting the data. Individual hospital reports are generated, which can be used to influence improvements both locally and on a national level. **Box 3.8** depicts some of the information that is collated.

Box 3.7   Other surgical procedures

Abdominal hysterectomy
Bile duct, liver or pancreatic surgery
Breast surgery
Cardiac surgery
Cranial surgery
Non-laparoscopic cholecystectomy
Gastric surgery
Large bowel surgery
Small bowel surgery
Spinal surgery
Vascular.

Source: Data from HPA, 2011.

Box 3.8 Some of the data collected for SSI surveillance

- Patient's full name, date of birth, NHS number, hospital number, height and weight
- Date of admission
- Operation date
- Indication for surgery
- Category of procedure
- Type of surgery (emergency or elective)
- Whether surgery was due to trauma
- ASA (American Society of Anesthesiologists) score (see Chapter 18)
- Wound class
- Grade of surgeon
- Whether a prosthesis was inserted and antibiotic cement was used
- Duration of surgery (time of incision and time of closure)
- Antimicrobial prophylaxis
- Record of patient and wound review (e.g. temperature, whether the wound is clean and dry, or any breakthrough on dressing)
- The date on which surveillance was discontinued and why
- Whether an SSI questionnaire was provided post discharge or whether the patient was contacted by telephone
- Whether the patient was given any information on SSIs
- If the patient developed an SSI – date of onset, how it was detected, the criteria for suspecting or diagnosing an SSI, the type of SSI, the specific site of infection and the causative organism.

Source: Data from HPA, 2011.

Chapter summary: key points

- All healthcare staff are involved in audit and surveillance activities.

- Auditing compliance with infection control practice is an integral part of any HCAI prevention programme.

- Audit results are only as good as the information obtained.

- Audit results should be fed back to staff promptly, and compliance with implementing recommended actions should be monitored.

- Surveillance enables the early identification of illnesses, infections and infectious diseases that can lead to outbreaks and assists in the identification of risk factors for the development of HCAIs.

- Done properly, audit and surveillance can be tools for change, leading to improvements in patient care both locally and nationally.

Further resources are available for this book, including interactive multiple choice questions. Visit the companion website at:

www.wiley.com/go/fundamentalsofinfectionprevention

References

Department of Health (DH) (2006). *Essential Steps to Safe, Clean Care: Self-Assessment Tools and Resources*. DH, London.

Gould I.M. (2005). The clinical significance of meticillin-resistant *Staphylococcus aureus*. *Journal Hospital Infection*. 61 (4): 277–282.

Health Protection Authority (HPA) (2010). List of causative agents. http://www.hpa.org.uk/Topics/InfectiousDiseases/InfectionsAZ/NotificationsOfInfectiousDiseases/ListOfCausativeAgents/ (accessed 2 March 2013)

Health Protection Agency (HPA) (2011). *Protocol for the surveillance of surgical site infections*. Surgical Site Infection Surveillance Service (SSISS), HPA, London.

Health Protection Agency (HPA) (2013a). Botulism. http://www.hpa.org.uk/Topics/InfectiousDiseases/InfectionsAZ/Botulism (accessed 2 March 2013)

Health Protection Agency (HPA) (2013b). Cholera. http://www.hpa.org.uk/Topics/InfectiousDiseases/InfectionsAZ/Cholera (accessed 2 March 2013)

Health Protection Agency (HPA) (2013c). Diphtheria. http://www.hpa.org.uk/Topics/Infectious Diseases/InfectionsAZ/Diphtheria/ (accessed 2 March 2013)

Health Protection Agency (HPA) (2013d). General information about Brucellosis. http://www.hpa.org.uk/Topics/InfectiousDiseases/InfectionsAZ/Brucellosis/GeneralInformation/bruc001GeneralInformation (accessed 2 March 2013)

Health Protection Agency (HPA) (2013e). Leprosy. http://www.hpa.org.uk/Topics/Infectious Diseases/InfectionsAZ/Leprosy (accessed 2 March 2013)

Health Protection Agency (HPA) (2013f). Malaria. http://www.hpa.org.uk/Topics/Infectious Diseases/InfectionsAZ/Malaria (accessed 2 March 2013)

Health Protection Agency (HPA) (2013g). Mandatory surveillance of *Escherichia coli* bacteraemia. http://www.hpa.org.uk/Topics/InfectiousDiseases/InfectionsAZ/EscherichiaColi/Mandatory Surveillance (accessed 2 March 2013)

Health Protection Agency (HPA) (2013h). Polio. http://www.hpa.org.uk/Topics/InfectiousDiseases/InfectionsAZ/Polio (accessed 2 March 2013)

Health Protection Agency (HPA) (2013i). Rabies. http://hpa.org.uk/Topics/InfectiousDiseases/InfectionsAZ/Rabies (accessed 2 March 2013)

Health Protection Agency (HPA) (2013j). Tetanus. http://www.hpa.org.uk/Topics/Infectious Diseases/InfectionsAZ/Tetanus (accessed 2 March 2013)

Health Protection Agency (HPA) (2013k). Yellow fever. http://www.hpa.org.uk/Topics/Infectious Diseases/InfectionsAZ/YellowFever/ (accessed 2 March 2013)

McCormick A. (1993). The notification of infectious diseases in England and Wales. *Communicable Disease Report*. 3 (2): R19–R24.

NHS Commissioning Board (2013). *Guidance on the Reporting and Monitoring of Arrangements and Post Infection Review Process for MRSA bloodstream infections from April 2013.* http://www.england.nhs.uk/ourwork/patientsafety/zero-tolerance/

World Health Organization (WHO) (2013a). *Haemorrhagic fevers, viral.* http://who.int/topics/haemorrhagic_fevers_viral/en/ (accessed 2 March 2013)

World Health Organization (WHO) (2013b). *Rabies.* http://www.who.int/topics/rabies/en (accessed 2 March 2013)

Further reading

Greenfeld K.T. (2006). *China Syndrome: The True Story of the 21st Century's First Great Epidemic*. Penguin. ISBN: 978-0141027531

McNeill H.M. (1976). *Plagues and Peoples*. Anchor Books Editions. ISBN: 0-385-121229

Quammen D. (2012). *Spillover: Animal Infections and the Next Human Pandemic*. Bodley Head. ISBN: 978-1847920102

Quinn T. (2008). *Flu: A Social History of Influenza*. New Holland Publishers (UK) Ltd. ISBN: 978-1845379414

Ziegler P. (2003). *The Black Death*. Sutton Publishing Ltd. ISBN: 978-0750932028

4

The investigation of clusters, periods of increased incidence and outbreaks of infection

Contents

Fundamentals of Infection Prevention and Control: Theory and Practice, Second Edition. Debbie Weston.
© 2013 John Wiley & Sons, Ltd. Published 2013 by John Wiley & Sons, Ltd. Companion Website: www.wiley.com/go/fundamentalsofinfectionprevention

Introduction

The investigation and subsequent management of clusters, periods of increased incidence (PIIs) and outbreaks of infection (or colonisation) are aspects of infection control work that many healthcare workers are likely to experience and be actively involved in. They can range from the relatively minor and easy to control (e.g. a cluster of ward-acquired meticillin-resistant *Staphylococcus aureus* [MRSA] colonisations on a medical ward, or a period of increased incidence of *Clostridium difficile* infection in a community hospital) to more serious and often larger outbreaks that affect public health in the wider context; outbreaks can affect a local population in a defined geographical area, or they can pose a global threat.

Whether it's a cluster, a PII or an outbreak, these 'incidents' can be extremely disruptive to the provision of healthcare services, costly and labour intensive, and cause undue anxiety and stress for patients, the public and the staff involved. They can, and often do, attract adverse publicity, and their duration can be prolonged. They can be devastating if lives are lost, and they can affect public confidence in the NHS and local services enormously. The consistent application of good infection control practice and compliance with policies and infection control and public health legislation means that many incidents are often avoidable; where non-compliance can be demonstrated to have caused, or contributed to, the incident, the potential implications can be far-reaching, and may lead to changes in practice not only locally but nationally too. They may also result in an investigation into practice and patient care (i.e. by the Care Quality Commission [CQC] and the Health and Safety Executive [HSE]), which can have legal implications that may result in litigation. The Stanley Royd *Salmonella* outbreak in 1984, for example, led to the eventual removal of crown immunity (immunity from prosecution for criminal liability) from NHS premises (see Fact Sheet 3.7 on the companion website).

This chapter aims to define clusters, PIIs and outbreaks for healthcare workers and provide a brief insight into the different factors that have to be taken into consideration and investigated in the event of a cluster, PII or outbreak. These factors apply to hospital, primary care and community settings.

Learning outcomes

After reading this chapter, the reader will be able to:

- Define the terms cluster, period of increased incidence and outbreak.

- List the general aspects of clinical practice that the Infection Prevention and Control Team will investigate.

Recognising a cluster, a period of increased incidence and an outbreak

Cluster

A cluster generally refers to a group of cases that are related in time and place, and that may or may not be greater than normal. A cluster may go on to become an outbreak. For example, there may be a cluster of patients on a hospital ward who have acquired MRSA since they have been in hospital. Whether or not a cluster is classed as, or leads to, an outbreak depends on various factors, including the time frame, whether other patients on the ward subsequently acquire the same infection and whether typing (see Chapter 7) identifies that the patients have the same strain.

Period of increased incidence

A period of increased incidence (PII) is an increased number of infections (or colonisations) occurring within a defined time. A PII can be declared for any organism, but it is most commonly associated with *C. difficile*, for which the Department of Health (DH) and the Health Protection Agency (HPA) (DH and HPA, 2008) provide the following definitions:

- *C. difficile* **period of increased incidence:** Two or more cases occurring more than 72 hours post admission (not relapses), in a 28-day period on a ward
- *C. difficile* **outbreak:** Two or more cases caused by the same strain, related in time and place over a defined period that is based on the onset of the first case.

Outbreak

The official definition of the word outbreak from the World Health Organization (WHO) is:

> the occurrence of cases of disease in excess of what would normally be expected in a defined community, geographical area or season. It may last for a few days or weeks, or for several years. A single case of a communicable disease long absent from a population or caused by an agent (e.g. bacterium or virus) not previously recognised in that community or area, or the emergence of a previously unknown disease, may also constitute an outbreak and should be reported. (WHO, 2013)

In healthcare settings, the general definition of an outbreak is 'an incident in which two or more people experiencing a similar illness are linked in time or place' (HPA, 2012). Nursing or medical staff may be the first to spot signs of illness or infections amongst their patients, such as rashes, chest infections, diarrhoea and/or vomiting, and signs of post-operative surgical site infection. These can all be an early indication of an impending outbreak, and if the Infection Prevention and Control Team (IP&CT) are alerted swiftly enough, control measures can be implemented more or less immediately and outbreak investigations initiated, and a full-blown outbreak may be avoided. Laboratory-based surveillance of microbiology results or notifications of infectious diseases may also indicate an outbreak. Surveillance is discussed in Chapter 3.

Fact Box 4.1   Community-acquired outbreak of Legionnaires' disease

The largest outbreak of Legionnaires' disease in the United Kingdom occurred in 2002 at Barrow-in Furness, Cumbria. Over a period of 10 days, 498 suspected cases were admitted to the local hospital (Smith *et al.*, 2005). Approximately 2500 people were considered to have been affected, of whom 180 were confirmed to have contracted Legionnaires' disease and seven died (Health and Safety Executive, 2002). The source of the outbreak was an air conditioning unit at an arts complex within Forum 28, the Town Civic Centre, which was run by Barrow-in-Furness Borough Council. Many of those affected reported walking down a lane between the Civic Centre and a shop, and anecdotal reports were received of large amounts of aerosol and water droplets issuing from an air-conditioning vent in the lane (Calvert and Astbury, 2002). The council and a council officer were convicted of health and safety offences at a trial lasting three months, and were eventually acquitted of seven counts of manslaughter. Outbreaks have also occurred in central London; one at the headquarters of the BBC in 1988 affected 79 people and resulted in the deaths of three (Department of Health, 2002).

Table 4.1 lists some of the microorganisms and infections that may cause outbreaks in hospitals and in primary care or community settings.

Table 4.1   Microorganisms that may cause outbreaks in hospital and in primary care or community settings

Hospital	Primary care or community
• MRSA, PVL (Panton Valentine Leukocidin) – S. aureus and PVL–MRSA (see Chapter 20) • *Clostridium difficile* (see Chapter 22) • Norovirus (see Chapter 23) • Respiratory TB (see Chapter 21) • *Legionella* (Legionnaires' disease) (see Fact Sheet 1.3 on the companion website) • Extended-spectrum β-lactamase (ESBL)-resistant organisms (see Chapter 10)	• MRSA, PVL–S. aureus and PVL–MRSA • *C. difficile* • Norovirus • Respiratory TB • *Legionella* (Legionnaires' disease) • Meningococcal meningitis (see Fact Sheet 3.4 on the companion website) • Measles (see Chapter 5) • Pertussis (see Fact Sheet 1.4 on the companion website) • Scabies (see Fact Sheet 3.6 on the companion website) • *Salmonella* and food poisoning (see Fact Sheet 3.7 on the companion website) • Influenza (see Chapter 1 and Chapter 5) • Invasive group A streptococcal disease (see Fact Sheets 3.3, 3.8 and 3.9 on the companion website).

Look-back exercise

Look-back exercises are respective reviews of individuals who may have been exposed to infection, or who may have been affected as a result of inadequate screening processes (e.g. breast or cervical cancer screening). Look-back exercises in relation to exposure to infections or potentially infectious microorganisms may be undertaken as part of outbreak control measures or they may lead to an outbreak being declared. Box 4.1 identifies instances whereby look-back exercises may be required

Box 4.1   Some common indications for look-back exercises

Respiratory TB in a healthcare worker who had been working whilst infectious and un-diagnosed

Patient with respiratory TB but had been in an open ward for a number of weeks prior to diagnosis

Failure to sterilise surgical instruments following disinfection (blood-borne virus exposure risk)

Failure to adequately decontaminate an endoscope after patient use (blood-borne virus exposure risk)

Endoscopic procedure undertaken on a patient at risk of or with possible symptoms of **Creutzfeldt–Jakob disease (CJD)** – endoscope reprocessed and used on other patients (see Fact Sheet 1.2 on the companion website).

Arranging a cluster, PII or outbreak control group meeting: who to invite and agenda planning

Once an incident has been recognised, who should attend the meeting very much depends on the nature and scale of the incident (the organism, location, number of patients and staff affected, severity of symptoms and mode of transmission) and its likely impact (spread to staff and members of the public, and effect on the provision of services). Most incidents within hospital settings are managed locally by the IP&CT, with the meeting chaired by the Director of Infection Prevention and Control (DIPC). The local Health Protection Unit (HPU) and the Clinical Commissioning Group (CCG) are usually notified as a matter of course, and the Consultant in Communicable Disease Control (CCDC) from the HPU and the Infection Control Lead from the Community IP&CT may attend the meeting depending on the type of incident. Certainly where the ramifications of the incident potentially extend beyond the hospital into the community (or vice versa), the CCDC will be in attendance and may even chair the meeting.

Box 4.2 and Box 4.3 provide examples of attendance lists for Acute Trust and community outbreak control group (OCG) meetings. These are not exhaustive lists, and there may be variations.

Once an incident has been recognised, and prior to the meeting being held, the IP&CT will undertake some investigations of their own (these may include audits of compliance with pertinent aspects of clinical practice, or environmental sampling) and collate information for

Box 4.2   Attendance at cluster, PII and outbreak meeting: Acute Trust

- The IP&CT
- Representation from the Executive Team (e.g. Chief Nurse) or nominated deputy
- Divisional and Directorate Head(s) of Nursing
- Ward Manager(s)
- Divisional and Directorate Matron(s)
- Hospital Manager and Bed Manager – if admissions, discharges and transfers are going to be affected and/or wards or beds are going to be closed
- Antimicrobial Pharmacist – if antimicrobial prescribing or stewardship needs to be reviewed
- Hotel Services and Facilities Manager – for cleaning issues
- Estates Department – if water quality and safety are to be discussed (e.g. *Legionella* or *Pseudomonas* outbreak)
- Occupational Health Consultant and Nurse Advisor – if there is an implication for staff health, such as screening, contact tracing or prophylaxis
- Representative from the Communications Team
- Consultant in Communicable Disease Control and Health Protection and Public Health Nurse from the local Health Protection Unit
- Infection Control Lead from the Community
- Community TB (Tuberculosis) Team – if the OCG meeting is to discuss TB

Box 4.3   Attendance at cluster, PII and outbreak meeting: Primary care or community

- Community Infection Control Team
- Consultant in Communicable Disease Control and Health Protection and Public Health Nurse from the local Health Protection Unit
- GP(s) or Practice Manager(s)
- Residential or Nursing Home Manager(s)
- Environmental Health Officer (in the event of a *Legionella* or food poisoning outbreak, when environmental sampling or investigation of premises is required)
- DIPC from Acute Trust (if outbreak will potentially affect the Trust, e.g. admissions to hospital or delayed discharges from hospital to community hospital or care facilities)
- Occupational Health Consultant or Nurse Advisor if there are implications for staff health
- Communications Team

discussion at the meeting. The time between the incident being identified or reported and a meeting being held is, by necessity, short and in the event of an outbreak it is a time of intensive activity.

In order to determine how and why the incident occurred and to prevent it from happening again, the IP&CT have to scrutinise every relevant aspect of infection control practice, and really drill down and look at practice and compliance within the clinical area concerned. Box 4.4 summarises some of the aspects of infection control clinical practice and compliance with policies that will be looked at as part of the investigative process, as well as some of the resource issues and other implications that have to be considered.

Box 4.4   The IP&CT – investigations and considerations

Patients: What is the risk to patients and what are the implications of cross-infection; is there an **index case** amongst current or past patients; what is or was this patient's location on the ward; and how is or was she or he managed?

Isolation or cohort nursing: How many single rooms are available on the ward for isolation purposes; are they fit for purpose (en-suite or observable?); are they used appropriately at all times or some of the time; were patients isolated or cohort nursed appropriately; if there were any difficulties regarding patient placement, were they escalated; were and are isolation room door signs available and appropriately displayed; and were and are isolation room doors kept closed (risk assessment documented if not)? (See Chapter 11.)

Personal protective equipment (PPE): Are gloves and aprons being worn and disposed of appropriately? (See Chapter 13.)

Hand hygiene: Are staff hand hygiene assessments up to date; what is the average weekly compliance for the ward observational hand hygiene audits; how compliant are staff with 'Bare Below the Elbows'; is alcohol hand rub available at the point of care; are sufficient facilities available for hand washing; do staff understand the application of the 5 Moments for Hand Hygiene, when to hand wash and when to use alcohol hand rub or gel; are patients encouraged to wash their hands or offered assistance? (See Chapter 12.)

Staff: staffing levels and skill mix; need to restrict staff movement (e.g. between wards); need for staff screening and Occupational Health involvement

Compliance with IC mandatory training: Have all clinical staff undertaken their mandatory annual or biennial infection control update; are training records available?

Training and competency: Have staff had their competency assessed regarding certain skills and procedures?

Cleaning (equipment): Is equipment being cleaned in between use; is the method of cleaning and decontamination appropriate; is there sufficient equipment; can equipment be dedicated to isolation rooms or cohort bays; is equipment being used for its intended purpose? (See Chapter 15.)

Cleaning (environment): Is the environment clean; what are the weekly and monthly cleaning scores; are there any concerns regarding cleaning and if so, how have these been escalated; is the cleaning resource sufficient; does the ward need to be deep-cleaned; is there sufficient storage; is the ward cluttered and untidy?

Documentation and communication: Are patient interventions documented; are Infection Control Patient Management Plans and Pathways completed; is the information recorded accurate; is there evidence that information recorded and relayed by the IP&CT has been acted upon? (See Chapter 2.)

Resources: time scale for action and response; need for additional staff; outside assistance (e.g. specialist input from HPA Reference Laboratory)

Financial: costs associated with additional cleaning; staffing; equipment; screening and environmental sampling; antibiotics and prophylaxis; financial penalties associated with cancellation of services, admissions, elective surgery and breaching of targets; penalties for exceeding trajectories (e.g. MRSA bacteraemia and *C. difficile*)

Reporting: Serious Untoward Incident (SUI) reporting; undertaking of a root cause analysis (RCA) (see Chapter 2).

Fact Box 4.2   Fungal contamination of wooden tongue depressors

In 1996, four babies on a neonatal unit in the United Kingdom developed fungal infections contracted from wooden tongue depressors that had been used as limb splints to secure vascular access devices. Two babies died; a third underwent a partial limb amputation. A fungus belonging to the *Rhizopus microsporus* group was subsequently isolated from 10% of the wooden tongue depressors found stored on a surgical trolley, but not from the tongue depressors stored in an unopened box (Public Health Laboratory Service, 1996).

The remainder of this section lists some of the specific information that will be collated by the IP&CT in relation to a cluster, PII or outbreak involving the following organisms:

- MRSA
- *C. difficile*
- *Legionella* (hospital or community)
- Respiratory tuberculosis.

The content given here is not exhaustive and is in addition to the investigations and considerations listed in Box 4.4.

Investigating a cluster of ward-acquired MRSA colonisations

Screening: compliance with admission and long-stay screening

MRSA-positive patients: How many patients have acquired MRSA during their admission over the previous two months or longer, and are these all colonisations or have there also been infections or bacteraemias; and what is the burden of MRSA on the ward (e.g. is there, or has there been, a high number of patients with MRSA requiring isolation or cohort nursing)?

MRSA decolonisation protocol: compliance with the timeliness of prescribing and administering the MRSA decolonisation (including staff competency).

Invasive devices (vascular access devices and urinary catheters): Are they managed according to Trust policy (e.g. completion of insertion records, recording of VIP scores and devices removed appropriately); is documentation relating to devices accurate; are staff competent in their insertion and management; is the skin being decontaminated appropriately prior to peripheral cannula insertion and blood culture collection; have staff taking blood cultures received training and been assessed as competent?

C. difficile – periods of increased incidence or outbreaks

Specimen collection: Were stool specimens collected appropriately?

Stool charts: Have stool charts been maintained consistently and accurately?

Isolation: Were the patients isolated promptly; and were any delays in isolation escalated appropriately and documented?

Antibiotic prescribing: Are antibiotics prescribed in accordance with local antibiotic-prescribing guidelines; is there evidence of antimicrobial stewardship; and are symptomatic patients being treated appropriately?

Hand hygiene: Are staff staffing washing their hands after patient contact or contact with the environment? Are patients encouraged to wash their hands, and are they offered assistance after using the toilet and before eating and drinking?

Commodes: Are commodes being cleaned in between every episode of patient use with a sporicidal agent? Are commodes being dedicated to patients if en-suite isolation facilities are not available? Are all commodes on the ward(s) clean, intact and in a good state of repair?

Legionella: hospital or community acquired (isolated case or outbreak)

Did the patient have healthcare contact within the incubation period? If yes, then both a community and hospital source will need to be considered and investigated until one can be effectively discounted.

Hospital source? If currently, or previously, an in-patient:

The ward: Did the patient use a shower or bath, and if so, which one, when and how frequently? Is the shower used at least daily? If the patient had a bath, is it an Arjo non-spa bath or Arjo spa bath? If it is a non-spa bath, is the water run for at least 2 minutes **and** is the bath cleaned in between each patient use (if the bath is not used at all, it should still be run in the morning and the evening to flush the system through)? Is there documentation to support that this is happening? If the bath is a spa bath, is it being **disinfected** twice a day (regardless of whether it is in use or not) **and** is it being disinfected in between each patient use? Is there documentation to support this?

If the patient was an out-patient: What department did he or she attend and when? Did the patient use the toilet facilities? If so, which ones? Is there any splash-back when the taps are run that could produce a spray? How frequently are that toilet and bathroom used?

Estates issues: Are there any 'dead legs' or areas of redundant pipe work; are the locations of all high-use or low-use water outlets known; is there a programme of flushing of low-use water outlets; is there a programme of daily flushing of all water outlets; and are there any toilets or bathrooms that are used as storage facilities, which impedes the use of the facilities for their intended purpose and restricts access for flushing?

Community: Need to establish the patient's travel and recreational history. In other words, travel abroad, hotel stay (air conditioning?) or use of whirlpool or spa bath in a hotel or leisure complex? Exposure to a water fountain? Proximity to a cooling tower?

Tuberculosis (smear positive): if the index case is, or was, a hospital in-patient

The patient: Dates of admission; location; symptoms on admission; was TB on the list of differential diagnoses? How infectious is or was the patient considered to be? Is the TB fully sensitive to anti-TB medication? Where is the patient now? Is he or she compliant with TB therapy?

Other patients: What was the length of exposure to the index case? Were any of the patient contacts likely to have risk factors that would increase their susceptibility? Where are these patients now (own home, other hospital or care facility)? How are they going to be contacted, and what is the time scale? What advice are they going to be given? If they need screening, how is this going to be done and by whom?

Staff contacts: Which staff groups have potentially been exposed to the index patient? How many are there? How are staff contacts going to be identified? How are they going to be contacted? How will they be screened?

If a member of staff is the index case:

- When did he or she first display symptoms, and when was TB confirmed?
- Was he or she working while probably infectious? What is the infectious period?
- Where was he or she working (type of ward or department, shift pattern and days of work, and nature of work undertaken)?
- Who are the staff contacts who need to be identified?
- Who are the patient contacts?

Note: A TB contact-tracing exercise will involve:

- Collating lists of in-patients exposed and potentially exposed to the index case
- Identifying those patients at risk
- Writing to the patients and their GPs
- Making arrangements for patient screening
- Identifying staff contacts
- Checking the Bacillus Calmette–Guérin (BCG) status of staff and identifying staff at risk (undertaken by the Occupational Health Department)
- Writing to staff
- Preparing a reactive press statement (patient and staff contacts should all be notified at the same time, e.g. letters sent out on the same day). A dedicated telephone help-line may need to be established.

At the meeting and after: actions and closure of the incident

Figure 4.1 provides an example of a draft cluster, PII or outbreak meeting agenda.

Title, date, time and venue

AGENDA

1. **Welcome, introductions and apologies**

2. **Confidentiality**

3. **Purpose of meeting, roles and responsibilities**

4. **History and background**, for example location, when the incident was first recognised and how, causative organism, numbers of patients and staff affected, and immediate actions

5. **Current situation**, for example number of patients and staff currently affected; and ward open or closed: effect on admissions, transfers and discharges

6. **Infection prevention and control report**, for example:

   - Isolation

   - Screening and sampling

   - Decolonisation

   - Antibiotic prescribing

   - Hand hygiene

   - PPE

   - Staffing

   - Equipment

   - Environment

Figure 4.1   Potential agenda items for a cluster, PII or outbreak meeting.

- Mandatory training

- Education

- Admissions, transfers and discharges

- Visitors

- Documentation

- Audit feedback

7. **Current control measures** – these may include a recap of the above points.

8. **Occupational Health Department** – if there are concerns regarding staff health; and need for screening and decolonisation, or prophylaxis.

9. **HPU** – the local HPU may have questions regarding management and control measures and/or may wish to make recommendations.

10. **CCG** – as above

11. **Communications** – depending on the nature of the incident, a reactive press statement may be required; this may involve liaison between the Trust, HPU and PCT communications teams.

12. **SUI reporting**

13. **Actions** – actions will be agreed and allocated to named individuals to be completed within a specified time frame.

14. **Any other business.**

15. **Date, time and venue of next meeting**

Figure 4.1   *Continued*

Reflection point

In the event of non-compliance with isolation, PPE and/or cleaning of patient equipment being identified at an Outbreak meeting, what do you think the actions will be? Who will be responsible for implementing them, and how will compliance be monitored?

At the meeting, following all of the necessary reporting, actions will be identified and allocated to individuals, who will be responsible for ensuring that they are implemented within a specified time frame. The actions may be displayed as an action plan, disseminated with the minutes, and if further meetings are required, the action plan will become a rolling agenda item for discussion and updating. The outcome of the meeting has to be fed back to staff, and the incident itself reported via the appropriate clinical governance and clinical risk channels, and to the Infection Control Committee. It may be reported as an SUI (Serious Untoward Incident). Whether further meetings are required or not depends on the scale of the incident, the type of incident (an outbreak may require meetings over a period of weeks to months), the effectiveness of control measures and whether there are any new cases. The IP&CT will declare the incident over when they are satisfied that control measures have been effective and sustained.

Chapter summary: key points

- Clusters, periods of increased incidence and outbreaks have numerous and potentially far-reaching implications.

- Clusters and periods of increased incidence may lead to an outbreak unless control measures are implemented swiftly.

- Look-back exercises may be undertaken as part of outbreak control measures or may lead to an outbreak being declared.

- Although clusters, periods of increased incidence and outbreaks are generally managed locally by the IP&CT, outside agencies are often involved.

- The IP&CT have to undertake in-depth investigations or observations regarding compliance with infection control policy and clinical practice.

- The management of outbreaks in particular is resource intensive.

- Clusters, periods of increased incidence and outbreaks are largely avoidable.

Further resources are available for this book, including interactive multiple choice questions. Visit the companion website at:

www.wiley.com/go/fundamentalsofinfectionprevention

References

Calvert N., Astbury J. (2002). Legionnaires disease outbreak in England. *Eurosurveillance*. 6 (32): ii–1904. http://www.eurosurveillance.org/ViewArticle.aspx?ArticleId=1904 (accessed 2 March 2013)

Department of Health (DH) (2002). *Getting Ahead of the Curve: A Strategy for Combating Infectious Diseases (including Other Aspects of Health Protection)*. Report by the Chief Medical Officer. DH, London.

Department of Health and Health Protection Agency (DH and HPA) (2008). *Clostridium difficile Infection: How to Deal with the Problem*. DH and HPA, London.

Health and Safety Executive (2002). *Report of the public meetings into the Legionella outbreak in Barrow-in-Furness*. http://www.hse.gov.uk/legionnaires/assets/docs/barrowreport.pdf (accessed 2 March 2013)

Health Protection Agency (HPA) (2012). *The Communicable Disease Outbreak Plan*. HPA, London.

Public Health Laboratory Service (1996). Invasive fungal infections and contaminated tongue depressors. *Communicable Disease Report Weekly*. 6 (17). 26 April: 145.

Smith A.F., Wild C., Law J. (2005). The Barrow-in-Furness legionnaires' outbreak: qualitative study of the hospital response and the role of the major incident plan. *Emerg Med J*. 22: 251–255.

World Health Organization (WHO) (2013). *Disease outbreaks*. http://www.who.int/topics/disease_outbreaks/en/ (accessed 2 March 2013)

5

Microbial classification and structure

Contents

Fundamentals of Infection Prevention and Control: Theory and Practice, Second Edition. Debbie Weston.
© 2013 John Wiley & Sons, Ltd. Published 2013 by John Wiley & Sons, Ltd. Companion Website: www.wiley.com/go/fundamentalsofinfectionprevention

Introduction

Microorganisms exist everywhere – in and on the bodies of both humans and animals, and in plants, soil and water. The medically important groups include bacteria, viruses, prions, fungi, helminths and protozoa (although only bacteria, viruses and prions are covered in this chapter and within the book). In order to understand how bacteria and viruses replicate, invade and establish themselves in the human host, resulting in colonisation or infection, a basic knowledge of their classification and structure is necessary. This chapter aims to provide the reader with a basic understanding of their properties and characteristics, particularly those which act as virulence factors and increase the organism's pathogenic potential, and relate these to the disease process.

Learning outcomes

After reading this chapter, the reader will be able to:

- Describe the main structure and components of a bacteria cell.

- Understand the difference between Gram-positive and Gram-negative bacteria, and give examples of each.

- Understand the key virulence factors of bacteria and their significance in the process of colonisation and infection.

- Understand how viruses differ from bacteria and how they cause infection and disease.

Bacteria

Fact Box 5.1   Bacteria

Bacteria are microscopically small organisms, measured in microns (1 micron = 1000th of a millimetre). While the majority of bacteria are not considered to be harmful to humans, there are at least 50 species that are considered to be pathogenic (Engelkirk and Duben-Engelkirk, 2011a) and therefore capable of causing a diverse spectrum of illness and disease, from colonisation to infection, and ranging from mild to life-threatening in a susceptible host. Other bacteria are opportunistic microorganisms, meaning that they cause infection only when the host's immune response is impaired.

Bacterial structure

Three important components of the bacterial structure are the cell membrane, cell wall and cytoplasm.

Cell membrane

The cell membrane, also known as the cytoplasmic or plasma membrane, is made up of proteins and lipids. It envelopes the cell, protecting its contents from the outside world, and controls the substances entering and leaving it.

The bacterial cell wall

The majority of bacteria have a cell wall, the exceptions being organisms called mycoplasmas, which have a cell membrane but no cell wall and so cannot be Gram-stained. The cell wall is essential for the survival of the bacteria, giving it shape, rigidity and strength and offering protection against the host's immune response and the effects of certain groups of antibiotics (Ryan and Drew, 2010). This does not mean that the cell wall cannot be breached, and Chapters 8 and 10 discuss in detail how the immune system and the actions of antibiotics destroy invading bacteria.

Fact Box 5.2   Peptidoglycan

The main component of the cell wall is peptidoglycan (or murein), which is a polymer (a long molecule consisting of structural units and repeating units) of peptidoglycan chains linked by smaller protein chains. The cross-linking of chains gives the cell wall its rigidity.

The thickness of the cell wall and its composition vary according to the species of the bacteria. A **Gram-positive bacterial cell wall** consists of two layers: an inner cytoplasmic membrane and an outer thick layer of peptidoglycan. The cell wall also contains other polymers including teichoic and lipoteichoic acids, a complex of sugar and phosphate, which act as surface antigens (molecules capable of inducing an immune response and reacting with antibodies and/or T lymphocytes [see Chapter 8], such as bacterial toxins or bacterial cells).

Gram-negative bacteria are much more complex. They also have an inner cytoplasmic membrane, but they have a much thinner layer of peptidoglycan which is covered by an outer membrane. This acts as a protective barrier, preventing or slowing the entry of antibiotics that may weaken or kill the bacteria. Coating the outer membrane is lipopolysaccharide (LPS), a complex of fatty acids, sugar and phosphate. LPS is the endotoxin component of the Gram-negative cell wall and consists of three parts – Lipid A, core polysaccharide and the O side chain.

Fact Box 5.3   Lipid A

Lipid A is the most significant component of LPS, impeding the effects of many antibiotics. It is also an antigenic determinant, inducing the formation of antibodies, and is toxic to the host when the cell lyses and the cell membrane breaks up, releasing Lipid A into the bloodstream (Ryan and Drew, 2010).

The process for identifying whether bacteria are Gram-positive or Gram-negative is described in Chapter 7.

Cytoplasm

The cytoplasm consists of water, enzymes, waste products, nutrients, proteins, carbohydrates and lipids, all of which are required for the cell's metabolic functions. Embedded within the cytoplasm is the cell's chromosome, its DNA molecule, which controls and initiates cell division and other cellular activities.

Bacterial classification

Bacterial classification is part of the process that enables rapid identification of the causative agent of illness or disease. Bacteria are classified according to:

- Their morphology or shape
- Their Gram-stain reaction (which identifies the differences in their bacterial cell wall and is of life-saving importance when it comes to diagnosis and treatment)
- Their growth requirements
- Spore formation
- Their name, which consists of two parts – the genus, followed by the species; for example, *Staphylococcus aureus*, *Streptococcus pyogenes*, *Clostridium difficile* and *Neisseria meningitidis*.

Chapter 7 discusses the staining of bacteria for identification and their growth requirements and reproduction in more detail.

Bacterial morphology

Bacteria adopt one of three basic shapes – round, rod shaped, and curved or spiral – and can occur in pairs, chains or clusters. Their shape can be revealed only by Gram-staining, and they need to be viewed under a compound light microscope which can magnify objects 1000 times smaller than the smallest objects which can be seen unaided by the human eye. Round bacteria are known as cocci, and can grow in pairs (diplococci), chains (streptococci) or grape-like clusters (staphylococci). Bacilli are rod-shaped and can also occur in pairs or chains, with very small bacilli referred to as coccobacilli, which may resemble cocci. Spiral-shaped bacteria are known as spirochaetes, and curved or 'comma'-shaped bacteria are called vibrios. Figure 5.1 illustrates the common bacterial shapes and arrangements.

Virulence factors: slime, capsules and biofilm

Some bacteria produce a thick layer of glycocalyx, a 'carbohydrate coat' outside of the bacterial cell wall which protects the cell surface (Willey *et al.*, 2011a).This may be in the form of either slime layers or capsules (Engelkirk and Duben-Engelkirk, 2011b).

Slime layers can facilitate motility and attachment to surfaces.

Capsules are seen in some important pathogens such as *Neisseria meningitidis* and *Salmonella typhimurium*, and their presence assists in the identification of bacteria. The capsule helps to protect the bacteria from the host's immune response as it makes it more difficult for cells of the immune system to adhere to it and inhibits phagocytosis (see Chapter 8).

Biofilm: Large numbers of encapsulated bacteria can congregate together and produce a biofilm, which consists of a matrix of thousands or millions of microorganisms all encased in capsular material, which may be of a pure culture originating from one species of bacteria or mixed.

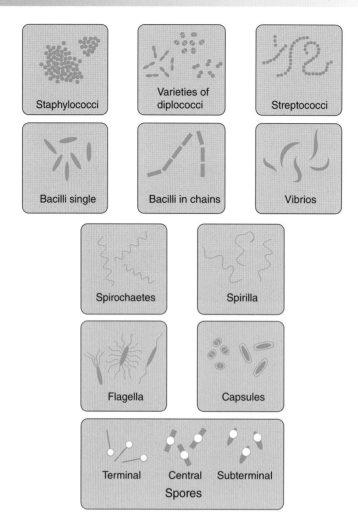

Figure 5.1   Common bacterial shapes and arrangements. (Wilson, 2003)

Fact Box 5.4   Biofilm activity

Biofilm have been defined as 'a community of micro-organisms irreversibly attached to a surface' (Lindsay and von Holy, 2006) and 'a complex, highly multi-cultural community with a level of activity within the biofilm that resembles a city' (Watnick and Koiter, 2000).

It is believed that there are five stages to their development (Petri *et al.*, 2010):

- Reversible, or transient, attachment
- Irreversible attachment
- Development of the biofilm architecture

- The development of micro-colonies, sub-divided by fluid-filled channels which carry nutrients and oxygen to the microorganisms and transport waste products away
- Dispersal of cells from the biofilm.

The clinical significance of biofilms

Bacterial biofilms are medically very significant as they are notoriously difficult for the host immune system to penetrate, have been reported to be at least 500 times more resistant to antibiotics than 'ordinary' bacterial cells (Petri *et al.*, 2010), are highly resistant to phagocytosis (Watnick and Koiter, 2000) and can cause persistent infections (Chen and Wen, 2011). While bacteria will adhere to virtually any available surface with the exception of plastic and glass, they are especially fond of indwelling devices such as intravenous cannulae and urethral catheters, as well as prosthetic implants. They can contaminate hot-water storage tanks, shower heads and air-conditioning units that use water, and develop on the surfaces of endoscope tubing (Petri *et al.*, 2010).

Spore formation

The formation of spores (known as endospores) by Gram-positive rods belonging to the bacterial genus *Bacillus* (*Bacillus anthracis*) or *Clostridium* (*Clostridium perfringens, Clostridium tetani, Clostridium botulinum* and *C. difficile*) can pose significant challenges for healthcare professionals. A spore is essentially a complex seed protected by a five-layered suit of armour. In adverse conditions that would not normally be conducive to an organism's survival, such as lack of nutrients, one cell produces one spore (a process known as sporulation) (Ryan and Drew, 2010), and the spore assumes a dormant, or hibernating, state. Once the environment improves (e.g. in the case of *C. difficile*, the spore is ingested via the faecal-oral route), it 'activates' and germinates into an active single bacterial cell. The significance of spores is discussed further in Chapter 22.

Fact Box 5.5   Spores

Spores are able to withstand ultraviolet and gamma radiation, desiccation, boiling and disinfectants. They are the organism's survival mechanism, and the spore is able to survive, potentially, for thousands of years, if not longer (Ryan and Drew, 2010; Willey *et al.*, 2011a).

Flagella

Flagella resemble long tails which are several times the length of the bacteria, and are essential for its motility (Gladwin and Trattler, 2004). There may be one to 20 flagella per bacteria, and their number and arrangement can be used to aid the identification and classification of certain bacterial species (Torres *et al.*, 2001). They may be sited all over the cell, clustered at one end of the cell or sited at both ends, or there may be just one solitary flagellum.

Fact Box 5.6   Flagella

Flagella make the bacteria move in a tumbling motion as they spin around, and they propel the cell towards or away from certain stimuli, such as movement towards a nutrient source, or away from phagocytes if the organism is attempting to evade the host immune response. This process of directed movement is known as chemotaxis, and it is not unique to bacterial cells. Flagella also assist the bacteria in attaching to surfaces (Willey *et al.*, 2011a).

Pili (fimbriae)

These are commonly seen on the surface of Gram-negative bacteria. There may be as many as 1000 pili on the surface of the bacterial cell wall (Willey *et al.*, 2011a), showing up as numerous hair-like protrusions or appendages. There are two forms of pili. Common pili are important virulence factors as they enable the bacteria to adhere and attach to host cells. The sex pili are involved in the transfer of genetic material through conjugation (see Chapter 10).

The production of invasive enzymes

- Some organisms produce a very potent cocktail of enzymes which facilitate penetration of the organism into the host's tissues, resulting in tissue damage.
- **Necrotising enzymes**, seen in **necrotising fasciitis**, cause rapid destruction of soft tissue.
- **Coagulase**, a protein produced by *S. aureus* (see Chapter 20), clots plasma which forms a sticky layer of fibrin around the bacteria, protecting it from phagocytes, antibodies and other host immune defences (Engelkirk and Duben-Engelkirk, 2011b). Sometimes, the host will cause a fibrin clot to form around the pathogen and wall it off in an attempt to prevent any further invasion and penetration of the tissues.
- **Kinases** have the opposite effect to coagulase, and they dissolve the fibrin clot. This means that kinase-producing bacteria such as staphylococcus and streptococcus are able to escape from these clots (Engelkirk and Duben-Engelkirk, 2011b).
- **Hyaluronidase**, often referred to as the 'spreading factor', enables pathogens to spread through connective tissue by breaking down hyaluronic acid which binds connective tissue together (Engelkirk and Duben-Engelkirk, 2011b). It plays an important role in the devastating tissue damage seen in necrotising fasciitis caused by *Streptococcus pyogenes*. *Streptococcus* and *Clostridia* are two pathogenic bacteria which secrete hyaluronidase.
- **Collagenase** breaks down collagen, which is found in tendons, cartilage and bone, enabling pathogens to invade tissue. *C. perfringens* secretes collagenase.
- **Haemolysins** damage the host's red blood cells (erythrocytes), causing them to burst and release iron (Engelkirk and Duben-Engelkirk, 2011c). This provides the pathogen with a source of iron which it utilises for microbial growth (Willey *et al.*, 2011b).

Toxin production

Bacteria have an impressive arsenal of weaponry at their disposal, but their ability to produce and release toxins, which are responsible for the signs, symptoms and complications of infection, is perhaps the most impressive. If the human host can survive the initial onslaught of toxins and mount an efficient immune response, they have every possibility of recovering.

Endotoxins are an integral part of the Gram-negative bacterial cell wall and not only are secreted or released when the cell is lysed or destroyed, but also are shed from living bacteria (Gladwin and Trattler, 2004). Septic shock (see Chapter 9) arising from Gram-negative endotoxins carries a high mortality rate.

Fact Box 5.7   Endotoxins and antibiotics

An unfortunate consequence of the administration of antibiotics to a patient with Gram-negative sepsis is that they can initially cause the patient's condition to worsen. This is because although the antibiotics cause the destruction of the bacteria, which is obviously the desired effect, this destruction also triggers the release of large quantities of endotoxin into the bloodstream.

Exotoxins are produced within the cell and secreted by Gram-positive and Gram-negative bacteria (with the exception of *Listeria monocytogenes*, a Gram-positive rod which causes meningitis in neonates and immunocompromised individuals, and which produces endotoxin) (Gladwin and Trattler, 2004). They are often named for the target organs that they affect (Engelkirk and Duben-Engelkirk, 2011a). For example:

Neurotoxins released by *C. botulinum* and *C. tetani* target the nervous system, blocking nerve impulses and often causing paralysis.

Enterotoxin is shed by *C. difficile* (Chapter 22) and *Salmonella* and *Campylobacter*, and it binds to and colonises the gastro-intestinal tract, causing diarrhoea.

Fact Box 5.8   Enterotoxin

Enterotoxin continues to be released until the pathogen is destroyed by the immune system or antibiotics, or the human host dies as a result of fluid loss, which may be severe. Enterotoxin can also be released by bacteria in food which, when ingested, results in rapid onset of diarrhoea and vomiting, as seen in *S. aureus* (see Chapter 20) and *Bacillus cereus*, both of which are very unpleasant causes of food poisoning.

Exfoliative or epidermolytic toxins, produced by some strains of *S. aureus*, affect the skin, resulting in sloughing of the epidermis (Engelkirk and Duben-Engelkirk, 2011a).

Panton–Valentine leukocidin (see Chapter 20) is a toxin produced by some strains of *S. aureus*, which destroys white blood cells and can cause devastating invasive infections such as necrotising pneumonia, which may be rapidly fatal (Morgan, 2005; Health Protection Agency, 2008).

Super-antigens are produced by bacterial species such as staphylococci and streptococci, as well as viruses. They are described as 'potent activators of CD4 T-lymphocytes' (Torres *et al*. 2001), over-stimulating the immune system through massive cytokine release (see Chapter 8) and causing fever, shock and potentially death (Proft and Fraser, 2003).

Plasmids

Plasmids are small, circular, extra-chromosomal DNA molecules which carry genes that can render bacteria drug resistant and give them new metabolic properties, enabling the bacteria to resist host defences or produce toxins and virulence genes (Ryan and Drew, 2010; see also Chapter 10). They offer bacteria an enormously competitive advantage in that the resistance genes and virulence factors that plasmids confer will ensure 'survival of the fittest' organisms.

Table 5.1 lists some common bacteria which are responsible for causing a wide range of infections, some of which are seen in healthcare settings, according to their Gram-stain reaction and shape.

Table 5.1   Bacteria according to Gram-stain and shape

Gram-positive	Morphology	Illness or disease
Staphylococcus: Staphylococcus aureus Staphylococcus epidermidis Staphylococcus saprophyticus	Cocci (clusters)	Skin infections (impetigo, cellulitis, abscesses and wound infection); intravenous (IV) line infections; pneumonia; food poisoning; osteomyelitis; acute endocarditis; septic arthritis; urinary tract infections
Streptococcus: Streptococcus pyogenes	Cocci (pairs)	Scarlet fever; 'strep' throat; post-streptococcal glomerulonephritis; skin infections; necrotising fasciitis; streptococcal toxic shock syndrome
Group B streptococci		Neonatal meningitis; pneumonia; sepsis
Streptococcus pneumoniae		Pneumonia; meningitis; otitis media
Bacillus: Bacillus anthracis Bacillus cereus	Rods (spore forming)	Anthrax Food poisoning
Clostridium: Clostridium botulinum Clostridium tetani Clostridium perfringens Clostridium difficile	Rods (spore forming)	Botulism Tetanus Gas gangrene Pseudomembranous colitis
Corynebacterium: Corynebacterium diptheriae	Rods (non-spore forming)	Diphtheria
Listeria: Listeria monocytogenes	Rods (non-spore forming)	Food poisoning; meningitis

Table 5.1   *Continued*

Gram-negative	Morphology	Illness or disease
Neisseria: *Neisseria meningitidis* *Neisseria gonorrhoea*	Diplococci	 Meningitis Gonorrhoea
Enterobacteriaceae: *Escherichia coli* *Klebsiella pneumoniae* *Proteus mirabilis* *Serratia* *Shigella:* *Shigella* dysenteriae *Shigella* flexneri *Shigella* boydi *Shigella* sonnei *Salmonella*	Rods	 Diarrhoea; urinary tract infections; sepsis Pneumonia; urinary tract infections Urinary tract infections Urinary tract infections Dysentery Dysentery Dysentery Dysentery Typhoid fever; gastroenteritis
Vibrionaceae: *Campylobacter jejuni* *Helicobacter pylori*	Curved	 Food poisoning Duodenal ulcer; gastritis
Pseudomonadacea: *Pseudomonas aeruginosa* *Haemophilus influenzae* *Bordetella pertussis* *Legionella pnemophila* *Yersinia pestis*	Rods	 Pneumonia; osteomylitis; sepsis; urinary tract infections; endocarditis; wound infections; corneal infections Meningitis; sepsis; septic arthritis Whooping cough Pontiac fever; Legionnaires' disease Bubonic plague
Chlamydia: *Chlamydia trachomatis* *Chlamydia psittaci*	Rods	 Conjunctivitis; infant pneumonia; pelvic inflammatory disease Atypical pneumonia
Spirochetes: *Treponema palladium* Leptospira	Spiral	 Syphilis Leptospirosis
Mycobacteria: *Mycobacterium tuberculosis* *Mycobacterium leprae*	Rods	 Tuberculosis Leprosy

Viruses

Fact Box 5.9   Viruses

Viruses are the smallest known infective agents, approximately 100 to 1000 times smaller than the cells they infect (Ahmad *et al.*, 2010a), and they are visible only via an electron microscope. Unlike bacteria, a virus is incapable of independent replication; it needs to access a host cell so that it can substitute its own nucleic acid for the cell's DNA. The ninth report of the International Committee on Taxonomy of Viruses (2009) has organised the virus community into 87 families, 19 sub-families, 349 genera and 2284 virus species (www.ictvonline.org; and see Willey *et al.*, 2010b).

Viruses are classified according to their shape, their capsid, their genetic material and whether or not they have an envelope. They may also be classified further according to their size; the host they affect, which may be human, plant, animal or bacteria (bacteriophages); and the effect which they have on the host (e.g. cell death, transformation of the cell into a state of malignancy, or latent infection which results in clinical illness at a later date).

Structure

The **virion** is the infectious particle of a virus and consists of single-stranded or double-stranded nucleic acid, which is either DNA (a molecule that contains all of the cell's genetic information) *or* RNA, which translates the genetic material into protein (Ahmad *et al.*, 2010a). The nucleic acid is surrounded by a coat of protein, called the capsid.

The **capsid** is symmetrical and tends to be either icosahedral, with 12 vertices, 30 sides and 20 faces which are each equilateral triangles; helical, with the nucleic acid tightly coiled; or complex, a combination of icosahedral and helical and therefore of a more complicated structure (Willey *et al.*, 2010c). The different viral structures are illustrated in Figure 5.2.

Capsomeres are protein units that make up the capsid, and they enable the virus to attach to a host cell (Collier *et al.*, 2011a). The number of capsomeres varies amongst viruses.

An **envelope** surrounds some viruses, which is acquired from the cell membrane of the host cell as the virus attaches and fuses to it (Ahmad *et al.*, 2010a). Those which do not have an envelope are referred to as non-enveloped, or naked.

Protein-receptor binding sites on the outer surface of the virus enable them to bind or attach to other cells with the same receptor, which explains why some viruses cause illnesses which affect only the respiratory or the gastro-intestinal tract.

Replication

There are several stages in the viral replication and infection process.

Collision and attachment

In order to initiate the beginning of the infective cycle, the virus has to 'collide' with the host cell, and virion attachment proteins on the virus and receptor molecules on the cell wall, which are

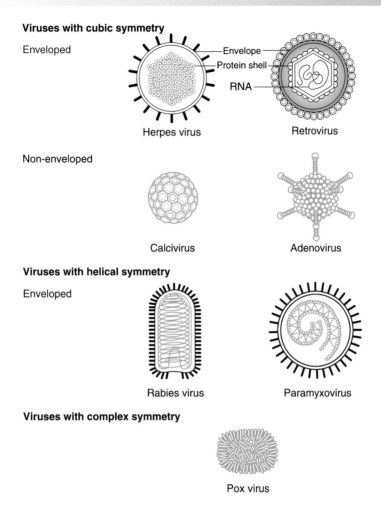

Viruses with cubic symmetry

Enveloped

Envelope
Protein shell
RNA

Herpes virus

Retrovirus

Non-enveloped

Calcivirus

Adenovirus

Viruses with helical symmetry

Enveloped

Rabies virus

Paramyxovirus

Viruses with complex symmetry

Pox virus

Figure 5.2   Different viral structures. (Wilson, 2003)

specific for each virus family, have to attach (Ahmad *et al.*, 2010a). For example, the human immunodeficiency virus (HIV) attaches to CD4 receptors on T lymphocytes (see Chapter 24). Because the virus–cell attachment is a highly specific reaction between the proteins and the receptors, not all collisions result in a successful infection, making collision and attachment 'hit-and-miss' events.

Uncoating, dismantling and 'injecting' of viral genes

Once the virus has attached to and penetrated the cell, it is protected from the immune system, and the process of uncoating begins, where the virus dismantles and injects its genetic material (Collier *et al.*, 2011a). DNA viruses inject their nucleic acid into the nuclei of the host cell; RNA viruses inject into the cytoplasm. Transcription, translation and replication take place as new virus particles are manufactured within the host cell. The host cell then bursts, releasing as many as 10 000 new virus particles (Collier *et al.*, 2011a), which go on to infect other host cells.

Some medically important viruses

This is not an exhaustive account of all medically important viruses, but offers a very brief description of some of the virus families and the viral infections that they result in which may be seen within the healthcare setting. Blood-borne viruses such as hepatitis B, hepatitis C and HIV, and other viral infections such as norovirus, are discussed in Chapters 23 (norovirus) and 24 (blood-borne viruses).

Adenoviridae

These are medium-sized, non-enveloped icosahedral viruses, containing a single piece of double-stranded DNA with 252 capsomeres (Collier *et al.*, 2011b). There are thought to be more than 100 different serotypes, with 51 known to cause infections in humans (Ahmad *et al.*, 2010b), and most individuals have been infected with several species of adenovirus by the time they reach adulthood. Adenoviruses cause acute febrile respiratory illnesses such as pneumonia and bronchiolitis, particularly in young children, as well as gastroenteritis and conjunctivitis. They spread readily by droplet infection, although faecal-oral transmission can also occur.

Herpesviridae

These are double-stranded DNA, enveloped, icosahedral viruses with 162 capsomeres (Ogilvie, 2004). Herpes viruses, of which there are in excess of 120 known species, include, amongst others, cytomegalovirus (see Fact Sheet 9.2 on the companion website), herpes simplex virus (HSV) 1 and 2, varicella zoster virus (VZV) and Epstein–Barr virus (EBV).

Herpes simplex virus: HSV can be shed in saliva and respiratory secretions, and primary infection generally occurs in childhood from contact with an infected older person (e.g. a parent) (Collier *et al.*, 2011c). It produces vesicles, seen as eruptions on the surface of the skin and mucous membranes, typically appearing on the lips as cold sores, and on the genital mucosa (genital herpes).

Picornaviridae

These are small enveloped icosahedrals, with single-stranded DNA and 32 capsomeres. This group consists of more than 70 enteroviruses (Burns, 2004), such as polioviruses, coxsackieviruses, echoviruses and rhinoviruses. Enteroviruses are found in the intestines and excreted in the faeces, causing a variety of illnesses. Infection with poliovirus can result in asymptomatic infection or a mild flu-like illness; the added involvement of the central nervous system gives rise to symptoms of meningitis, or paralysis. Polio is preventable only through immunisation (see http://www.who.int/topics/poliomyelitis/en/). Infection with coxsackieviruses and echoviruses can result in meningitis, upper respiratory tract infections, gastroenteritis, pleurisy and pericarditis. Rhinoviruses are the culprits responsible for the 'common cold'.

Hepadnaviridae

These are small enveloped icosahedrals with 180 capsomeres and double-stranded DNA. Hepatitis B virus (HBV) is discussed in detail in Chapter 24.

Paramyxoviridae

Enveloped, helical, single-stranded RNA. The viruses in this group include the para-influenza virus, which is associated with croup and bronchiolitis in children, and minor upper respiratory tract infections, and the mumps and measles viruses (Collier *et al.*, 2011d). The **mumps virus** is generally an illness of childhood and causes pain and swelling of the parotid salivary glands. It is spread by droplet infection, with an incubation period of 14–18 days, with individuals considered to be infectious from 12 to 25 days after exposure. Peak **incidence** is in the winter and spring. Aseptic (viral) meningitis and orchitis are common complications, along with deafness and encephalitis.

Measles: Measles is a serious disease, responsible for one million deaths among children worldwide each year (http://www.hpa.org.uk/Topics/InfectiousDiseases/InfectionsAZ/Measles). It has an incubation period of 10–12 days and begins with a flu-like prodromal illness, with a hacking cough and conjunctivitis. A widespread macropapular rash usually appears after four days, beginning on the forehead and spreading down the body. Although it is usually a childhood infection, it can affect any age group, and complications includes pneumonia, otitis media (ear infection) and post-measles encephalitis (Collier *et al.*, 2011d). It became a notifiable disease in England and Wales in 1940 (Department of Health, 2011).

Measles–mumps–rubella (MMR) vaccination

MMR can be given at any age, but it is recommended that the first vaccination is given at around 13 months, and the second before the child begins at school to capture those children in whom the first vaccination did not generate a full immune response (http://www.hpa.org.uk/Topics/InfectiousDiseases/InfectionsAZ/MMR/).

Controversy in recent years over a suspected link between the MMR vaccine and autism and Crohn's disease has led to a decrease in MMR uptake and subsequent fears of a measles epidemic. This has now become something of a reality with almost 2000 cases of measles reported in 2012 (reported by Public Health England and the DH as a 'record high'), plus a further 587 cases in the first quarter of 2013. This increase, which has seen 108 affected individuals admitted to hospital during January – March 2013 (15 with complications) has been attributed to 10–16 years who were not vaccinated during the late 1990s onwards and who were therefore unprotected. Information on the safety of the vaccine and the importance of vaccination is available on the immunisation pages of the Department of Health website (www.dh.gov.uk).

Fact Box 5.10   MMR vaccine

A single vaccine against measles became available in 1968, but it wasn't until the combined MMR vaccine was introduced in 1988 that the number of epidemics occurring among children of school age and younger fell dramatically. In April 2013, Public Health England, NHS England and the DH announced a national MMR vaccination 'catch-up' campaign to decrease the pool of unprotected children, amid estimates that approximately one third of a million children are currently unvaccinated, and that there are a further one third of a million who are partly vaccinated.

Togaviridae

The **rubella virus** (Rubivirus) belongs to the family of viruses known as Togaviridae, which are enveloped viruses with single-stranded DNA. Rubella (also known as German measles) is spread via respiratory secretions. Symptoms include enlargement of the lymph nodes behind the ears, in the neck and axillae, along with a pyrexia, malaise, conjunctivitis and a rash which affects the head and neck initially before spreading to the trunk (Collier *et al.*, 2010e). Although it is generally a mild infection, it can have serious implications for pregnant women, particularly in the first 8–10 weeks of pregnancy when there is a significant risk of severe foetal abnormalities. Rubella is preventable through vaccination, which is given through the combined MMR vaccine.

Caliciviridae

These are spherical, non-enveloped, single-stranded RNA viruses, with 32 cup-shaped depressions on their capsid (Collier *et al.*, 2011f). They are the main causative agents of viral diarrhoea and vomiting. Norovirus is by far the most notorious member of the caliciviruses and is discussed in detail in Chapter 23.

Coronaviridae

These are complex, enveloped, single-stranded RNA viruses, 60–220 nm in diameter. They have a 'crown-like' appearance (corona), which creates a halo effect around the virus. They are primarily responsible for causing upper respiratory tract infections, along with viral gastroenteritis, in humans, but they are also pathogens in animals and have been known to mutate and infect new species (McIntosh and Anderson, 2004).

SARS

As mentioned in Chapter 1, severe acute respiratory syndrome (SARS) was the first new disease threat of the twenty-first century, and was caused by a novel coronavirus. Early in November 2002, when the first cases of SARS emerged in Guangdong Province, China, there were reports that some of those affected had been exposed to live wild game animals in markets. Some of these animals were subsequently tested and were found to carry a virus that was very similar to the human SARS coronavirus, most notably the Himalayan palm civet cat (*Paguma larvata*) (73% of the market traders primarily trading in palm civet cats were found to be seropositive), the raccoon dog (*Nyclereutes procyonoides*) and the Chinese ferret badger (*Melogale moschata*) – all regarded as delicacies in southern China. The virus was therefore presumed to be zoonotic in origin, arising from the animal kingdom with the palm civet cat as the most important animal reservoir (Donnelly *et al.*, 2004).

Fact Box 5.11   SARS – virus amplification

The live market setting, offering a diversity of animal species, is believed to have given the virus ample opportunity to amplify and over a period of time jump hosts, eventually infecting humans and resulting in human-to-human transmission. In September 2005, a study from China confirmed that 40% of horseshoe bats near Hong Kong were infected with a coronavirus similar to SARS, raising the question 'Did the horseshoe bats infect the palm civet cats?'

Orthomyxoviridae

These are 80–120 nm, helical, enveloped, single-stranded RNA viruses. This group consists of the influenza viruses. There are three serotypes which are based on antigenic differences and differences in genetic makeup, structure, host susceptibility, epidemiology and clinical features. Influenza A viruses, while mostly prevalent among humans, also circulate among many mammalian and avian species, and it is this ability to jump the species barrier that makes this serotype the biggest threat in terms of the evolution of new influenza viruses with pandemic potential, as seen with the emergence of H1N1 (2009) 'swine flu', which originated in Mexico and spread globally (the pandemic was declared over by the World Health Organization in 2010). While influenza B can cause severe disease in 'at-risk' groups, and influenza C causes mild disease throughout the year, neither of these serotypes have been linked to previous pandemics, although that does not rule out the possibility of a new B or C strain evolving that has pandemic potential.

The virus is covered with surface projections or spikes, which consist of two types of antigen – hemoglutinin (HA) antigen and neuraminidase (NA) antigen. HA antigen plays an important role in initiating infection by enabling the virus to attach to receptor sites on the respiratory cell surface in the host. NA antigens assist fusion of the viral cell envelope with the surface of the host respiratory cell and aid the release of newly formed virus particles from infected cells, which go on to enter and replicate within other cells. Influenza viruses are able to mutate and swap genes, undergoing frequent changes in their surface HA and/or NA antigens which may be minor (antigenic drift) or major (antigenic shift).

Fact Box 5.12   Antigenic drift

Antigenic drift, caused by a single mutation in the viral RNA, occurs constantly among influenza A viruses and is responsible for annual flu epidemics, with new strains emerging every year. Generally, with antigenic drift there is some kind of serological relationship between the new and old HA and NA antigens, so although the virus is 'drifting' and changing subtly, it does not differ too drastically from previous strains. Some of the population will have immunity to the virus, and vaccination is a preventative measure in those with no immunity or who are in at-risk categories.

Fact Box 5.13   Antigenic shift

Major changes to actual gene segments on the surface antigens lead to the creation of a 'new' virus. Immunity will be virtually non-existent. Antigenic shift can occur either as a sudden 'adaptive' change during replication of a normal virus, or from genetic exchange between a human and an animal strain of influenza A. With genetic exchange, an animal is co-infected with both a human and an animal strain and serves as a 'mixing vessel' for the virus, allowing it to genetically 're-assort' itself and create a new virus capable of causing disease in humans.

Retroviridae

These are 80–100 nm, complex, enveloped, single-stranded RNA viruses. Retroviruses cause HIV (see Chapter 24 for more details).

Prions

During the 1990s, an outbreak of disease among cattle which had begun in the United Kingdom in 1986 reached epidemic proportions. Bovine spongiform encephalopathy (BSE), or 'mad cow disease' as it was commonly called, has affected more than 170 000 cattle and led to the slaughter of 4.7 million. It devastated the cattle and meat export industry, and ruined the livelihood of thousands of farmers in the process. The government denied that the outbreak posed any significant threat to public health, assuring the worried public that it was safe to eat beef, but that changed in 1996 when the Secretary of State for Health, Stephen Dorrell, announced that 10 young people in the United Kingdom had developed a variant form of Creutzfeldt–Jakob disease (called new variant Creutzfeldt–Jakob disease, or vCJD). Both BSE and vCJD are caused by transmissible spongiform encephalopathies (TSEs), otherwise known as prion diseases, which fatally affect the central nervous system in animals and humans. Prions, or proteinaceous infectious particles (PrPs), were first identified by Stanley Prusiner (1982), an American neurologist and biochemist, as the causative agents of a group of fatal degenerative neurological diseases which affect animals – the TSEs – causing scrapie in sheep and goats and BSE in cattle. They are thought to be naturally occurring proteins derived from normal body proteins which undergo a rare spontaneous process, affecting normal protein synthesis in the individual, and creating microscopic vacuoles (holes) in the grey matter of the brain, giving it a sponge-like appearance. They are unconventional infectious agents which do not induce an immune response (Belay and Schonberger, 2005), replicate by converting natural prion protein into the abnormal form and are distinguished from viruses and viroids as they have no detectable nucleic acid.

Fact Box 5.14   The medical significance of prions

Prions are virtually impossible to inactivate or eliminate as they are extremely, and unusually, resistant to conventional decontamination methods (both physical and chemical), high doses of ionising and ultraviolet radiation, and sterilisation (infectivity persists after standard autoclaving at 134 °C for three minutes).

Chapter summary: key points

- The medically important groups of microorganisms include bacteria, viruses, prions, fungi, helminths and protozoa.

- The surface of the human body consists of 10 times more microorganisms on the skin than it does cells.

- It is estimated that there are between 500 and 1000 different species of bacteria that inhabit the body.

- There are 50 species of bacteria that are known to cause infection or disease in humans. Others are opportunistic, causing infection when host immune defences are breached.

- Bacteria are identified according to their shape, cell wall, Gram-stain reaction and virulence factors.

- The production of invasive enzymes helps the organism penetrate into the host's tissues, causing tissue damage.

- The production and release of toxins are responsible for many of the signs and symptoms, or clinical features, of infection.

- Resistance to antibiotics, and virulence factors such as toxin genes, can be carried on plasmids and transmitted between different strains of the same bacteria, or between different bacterial species.

- Viruses are the smallest known infective agents, approximately 100 to 1000 times smaller than the cells they infect.

- A virus is incapable of independent replication; it needs to access a host cell so that it can substitute its own nucleic acid for the cell's DNA.

- Viruses are classified according to their shape, their capsid, their genetic material, the presence of a viral envelope, the host they affect (human, plant, animal or bacteria) and the effect which they have on the host.

- Once a host cell has been infected by a virus it bursts, releasing as many as 10 000 new virus particles which go on to infect other host cells.

Reflection point

Does an understanding of the virulence factors of bacteria and viruses, particularly those associated with the bacterial cell wall and toxin production, make healthcare staff more likely to appreciate and understand the importance of compliance with infection control standard precautions?

 Further resources are available for this book, including interactive multiple choice questions. Visit the companion website at:

www.wiley.com/go/fundamentalsofinfectionprevention

References

Ahmad N., Ray C.G., Drew W.L. (2010a). The nature of viruses. In: Ryan K.J., Ray G.C. (Eds.), *Sherris Medical Microbiology*. 5th ed. McGraw-Hill Medical, New York: 101–135.

Ahmad N., Ray C.G., Drew W.L. (2010b). Influenza, parainfluenza, respiratory syncytial, adenovirus and other respiratory viruses. In: Ryan K.J., Ray G.C. (Eds.), *Sherris Medical Microbiology*. 5th ed. McGraw-Hill Medical, New York: 167–188.

Belay E.D., Schonberger L.B. (2005). The public health impact of prion diseases. *Annual Review of Public Health*. 26: 191–121.

Burns S.M. (2004). Picornaviruses. In: Greenwood D., Slack R.C.B., Peutherer J.F. (Eds.), *Medical Microbiology. A Guide to Microbial Infections: Pathogenesis, Immunity, Laboratory Diagnosis and Control*. 16th ed. Churchill Livingstone, London: 455–467.

Chen L., Wen Y. (2011). The role of bacterial biofilm in persistent infections and control strategies. *International Journal of Oral Science*. 3: 66–73.

Collier L., Kellam P., Oxford J. (2011a). General properties of viruses. In: Collier L., Oxford J., Kellam P. (Eds.), *Human Virology*. 4th ed. Oxford University Press, Oxford: 8–16.

Collier L., Kellam P., Oxford J. (2011b). Upper respiratory tract and eye infections due to adenoviruses, coronaviruses (including SARS CoV) and rhinoviruses. In: Collier L., Oxford J., Kellam P. (Eds.), *Human Virology*. 4th ed. Oxford University Press, Oxford: 74–84.

Collier L., Kellam P., Oxford J. (2011c). The herpesvirus: general properties. In: Collier L., Oxford J., Kellam P. (Eds.), *Human Virology*. 4th ed. Oxford University Press, Oxford: 165–169.

Collier L., Kellam P., Oxford J. (2011d). Infections caused by the paramyxoviruses. In: *Human Virology*. 4th ed. Oxford University Press, Oxford: 86–97.

Collier L., Kellam P., Oxford J. (2010e). Rubella: postnatal infections. In: *Human Virology*. 4th ed. Oxford University Press, Oxford: 122–126.

Collier L., Kellam P., Oxford J. (2011f). Gastroenteritis viruses. In: *Human Virology*. 4th ed. Oxford University Press, Oxford: 111–120.

Department of Health (2011). *Immunisation against Infectious Disease*. Department of Health Green Book. Department of Health, London. http://media.dh.gov.uk/network/211/files/2012/07/Green-Book-original-2006.pdf (accessed 26 February 2013)

Donnelly C.A., Fisher M.C., Fraser C., Ghani A.C., Riley S., Ferguson N.M., Anderson R.M. (2004). Epidemiological and genetic analysis of severe acute respiratory syndrome. *The Lancet Infectious Diseases*. 4 (November): 672–683.

Engelkirk G., Duben-Engelkirk J. (2011a). Microbiology: the science. In: *Microbiology for the Health Sciences*. 9th ed. Lippincott Williams and Wilkins, Philadelphia: 1–12.

Engelkirk G., Duben-Engelkirk J. (2011b). Cell structure and taxonomy. In: *Microbiology for the Health Sciences*. 9th ed. Lippincott Williams and Wilkins, Philadelphia: 24–39.

Engelkirk G., Duben-Engelkirk J. (2011c). Pathogenesis of infectious diseases. In: *Microbiology for the Health Sciences*. 9th ed. Lippincott Williams and Wilkins, Philadelphia: 238–250.

Gladwin M., Trattler B. (2004). Cell structure, virulence factors and toxins. In: *Clinical Microbiology Made Ridiculously Simple*. 3rd ed. MedMaster Inc., Miami: 8–15.

Health Protection Agency (2008). *Guidance on the Diagnosis and Management of PVL-Associated Staphylococcus aureus (PVL-SA) Infections in England*. Report prepared by the PVL sub-group of the Steering Group on Healthcare Associated Infections. 2nd ed. November. Health Protection Agency, London.

Lindsay D., von Holy A. (2006). Bacterial biofilms within the clinical setting: what healthcare professionals should know. *Journal of Hospital Infection*. 65 (4): 313–325.

McIntosh K., Anderson L.J. (2004). Coronaviruses, including severe acute respiratory syndrome (SARS)-associated coronavirus. In: Mandell G.L., Bennett J.E., Dolin R. (Eds.), *Mandell's Principles and Practices of Infectious Diseases*. 6th ed. Churchill Livingstone, London.

Morgan M. (2005). Editorial. *Staphylococcus aureus*, Panton-Valentine leukocidin and necrotising pneumonia. *British Medical Journal*. 331 (7520): 793–794.

Ogilvie M.M. (2004). Herpes viruses. In: Greenwood D., Slack R.C.B., Peutherer J.F. (Eds.), *Medical Microbiology. A Guide to Microbial Infections: Pathogenesis, Immunity, Laboratory Diagnosis and Control*. 16th ed. Churchill Livingstone, London: 399–420.

Petri W.A., Mann B.J., Huston C.D. (2010). Microbial biofilm: In: Mandell G.L., Bennett J.E., Dolin R. (Eds.), *Mandell's Principles and Practices of Infectious Diseases*. 6th ed. Churchill Livingstone Elsevier, London. http://expertconsult.com (accessed 28 February 2013)

Proft T., Fraser J.D. (2003). Bacterial superantigens. *Clinical and Experimental Immunology*. 133: 299–306.

Prusiner S.B. (1982). Novel proteinacious infectious particles cause scrapie. *Science*. 216 (9): 136–144.

Ryan K.J., Drew W.L. (2010). The nature of bacteria. In: Ryan K.J., Ray G.C. (Eds.), *Sherris Medical Microbiology*. 5th ed. McGraw-Hill Medical, New York: 347–387.

Torres B.A., Kominsky S., Perrin G.Q., Hobeika A.C., Johnson H.W. (2001). Superantigens: the good, the bad and the ugly. *Experimental Biology and Medicine*. 226: 164–176.

Watnick P., Koiter R. (2000). Biofilm, city of microbes. *Journal of Bacteriology*. 182 (10): 2675–2679.

Willey J.M., Sherwood L.M., Woolverton C.J. (2011a). Bacteria and archaea. In: *Prescott's Microbiology*. 8th ed. McGraw-Hill Medical, New York: 46–87.

Willey J.M., Sherwood L.M., Woolverton C.J. (2011b). Infection and pathogenicity. In: *Prescott's Microbiology*. 8th ed. McGraw-Hill Medical, New York: 739–759.

Willey J.M., Sherwood L.M., Woolverton C.J. (2011c). The viruses. In: *Prescott's Microbiology*. 5th ed. McGraw-Hill Medical, New York: 616–643.

6

The collection and transportation of specimens

Contents

Fundamentals of Infection Prevention and Control: Theory and Practice, Second Edition. Debbie Weston.
© 2013 John Wiley & Sons, Ltd. Published 2013 by John Wiley & Sons, Ltd. Companion Website: www.wiley.com/go/fundamentalsofinfectionprevention

Introduction

In order to accurately diagnose a patient's infection and disease and prescribe the appropriate antimicrobial agent(s), the collection of the appropriate clinical specimen is essential. Unfortunately, many specimens received in the laboratory are substandard and therefore are not considered viable for a number of reasons that can, and should, easily be avoided. This chapter identifies the most commonly requested specimens that healthcare staff are required to collect for examination in the laboratory, and looks at the recommended methods of collection together with the health and safety issues that need to be taken into account to protect both the staff obtaining and transporting the specimen, and the laboratory staff who process it.

Learning outcomes

After reading this chapter, the reader will be able to:

- Understand the basic principles of specimen collection, taking into account health, safety and infection control precautions.

- Be able to obtain or assist in the collection of clinical specimens commonly requested for the detection of infections – urine, sputum, wound swabs, faecal specimens, throat swabs, nasal swabs, cerebral spinal fluid and blood.

General points

A clinical specimen can be defined as any bodily substance, solid or liquid, that is obtained for the purpose of analysis. In order to accurately diagnose the patient's infection or disease and prescribe the appropriate antimicrobial agent(s), the collection of the appropriate clinical specimen is essential (Thys *et al.*, 1994). The quality of the result achieved from a specimen is directly related to the quality of the specimen itself, meaning that the *correct* specimen has to be obtained from the *correct* site using the *correct* technique in order to avoid a false-negative result (Murray and Witebsky, 2010).

Bearing in mind that the person collecting the specimen is responsible for its quality, it is imperative that healthcare workers possess the necessary knowledge to enable them to obtain specimens appropriately. This chapter identifies the most commonly requested specimens that healthcare staff are required to collect for examination in the laboratory, and looks at the recommended methods of specimen collection together with the health and safety issues that need to be taken into account in order to protect both the staff obtaining and transporting the specimen, and the laboratory staff who process it. Chapter 7 examines how these specimens are cultured.

Specimens must be collected in the appropriate container

A variety of specimen containers are available in all wards, departments, GP surgeries and health centres, and advice on the correct container and collection of the specimen can be sought from the medical microbiology laboratory where the specimen will be processed.

The containers must be shatterproof, not overfilled, the lid secured tightly and the specimen placed in a specimen bag, which is then sealed to prevent leakage. If there is any contamination on the outside of the container (e.g. with blood or body fluids), this must be removed before the container is put into the bag. The request form should then be placed into a separate sleeve on the bag to prevent it from becoming contaminated.

For specimens that are being transported by road to a laboratory, either by car (e.g. a taxi, a courier or the District Nurse's own vehicle) or designated pathology transport van, the container must be transported in a secure, rigid, unbreakable container or transport box and clearly labelled. The transportation of specimens must be compliant with the Carriage of Dangerous Goods Act 2004.

Taking the correct specimen

The correct specimen for the diagnosis of illness or disease needs to be collected from the appropriate body site using an aseptic technique in order to avoid inadvertently contaminating the sample. The results of the laboratory investigation could then be misleading, and the patient may not receive the correct treatment.

Fact Box 6.1   Contamination of clinical specimens

Contamination can arise from the patient's own body flora if due care isn't taken when collecting the specimen, from the flora of the person collecting the specimen or from a non-sterile specimen container.

Obtaining a specimen at the correct time

Where possible, specimens should be obtained *before* the patient commences antibiotics, as treatment with antibiotics before the causative organism has been identified may inhibit its growth, and it may not be detected in the laboratory. In addition, the antimicrobial agent prescribed may not have actually been effective in treating the infection. However, there are some conditions such as meningitis where antibiotic therapy needs to commence immediately, and delays in waiting for the results of any laboratory tests can mean the difference between life and death. In situations such as this, treatment with antibiotics **must not** be delayed or withheld.

The labelling of specimens and the specimen request form

Poorly completed specimen request forms, and poorly labelled specimens, are likely to result in the specimen **not** being processed by the laboratory staff and the specimen being discarded. This delays diagnosis and treatment, may increase the risk of cross-infection by delaying recognition of the need for patient isolation, and inconveniences the patient who has to go through the process again. It also wastes valuable healthcare worker time and money.

Apart from the obvious information such as the patient's name, hospital number and date of birth and the ward or department that the result needs to go back to, there is a lot of other essential information which is required but which is often incomplete.

Specimen type and site

Sending a swab merely labelled 'wound' from a patient who may have more than one wound site is far from helpful. Different areas of the body are home to different resident body flora (see Chapter 8), and a poorly labelled clinical specimen will make it harder for the laboratory staff to differentiate between organisms which could normally be expected to reside at a particular site, and those organisms which should not be there. It may also make it harder for the right diagnostic investigation to be performed.

Date and time that the specimen was collected

The 'age' of the specimen is important – some organisms are fragile and will die once they leave the body, which will obviously make their identification difficult. Additionally, if there is a mixed growth of organisms in the specimen, or the specimen was contaminated during the collection process, some organisms may overgrow, making it difficult to single out the particular organism that is causing the problem.

Relevant clinical information

This highly useful and very important section is all too often either left blank or inadequately completed. Its completion really is essential and will help the laboratory staff and the microbiologist interpret the results.

Box 6.1 identifies the clinical information that should be provided on the specimen request form where relevant or applicable.

Box 6.1   Clinical information to be included on the specimen request form

- Any relevant clinical signs and symptoms
- Date of surgery
- Recent history of foreign travel (details of countries visited must be included) and any vaccinations
- Whether the patient is immunocompromised as a result of other illness, as immunocompromised patients are highly susceptible to infection by opportunistic and 'non-pathogenic' organisms
- Whether the patient is receiving steroids or immunosuppressive drugs which can depress the inflammatory response
- Current or recently completed antibiotic treatment – if antimicrobial agents are present in the specimen at the time of collection, they will inhibit the growth of any pathogens.

The investigation required

Sometimes, requesting microscopy, culture and sensitivity (MC&S) is sufficient but it will not detect all pathogens. If stool specimens are being obtained from a ward during a norovirus outbreak, for example, the laboratory staff need to know what they are looking for. Giving all relevant information on the request form relating to the patient's symptoms, and a request for electron microscopy for example, will ensure that the right investigation is carried out. A different request form is normally required for specimens which have been obtained for the detection of viruses.

'Danger of Infection' labelling

Specimens from patients known, or strongly suspected, to have tuberculosis (Chapter 21), or a blood-borne virus infection (Chapter 24), must be labelled with a 'Danger of Infection' sticker to alert staff transporting the specimen, and the laboratory staff.

Microorganisms are categorized according to the level of risk that they may pose, and where specific pathogens are suspected, the specimen will be classified as hazardous and processed under laboratory conditions accordingly. With regard to blood-borne viruses, although all blood and body fluids should be treated as potentially infectious and exposure to them managed using standard precautions, additional precautions will be taken in the laboratory, and post-exposure prophylaxis may be required in the event of an inoculation injury.

Prompt delivery to the laboratory

Finally, the specimen must be transported to the laboratory as soon as possible. Some pathogens may die rapidly when they have left the host and may not be detected if the specimen has been left sitting at room temperature on the ward for several hours waiting to be collected. Normal body flora within the specimen may proliferate and overgrow, inhibiting or killing the pathogen. The clinical specimens that can be refrigerated overnight only if necessary are identified in Box 6.2.

Box 6.2   Specimens that can be refrigerated overnight

Wound swabs
Urine (boric acid in the container will preserve white blood cells and prevent the overgrowth of bacteria)
Faeces
Throat swabs
Meticillin-resistant *Staphylococcus aureus* (MRSA) swabs and screens.

Blood cultures and specimens of cerebral spinal fluid (CSF) are always treated as urgent and must be sent to the laboratory *immediately*. Arrangements are always in place for those specimens requiring processing and urgent analysis out of hours, as the results are often of life-threatening importance.

Sputum specimens can be stored at room temperature for no longer than 24 hours; they must not be refrigerated as this will destroy fragile organisms such as *Streptococcus pneumoniae*.

Healthcare workers should be aware that there are various acts and regulations that govern the safe collection, handling and transportation of clinical specimens (see Box 6.3).

Box 6.3   Acts and regulations regarding the safe collection, handling and transportation of specimens

The Health and Safety at Work Regulations 1974

The Health and Safety (Dangerous Pathogens) Regulations 1981

The Carriage of Dangerous Goods and the Use of Transportable Pressure Equipment Regulations 2004

The Management of Health and Safety at Work Regulations 1992

Reporting of Injuries, Diseases and Dangerous Occurrences Regulations (RIDDOR) 1995: Under RIDDOR, employers are required to report accidents, dangerous occurrences and cases of ill health amongst employees to the Health and Safety Executive (HSE). This includes accidents or occurrences that are relevant to clinical laboratories where infections are attributable to working with microorganisms (e.g. hepatitis and TB); exposure to an agent, toxin or infectious material resulting in an acute illness that requires medical treatment; release of a biological agent with the potential to cause severe harm or infection or exposure to a biological agent involving loss of consciousness.

The Control of Substances Hazardous to Health (COSHH) Regulations 2000: Substances that are hazardous to health and covered under COSHH regulations include chemicals and products containing chemicals; fumes, dust and vapours; mists; gases and asphyxiating gases; nanotechnology and 'biological agents'. Biological agents are defined by COSHH as 'any micro-organism, parasite, microscopic infectious form of larger parasite, including any which have been genetically modified, which may cause an infection, allergy, toxicity or otherwise create a hazard to human health'. Biological agents therefore include bacteria, viruses, parasites, fungi, protozoa and prions.

They are categorized into four hazard groups according to whether they are pathogenic for humans, hazardous to employees and/or transmissible to the community and whether effective treatment or prophylaxis is available:

- Hazard Group 1 – This group is unlikely to cause human disease.
- Hazard Group 2 – These hazards can cause human disease and may be a hazard to employees, but are unlikely to spread to the community; treatment or prophylaxis is available.
- Hazard Group 3 – This group can cause severe human disease and may present a severe hazard to employees; it may also spread to the community, but treatment or prophylaxis is available. The majority of the microorganisms discussed in this book belong to Hazard Groups 2 and 3.
- Hazard Group 4 – These hazards cause severe human disease and may be a severe hazard to employees; they are likely to spread to and within the community, and there is usually no effective treatment or prophylaxis. Hazard Group 4 agents include the viral haemorrhagic fevers (VHFs) (see Fact Sheet 3.12 on the companion website). Patients with infections caused by a Group 4 agent will be cared for in a High Security Infectious Diseases Unit.

  Further information regarding biological agents and hazard categories can be found in the Health and Safety Executive and Advisory Committee on Dangerous Pathogens (2004) publication *The Approved List of Biological Agents*.

Commonly requested clinical specimens

- Urine
- Sputum
- Wound swabs
- Faeces
- Throat swabs
- Nasal swabs
- Blood culture
- CSF.

Urine

See also Chapter 17, which discusses urinary tract infections in greater detail.

Indications for collection

- Urinary tract infection
- Sepsis screen
- Pyrexia of unknown origin (PUO)
- *Legionella* infection (see Fact Sheet 1.3 on the companion website)
- Tuberculosis (see Chapter 21).

Urine for MC&S is one of the most frequently requested laboratory tests (Murray and Witebsky, 2010). Bladder urine is sterile, but infection may arise as a result of perineal or bowel flora ascending the urethra.

In an un-catheterised patient, a urine specimen may become contaminated during urination by the normal flora found at the distal urethra, which is the part of the urethra furthest from the bladder. In order to reduce the risk of a contaminated sample, the urine should be obtained as either 'a clean-catch' into a sterile container (i.e. for children) or a mid-stream specimen (MSU). In babies, a self-adhesive urine collection bag can be used. There is very little evidence to suggest that meatal perineal cleansing prior to obtaining the specimen is of any real benefit in preventing contamination of the urine sample with genital flora, although in patients with poor personal hygiene washing the perineum with soap and water before the MSU is collected may be of some value and is often preferred.

Obtaining an MSU

When an MSU is obtained, the first portion of urine is voided directly into the toilet or a bedpan, so that the organisms that normally reside within the distal urethra are flushed out. The patient must then have sufficient bladder control to be able to void the mid-stream into a sterile container, and then the remainder into the toilet or bedpan again. Collecting an uncontaminated specimen is sometimes difficult, and so the specimen request form should state the method by which the urine specimen has been obtained.

Obtaining a catheter specimen of urine (CSU)

In catheterised patients, urine should be sent for laboratory culture **only** if the patient has clinical sepsis, **not** because the appearance or smell of the urine suggests that bacteria are present in the urine (bacteriuria) (Scottish Intercollegiate Guidelines Network, 2006) (see Chapter 17).

If the patient is catheterised (with either a urethral or supra-pubic catheter), a urine specimen must be obtained via the catheter sampling port using an aseptic technique (see Box 6.4). It must **never** be obtained directly from the catheter bag as the stagnant urine within the bag will be contaminated from a heavy growth of microorganisms.

Once collected, urine specimens must be sent to the laboratory within two hours of collection; if that is not possible, they must be refrigerated at 4 °C for no longer than 24 hours. If the specimen is not refrigerated and is left at room temperature, bacteria within the sample will multiply and the detection and identification of any pathogen will be difficult. Universal urine specimen containers which contain borate, a preservative, are widely used, and mean that urine can be refrigerated overnight. However, their use has been shown to adversely affect the result of urine culture and the clinical interpretation of the results (Gillespie *et al.*, 1999).

Sputum

The function of sputum is to trap an inhaled foreign material, which includes bacteria, and it is produced in excess when the lower respiratory tract becomes inflamed. Sputum produced as a result of infection is generally purulent, and a good sample can yield a high bacterial load. Unfortunately, however, as the mouth and pharynx are home to a large number of normal resident flora (see Chapter 8), this can make the detection of the pathogen hidden among them far from easy. Too many of the 'sputum' specimens sent to the laboratory are actually saliva, which is of no benefit at all as it will not yield any clinically relevant results.

Box 6.4   Procedure for collecting a catheter specimen of urine (CSU)

1. Explain and discuss the procedure with the patient.
2. Screen the bed.
3. Decontaminate hands using alcohol hand rub or by handwashing with liquid soap.
4. Put on a disposable plastic apron (to protect uniform).
5. Put on examination gloves (contact with blood or body fluids).
6. Clean the access port on the catheter bag with an isopropyl alcohol 70% and chlorhexidine 2% 'steret'. Allow 30 seconds to dry.
7. Using a sterile syringe, aspirate the required amount of urine from the access point.
8. Decant the specimen into a sterile container.
9. Remove gloves and decontaminate hands using alcohol hand rub or by handwashing with liquid soap.
10. Label the container and dispatch with the request form in a specimen bag.

Obtaining a sputum specimen

It is important that the patient is instructed to give a deep cough in order to produce a good specimen, and often the best specimen is produced first thing in the morning. In situations where it is difficult to obtain a sputum specimen, either because the patient is physically unable to produce a sputum specimen, or because there is no productive cough, sputum production can be induced by the administration of nebulized saline, or by bronchoscopy and lavage. The generation of sputum via nebuliser is an aerosol-generating procedure that should be undertaken in a single room with the door closed, and the physiotherapist should wear respiratory protection (see Chapter 13 on personal protective equipment).

For tuberculosis, three separate sputum specimens over three days are required – this is because the number of bacilli present in a clinical specimen can vary by the hour, so generally the more specimens collected, the higher the chance of detection. Ideally, specimens should be obtained prior to the commencement of anti-tuberculosis therapy, but where there is clear clinical evidence of respiratory disease, a decision may be made to initiate treatment before any specimens have been obtained or the microbiology results are available. Attempts should still be made to obtain a specimen, which can be sent for microscopy and culture within seven days of treatment commencing.

Fact Box 6.2   Respiratory pathogens

Respiratory pathogens do not tend to survive for long once they have left the host and should either be sent to the laboratory immediately or refrigerated for no longer than 24 hours.

Wounds

Wound swabs should be taken only if there are clinical signs of infection (see Chapter 18), and routine wound swabs should be avoided, particularly from chronic wounds such as leg ulcers. These are often heavily colonised with skin flora, and if there is no evidence of cellulitis and/or fever, a swab will be of little value. Although most wound infections do arise as a result of infection from the patient's own resident skin flora, care must be taken to ensure that the specimen is obtained directly from the site of inflammation or infection, and not from the surrounding skin.

Obtaining a wound swab

In order to obtain a 'good' sample, the swab should be moved over the surface of the wound in a zigzag rolling fashion. If the wound is dry, the tip of the swab should be moistened with normal saline to make it more absorbent and increase the survival of any pathogens present prior to culture. Any loose debris on the surface of the wound should be removed before the swab is taken as this may contain high numbers of bacteria but will not be representative of the infecting organism. If pus is present, it should be aspirated using a sterile syringe and decanted into a sterile specimen pot – do not send syringes containing pus to the laboratory. As discussed in this chapter, the site and nature of the wound must be clearly indicated on both the swab and the request form.

Faeces

The gut is home to huge numbers of enteric pathogens, along with resident bowel flora. Faecal specimens are requested for the detection of gastro-intestinal infections caused by a large number of pathogens (Health Protection Agency, 2007):

- *Clostridium difficile* (see Chapter 22)
- *Salmonella* spp.
- *Campylobacter*
- *Staphylococcus aureus* toxin (see Chapter 20)
- *Escherichia coli* 0157
- *Cryptosporidium* (www.hpa.org.uk/Topics/InfectiousDiseases/InfectionsAZ/Cryptosporidium)
- *Bacillus cereus* (www.hpa.org.uk/Topics/InfectiousDiseases/InfectionsAZ/BacillussppFoodPoisoning)
- Rotavirus
- Norovirus (see Chapter 23)
- *Giardia* (www.cdc.gov.uk/parasites/giardia)
- *Entamoeba histolytica* (www.cdc.gov.uk/parasites/amebiasis).

Fact Box 6.3 Faecal specimens

Faecal specimens should ideally be obtained within the first 48 hours of illness as the chances of successfully identifying the pathogen diminish once the acute stage of the illness passes. In patients admitted to hospital with diarrhoea, or in whom diarrhoea develops within 72 hours of admission, it is important that a stool specimen is obtained at the earliest opportunity in order to determine not only the cause, but also whether the infection is community acquired (onset within 72 hours of admission) or hospital acquired (onset > 72 hours of admission).

They should reach the laboratory on the same day, although they can be refrigerated overnight. Where faecal specimens are required for the detection of infections caused by intestinal protozoa, a fresh or 'hot' stool is required as the protozoa are more likely to be mobile and therefore more easily identified live in a warm stool.

Obtaining a stool specimen

The stool should be passed into a bedpan or commode, as faecal specimen pots have a handy 'scoop' attached to the inside of the lid. If an intestinal protozoa infection is suspected, the stool specimen must reach the laboratory within minutes of being passed. It is acceptable to obtain a stool specimen from a patient with faecal incontinence using the scoop from the faecal specimen pot; contrary to popular belief, stool specimens can be sent to the laboratory even if mixed with urine. The specimen request form should state if this is the case.

Rectal swabs

Rectal swabs are required for the detection of carbapenemase-producing coliforms (see Chapter 10) and must be taken using charcoal swabs (there is no need to moisten the swab with normal saline). The swab must be gently inserted through the rectal sphincter, rotated through one full turn and then withdrawn. Rectal swabs can seem particularly intrusive, and the procedure needs to be explained with care.

Throat swabs

Although the majority of sore throats are due to viral infections, group A streptococcus (*Streptococcus pyogenes*) is the most common bacterial cause of sore throats (see Fact Sheet 3.9 on the companion website). *Neisseria meningitidis*, the causative agent of meningococcal meningitis, is a normal inhabitant of the human nasopharynx, and patients with meningitis and their close contacts will have throat swabs taken for the detection of meningococci (see Fact Sheet 3.4 on the companion website).

Obtaining a throat swab

The swab should be rolled over any areas of exudate or inflammation, or over the tonsils and posterior pharynx. Care must be taken on withdrawing the swab so that it does not touch the cheeks, teeth, tongue or gums as the specimen will become contaminated by the resident flora. For bacterial culture, swabs are supplied with charcoal transport medium. For virus detection, the swab should be placed in viral transport medium and transported to the laboratory as soon as possible.

MRSA screen (nose and axillae)

The most common indication for taking a nasal swab is generally as part of an MRSA screen, which may also involve screening the axillae, as opposed to routinely screening the groin or perineum, using an enrichment broth (see Box 6.5). **Note:** In laboratories where screening using enrichment is not undertaken, and/or if groin or perineal swabs form part of MRSA screening, charcoal swabs must be used (the tip of the swab should be moistened with the transport medium or with normal saline). For nasal screening using charcoal swabs, the swab should be inserted just inside the anterior nasal nares with the tip directed upwards and then gently rotated.

Blood culture

Blood cultures are indicated if the patient displays systemic signs of infection or has pyrexia of unknown origin, and should be taken when the patient's temperature spikes, as the numbers of bacteria circulating within the bloodstream will be at their greatest then. 20–30 mL of blood is drawn which is inoculated into separate culture bottles containing liquid culture media, one for aerobic and one for anaerobic incubation, and it should be transported to the laboratory immediately.

Box 6.5   Protocol for undertaking MRSA screens (nose and axillae): broth method

2 × plastic tipped swabs (supplied with the broth)
1 × broth (**Note**: 1 broth bottle per patient screen)
1 × printed label (patient details)

- Hands must be decontaminated prior to undertaking the procedure (gloves are not strictly necessary, but non-sterile examination gloves may be worn).
- Swab *both nostrils* with *1 x plastic-tipped swab*.
- Open the broth bottle and swirl the plastic-tipped swab in the broth for *5 seconds*.
- Discard the swab as clinical waste; replace the lid on the broth.
- Swab *both axillae* with *1 x plastic-tipped swab*.
- Open the broth bottle and swirl the plastic-tipped swab in the broth for *5 seconds*.
- Discard the swab as clinical waste; replace lid on the broth.
- Decontaminate hands.
- Fix printed label to the broth bottle; complete and print the Specimen Request Form.

Fact Box 6.4   Blood culture collection

Blood culture collection is a skilled procedure and must be undertaken **only** by Nurses, Phlebotomists and Medical Staff who have received training **and** passed a competency assessment (this should be undertaken annually and form part of mandatory training). If the skin is not decontaminated appropriately prior to drawing the blood, the culture may become contaminated with skin flora such as coagulase-negative staphylococci (Marwick *et al.*, 2006; Murray and Witebsky, 2010). The isolation of MRSA from a blood culture is not necessarily clinically significant if the patient is systemically well, and may indicate contamination as opposed to clinical infection. However, contaminated blood cultures will be reported as avoidable.

Contaminated blood cultures are by and large preventable through sound aseptic technique and optimal skin decontamination (Department of Health [DH], 2007; Rowley and Clare, 2011). The DH (2007) published *Taking Blood Cultures: Summary of Best Practice* as guidance for NHS Trusts in order that they could effectively review their policies and practices and reduce the risk of, and number of, contaminated cultures. Box 6.6 lists the indications for blood culture collection, and Box 6.7 lists the best practice for the prevention of contaminated blood cultures.

Box 6.6   Indications for blood culture collection

Core temperature out of normal range (>38°C)
Focal signs of infection
Other signs of septic shock, such as acute circulatory failure, low blood pressure and/or increased respiratory rate
Chills and/or rigors within the previous 24 hours
Raised or very low white cell count
New or worsening confusion

Data from DH, 2007.

Box 6.7   Best practice: prevention of contaminated blood cultures

- **Only** staff who have been assessed as competent in blood culture collection should be permitted to undertake the procedure (mandatory annual training and competency assessment).
- Use a dedicated blood culture collection pack.
- If blood is being collected for other tests, collect the blood culture **first**.
- **Do not** use existing cannulae or sites immediately above existing cannulae. If a central venous catheter (CVC) is in situ, blood can be taken from the CVC **but** the hub must be disinfected using a 2% chlorhexidine in 70% alcohol swab, **and** blood must be taken from a separate peripheral venous stab **first**.
- **Never** take a blood culture from a femoral stab due to the high risk of contamination. Blood may be taken from a newly sited cannula **after** disinfecting the hub with a 2% chlorhexidine in 70% alcohol swab **as long as** the skin was decontaminated with 2% chlorhexidine in 70% alcohol **prior to** the cannula being inserted.
- Decontaminate hands **prior** to decontaminating the patient's skin, **prior** to putting on examination gloves (which should be just before attaching the winged blood culture collection set to the blood collection adaptor cap), and **after** removing gloves (once the winged blood collection set has been discarded into the sharps container).
- Use 2% chlorhexidine in 70% alcohol to decontaminate the patient's skin, and allow to dry; do not re-palpate the skin.
- Always make a fresh stab in patients with suspected bacteraemia (it is recommended that two sets of cultures are taken at different times from different sites).

- Use a 2% chlorhexidine gluconate in 70% alcohol swab to decontaminate the blood culture bottle tops (these are clean but not sterile), and allow to dry (approximately 30 seconds) before inoculating the bottles.
- **Document the procedure** in the patient's notes – indication for blood culture; date and time; site of blood culture; signature and print name; and bleep and telephone number. **Note**: Completion of a pre-printed 'Record of Blood Culture Collection Label,' containing the above information and a statement that the blood culture has been collected according to Trust policy by a healthcare worker who is competent to undertake the procedure, helps to provide assurance that best practice has been followed. In the event of the patient being found to have an MRSA bacteraemia, the person who took the blood culture should be contacted by the Infection Prevention and Control Team and asked to (1) describe step by step the procedure that he or she used and (2) provide evidence that he or she has completed the appropriate training and passed the competency assessment.

Source: Data from DH, 2007.

Reflection point

How is compliance with blood culture training and blood culture collection audited within your place of work?

Cerebral spinal fluid

CSF is obtained by lumbar puncture for the diagnosis of meningitis and encephalitis. A lumbar puncture is performed using strict aseptic technique, and the skin is thoroughly decontaminated with chlorhexidine to prevent the introduction of organisms during the procedure, and contamination of the CSF with resident flora. It is collected into three sterile bottles and examined with regard to its appearance (which should be clear and colourless), glucose, protein, cell count and the presence of bacteria, viruses and fungi. Specimens of CSF should be dealt with by the laboratory as an emergency and maintained at room temperature and cultured within two hours of collection.

Chapter summary: key points

- The correct specimen has to be taken obtained at the correct time from the correct site using the correct technique.
- The quality of the result achieved from a specimen is directly related to the quality of the specimen itself.

Continued

- An aseptic technique has to be used to avoid contamination of the specimen. Specimens should be taken only by staff who are competent to undertake the task.

- Although clinical specimens should ideally be taken before antibiotic treatment commences, treatment should not be unnecessarily delayed; it may be of life-saving importance in the case of certain infections and infectious diseases, where treatment is the priority, not taking the specimen.

- Relevant clinical information must be provided on the Specimen Request Form. This will help the Laboratory Staff and Microbiologist interpret the results.

- Healthcare staff should be aware of the acts and regulations regarding the safe collection, handling and transportation of specimens.

Further resources are available for this book, including interactive multiple choice questions. Visit the companion website at:

www.wiley.com/go/fundamentalsofinfectionprevention

References

Department of Health (2007). *Taking Blood Cultures: A Summary of Best Practice*. Department of Health, London.

Gillespie T., Fewster J., Masterton R.G. (1999). The effect of specimen processing delay on borate urine preservation. *Journal of Clinical Pathology*. 52: 95–98.

Health Protection Agency (2007). *Infectious Diarrhoea. The Role of Microbiological Examination of Faeces: Quick Reference Guide for Primary Care*. Health Protection Agency, London.

Marwick C.A., Ziglam H.M., Nathwani D. (2006). Your patient has a blood culture positive for *Staphylococcus aureus* – what would you do? *Journal of the Royal College Physicians Edinburgh*. 36: 350–355.

Murray P.R., Witebsky F.G. (2010). The clinician and the microbiology laboratory. In: Mandell G.L., Bennett J.E., Dolin R.D. (Eds.), *Mandell's Principles and Practices of Infectious Diseases*. 6th ed. Churchill Livingstone Elsevier, London. Expert Consult online: http://expertconsult.com (accessed 14 January 2012)

Rowley S., Clare S. (2011). ANTT: an essential tool for effective blood culture collection. *British Journal of Nursing*. 20 (14; Suppl.): 9–14.

Scottish Intercollegiate Guidelines Network (2006). *Management of Suspected Bacterial Urinary Tract Infections in Adults. A National Clinical Guideline*. SIGN Publication 88. Scottish Intercollegiate Guidelines Network, Edinburgh.

Thys J.P., Jacobs F., Bye B. (1994). Microbiological specimen collection in the emergency room. *European Journal of Emergency Medicine*. 1 (1): 47–53.

Further reading

Advisory Committee on Dangerous Pathogens (ACDP) (2003). *Infection at Work: Controlling the Risks – a Guide for Employers and the Self-employed on Identifying, Assessing and Controlling the Risks of Infection in the Work Place*. ACDP, London.

Advisory Committee on Dangerous Pathogens (ACDP) (2006): *BSE – Occupational Guidance*. ACDP, London.

Department of Health (2007). *Transport of Infectious Substances: Best Practice Guidance for Microbiology Laboratories*. Department of Health, London.

Health and Safety Executive (HSE) (2001). *Blood-borne Viruses in the Work Place. Guidance for Employers and Employees*. Health and Safety Executive, London.

Health and Safety Executive (1991). *Safe Working and the Prevention of Infection in Clinical Laboratories and Similar Facilities*. www.hse.gov.uk (accessed 17 March 2013)

7

The microbiology laboratory

Contents

Fundamentals of Infection Prevention and Control: Theory and Practice, Second Edition. Debbie Weston.
© 2013 John Wiley & Sons, Ltd. Published 2013 by John Wiley & Sons, Ltd. Companion Website: www.wiley.com/go/fundamentalsofinfectionprevention

Introduction

In order to detect, identify and treat bacterial and viral infections, the infecting microorganisms need to be grown under laboratory conditions which mimic the conditions in which they would grow optimally within the human host. Focussing predominantly on bacteria, this chapter looks at some of the work undertaken in the microbiology laboratory and describes how bacterial cell division and growth occur. Techniques for culturing and identifying bacteria are described, along with some other commonly used laboratory investigations. The reader should note that these investigations can vary according to the facilities available within individual laboratories, and some specimens may have to be sent to other laboratories.

Learning outcomes

At the end of this chapter, the reader will:

- Understand how bacteria grow and divide.

- Understand the culture and staining techniques used to grow and identify bacteria.

- Understand the basic principles of polymerase chain reaction, immunofluorescence, serology and tissue culture in aiding bacterial and viral detection.

Bacterial growth

Bacterial growth involves an increase in both the size and number of organisms, resulting in an increase in its total mass, or biomass (Barer, 2007). This growth is dependent upon various environmental factors; if the environmental conditions are not optimal, the organism will not survive.

Nutrients

An adequate supply of nutrients is essential for the bacteria's survival, many of which the bacteria break down to derive energy from. In addition to the basic necessities such as water, oxygen, carbon dioxide, iron and carbohydrates, trace elements such as copper, zinc, magnesium, cobalt, nitrogen and nickel are also required.

Temperature

All organisms have an optimum growth temperature, at which they will be growing at their optimum rate. Temperature is important as bacteria will cease to grow below their minimum growth temperature, and will die in environments where the temperature is above the maximum.

Fact Box 7.1   Temperature control and the growth of *Legionella*

Legionella bacteria thrive in water temperatures of 20–50 °C, but are unable to withstand temperatures of 60 °C or above, where they die rapidly. Therefore the growth of *Legionella* in man-made water systems can be controlled by maintaining the cold water temperature below 20 °C and the hot water temperature above 60 °C. Pathogenic bacteria that grow on or in the body have to be able to grow within 20–40 °C (Barer, 2007).

(See Fact Sheet 1.3 on companion website.)

Fact Box 7.2   The benefit of pyrexia

The pyrexia which often accompanies many illnesses is useful in combating infections and is actually a protective response, given that most pathogens replicate best and achieve their optimum growth at temperatures of 37 °C or below.

Moisture

As 70–95% of the bacterial cell consists of water, the majority of bacteria will die without an adequate moisture supply, although some bacteria form spores which protect them when the moisture or nutrient supply is low (see Chapter 5). An example of a spore-producing organism is *Clostridium difficile* (see Chapter 22). The spores enable the bacteria to survive for long periods in the environment in a dormant state, and then reactivate when the environmental conditions are right.

Oxygen

The human body provides a mix of aerobic and anaerobic environments, and the ability of an organism to grow and replicate in either environment is advantageous for many pathogens (Barer, 2007; Levinson, 2010). Strict, or obligate, aerobic bacteria can grow only in the presence of oxygen, and can be found on the surface of wounds or within the lung fields, for example (e.g. *Pseudomonas aeruginosa* and *Mycobacterium tuberculosis* – see Chapters 10 and 21). Strict or obligate anaerobes, however, cannot grow in an oxygen-rich environment and thrive deep in wounds where the tissue is dead (i.e. *Clostridium perfringens*). They do not survive long in clinical specimens and therefore can be difficult to isolate in the laboratory. Facultative organisms can grow with or without oxygen but achieve their optimum growth in an oxygen-rich environment (e.g. *Staphylococcus aureus* and *Escherichia coli* – see Chapters 10 and 20).

Cell division

The process of bacterial cell division is also known as **binary fission**, where one bacterial cell (called a parent cell) divides in half to produce two daughter cells (Levinson, 2010). Before cell division begins, the cellular DNA is replicated so that each daughter cell will contain the same genetic material as the original parent cell. This means that each subsequent division of the cell should therefore result in the precise replication of the DNA. However, with millions of cell divisions occurring, it is inevitable that this process can sometimes go wrong, resulting in cell mutations.

Fact Box 7.3   Cell mutations

Although most cell mutations will cause the cell to die, there are instances where mutations can actually make the cell more adaptable and it can thrive in circumstances that would normally destroy it. These mutations are one of the factors that contribute to antibiotic resistance, which is discussed in Chapter 10.

The growth of bacteria is demonstrated in the laboratory on culture media where the number of cells increases exponentially with time, and this stage of the bacterial growth cycle is known as the exponential or log phase of growth (Barer, 2007). The amount of time taken for the cell to divide is known as the generation or doubling time, which varies amongst bacterial species.

Fact Box 7.4   Bacterial cell division

Bacteria such as *Pseudomonas* and *Clostridium* have a short generation time of 10 minutes. A single cell of *E. coli* can produce one million cells in seven hours (Levinson, 2010), or 10 million cells in eight hours if grown in the right culture medium (Strohl *et al.*, 2001). *M. tuberculosis* is a slow grower and divides once within 18–24 hours (Strohl *et al.*, 2001; Barer, 2007). Given the short generation time of some organisms, it is easy to see that if an antibiotic-resistant mutant occurs during cell division, it can rapidly become the dominant organism.

As the nutrient supply becomes depleted, toxic waste products build up, the culture media become over-populated, and bacterial growth enters the stationary or lag phase as growth eventually slows down and then ceases altogether (Barer, 2007). If the bacteria are inoculated onto fresh media, exponential growth will continue after a lag phase. If the stationary period is extended, the bacteria will eventually die.

Bacterial culture

The principle aim of bacterial culture is to grow a population of bacterial cells which will be visible as a colony on a plate of media. This population of cells is referred to as a culture, and the visible mounds of bacterial mass seen on the surface of solid (agar) culture media are called colonies, which are the product of 20–30 cell divisions of a single cell (Barer, 2007). If there are different species or strains of bacteria in the culture, the colonies produced will be of different shapes and sizes as a result of different growth rates and their response to the nutrients within the media.

Culture media

Culture media come in either solid or liquid form, and generally consist of water, sodium chloride and electrolytes, peptone, meat and yeast extracts and blood. Solid culture media consist of agar (which is derived from seaweed) and are cultured on Petri dishes, which are 90 mm in diameter and have a vented lid. Various nutrients can be added to the agar to create the optimum environment for supporting bacterial growth. In order to select the most appropriate culture media, the laboratory staff need to be provided with the relevant information in relation to the clinical specimen which is being tested (see Chapter 6).

The type of culture media used may vary widely between laboratories but broadly comes under the headings of enrichment, selective and indicator media. **Enrichment media** are used to encourage and amplify the growth of fastidious fragile pathogens in sufficient numbers so that they are readily detectable. These can take the form of either solid agar or nutrient broth.

Blood agar, which contains nutrient agar plus 5% horse blood, will support the growth of most Gram-positive and Gram-negative bacteria.

The upper respiratory tract and the gastro-intestinal tract have abundant resident flora (see Chapter 8), and detecting a pathogen in a body site where there is a heavy population of mixed flora is not always easy. **Selective media** have inhibitors such as bile salts or antibiotics added, to inhibit the growth of some bacteria and therefore encourage the growth of others, and are used to culture organisms within throat swabs and faecal specimens (Barer, 2007).

MacConkey agar inhibits the growth of most Gram-positive bacteria but supports the growth of most Gram-negative rods. Colonies of pathogens grown on selective media may be further identified by culture using indicator media, which differentiates between species by effecting a colour change.

Inoculation of culture media

Petri dishes containing the nutrient agar are inoculated with the clinical specimen using a strict aseptic technique to avoid contamination (Health Protection Agency, 2011a). Box 7.1 describes the procedure for inoculating an agar plate.

Clinical specimens that are likely to contain only small numbers of organisms, such as cerebral spinal fluid or blood, may be cultured using **nutrient broth**, a liquid suspension without the addition of any setting agents. The broth is inoculated with the specimen using a sterile loop.

Once the specimen has been plated, or inoculated into a liquid medium, it is incubated either aerobically or anaerobically at 35–37° C for 24–48 hours and then 'read' or visually observed for growth. Millions of bacterial cells will be visible on the agar plate as colonies along the inoculation lines after 24 hours, unless the organism happens to be a slow grower with a long generation time, in which case there will be no visible growth. In the case of nutrient broth, it will become increasingly cloudy or turbid due to the growth of bacteria. **Obligate aerobes** tend to grow on the surface of nutrient broth, while **obligate anaerobes** will be hidden in the depths of the media, away from the surface.

Culture plates normally grow a mix of bacteria, including normal body flora. So that a 'pure culture' of only one type of bacteria is grown, the colonies can be inoculated onto another culture plate containing a culture medium that is more selective. The colonies for subculture are picked out using a sterile wire or loop and plated out using the same method as before.

Bacteria grown in nutrient broth are inoculated onto solid culture medium for bacterial identification. Serial dilutions of the broth are prepared in either 0.1 mL or 1.0 mL portions, inoculated onto an agar plate and incubated overnight. The colonies are then counted, and the

Box 7.1 Procedure for inoculating an agar plate

- A sterile inoculating loop is used to apply the specimen to the culture medium, which is dragged or streaked over the surface of the agar plate.
- The lid of the Petri dish is replaced to prevent airborne contamination of the plate.
- The loop is then 'flamed' by passing it through the flame of a Bunsen burner until the loop reaches 'red heat' to remove any residual bacteria.
- The lid is then removed.
- The plate is streaked a second time, with this second streak overlapping the first but finishing independently of it.
- The lid is replaced.
- The loop is flamed yet again.
- The lid is removed, and a third streak is made.
- Each streak reduces the initial inoculum. Bacteria that are well separated from others will grow as isolated colonies and can be assumed to have arisen from a single organism, or an organism cluster which is known as a colony-forming unit.

total number of bacteria present in the original sample is calculated by multiplying the number of colonies grown by the dilution factor.

Culturing viruses

As viruses replicate only within living cells, living cell cultures that support their replication are the primary method of detecting them. Viral growth will be shown as either changes in cellular morphology or cell death.

Gram-staining

When viewed under the microscope, bacteria are colourless and transparent and it is impossible to identify them. Gram-staining differentiates between Gram-positive and Gram-negative bacteria according to the makeup of their cell wall, and also reveals their shape (see Chapter 5). As prompt identification of any infecting organism is of potentially lifesaving importance, Gram-staining (see Box 7.2) can be used to guide the choice of antimicrobial therapy until definitive identification of the organism has been made.

Processing specimens

In order to give the reader a brief insight into how meticillin-resistant *S. aureus* (MRSA; see Chapter 20), *M. tuberculosis* (see Chapter 21) and *C. difficile* (see Chapter 22) are detected, this next section briefly describes how wound, sputum and stool specimens are processed. **It is not intended to give a definitive account, as the techniques and type of media used can vary slightly between laboratories, and the reader is advised to seek further information and guidance from their Microbiology Laboratory.**

Box 7.2   Gram-staining technique

The specimen is 'heat-fixed' onto a glass slide. Methods of heat fixing may vary but they traditionally involve passing the slide through the flame of a Bunsen burner several times.

The slide is flooded with a blue dye (crystal violet) and left for 30 seconds; iodine is then poured onto the slide to wash away the stain, and then the slide is flooded with fresh iodine and left for 30 seconds.

The iodine is washed off of the slide with either ethanol or acetone until the colour has run out of the slide.

The slide is rinsed with water, and a counter stain is applied by flooding the slide with a counterstain (neutral red, safranin or carbol fuchsin) and leaving it to act for approximately two minutes.

The slide is washed with and then blot dried using blotting paper.

- **Gram-positive bacteria retain the blue (crystal violet) dye and are stained blue-black.**
- **Gram-negative bacteria are stained red-pink, as they retain the red safranin dye.**

Source: Data from HPA, Health Protection Agency, 2011b.

MRSA

Culture

Enrichment media, either solid or nutrient broth (see Chapter 6 for a broth-screening technique), are generally used for the culture of *S. aureus* (Health Protection Agency, 2012a). If the specimens have been obtained using charcoal swabs, the swabs are cultured (plated) onto a chromogenic selective MRSA medium and incubated aerobically for 18–48 hours at 37 °C. If nutrient broth has been used, the broth is incubated aerobically for 18–24 hours at 30 °C and then sub-cultured (plated) onto a chromogenic selective medium and incubated for a further 18–48 hours. The culture plates are 'read' daily. Individual colonies are 2–3 mm in diameter, circular, with a smooth shiny appearance and a golden-yellow or creamy colour. In order to distinguish MRSA from a sensitive *S. aureus*, or *Staphylococcus epidermidis* (coagulase-negative staphylococci), further identification and sensitivity testing need to be undertaken.

Coagulase test

S. aureus has the ability to clot plasma through the production of an extracellular enzyme called coagulase, and the coagulase test (Health Protection Agency, 2010) is the definitive test for distinguishing between *S. aureus* and other staphylococci. This can be carried out using either a glass slide or a test tube, and involves the use of either human or rabbit plasma. In the slide coagulase test, a drop of distilled water is placed on the slide and the specimen is emulsified to produce a thick homogeneous suspension. The plasma is added to the slide using an inoculating loop or wire. A positive result sees visible clumping of the cells within 10 minutes. The tube coagulase test gives a positive result in approximately four hours. A test tube containing 1 mL of plasma, diluted according to the manufacturer's instructions, is prepared, and then a sample from the test strain is added. It is then incubated at 35–37°C and examined hourly for four hours. If a clot forms during that time, the result is positive.

Antibiotic susceptibility

In order to determine the antibiotic susceptibility of organisms and choose the correct therapeutic agents to treat the infection, antibiotic susceptibility and sensitivity testing is required. Isolated colonies are selected from the primary culture plate for testing. The most widely used technique is the disc diffusion method. Using an aseptic technique, an agar plate is inoculated with the test organism and paper discs containing the antibiotic placed on the agar plate using either cooled, flamed forceps or a disc dispenser. The discs are applied no longer than 15 minutes after the agar plate has been inoculated with the specimen, otherwise the organisms may grow, which will affect the zone sizes that form around the discs.

The antibiotic begins to diffuse into the agar immediately, and if it inhibits bacterial growth, a zone of inhibition will become apparent around the antibiotic disc. This means that the organism is sensitive to the antibiotic, and infection can be treated with that antimicrobial agent at the therapeutic dose recommended for treatment of the organism. If it is resistant to the antibiotic, the organism will grow right up to the edge of the disc.

If the strain of *S. aureus* grown is an MRSA, it will be resistant to the beta-lactam agents (penicillins and cephalosporins). There may be other differences in antibiotic susceptibility which may indicate whether the MRSA is a hospital-acquired or a community-acquired strain. For example, EMRSA-16, a strain of MRSA common in healthcare settings, is susceptible to ciprofloxacin; community-acquired strains of MRSA are generally ciprofloxacin sensitive. MRSA is discussed in detail in Chapter 20.

Mycobacterium tuberculosis

Sputum

The definitive method for detecting whether or not a patient has infectious respiratory tuberculosis (see Chapter 21) is to examine a sputum specimen for the presence of rod-shaped bacilli (Health Protection Agency, 2012b). A mucolytic agent is added to the sputum to break it up, and it is then 'spun' or centrifuged to further break down any deposits and leave a 'pure' specimen. The bacterial cell walls of Mycobacteria have a high lipid content and generally stain poorly as a result. However, they can be stained through the prolonged application of concentrated dyes, facilitated by heat. Once stained, the lipids in the cell wall do not dissolve when the stain is washed off with acid–alcohol, hence the name 'alcohol–acid fast bacilli' (AAFB), and they retain the fluorescent stain. There are two staining methods, auramine–phenol and Ziehl–Nelson (ZN), and the latter is discussed here.

Ziehl–Nelson stain

A thin smear is placed onto a glass slide which is flooded with a strong solution of carbol fuchsin, heated gently until it starts to steam and then left to rest for 3–5 minutes, following which it is rinsed thoroughly with water. It is then decolourised for approximately 2–3 minutes with an acid–alcohol solution, which is then rinsed and reapplied for 3–4 minutes until the slide is a faint pink colour. The slide is rinsed thoroughly with water again and counterstained with either methylene blue or malchamite green for 30 seconds, then rinsed with water and allowed to air dry before being examined under the microscope.

If red bacilli are seen against the contrasting background colour, the result is commonly reported as 'AAFB smear positive'. A diagnosis of 'open' respiratory tuberculosis is made if 5000–10000 acid-fast bacilli are detected in 1 ml of sputum (Pratt *et al*., 2005; Fitzgerald *et al*., 2010).

A negative sputum smear does not mean that the patient does not have respiratory tuberculosis, although it does mean that their infectivity is likely to be low. The sputum specimen will need to be sub-cultured onto special culture media to see if *M. tuberculosis* can be grown. The specimen is decontaminated in the first instance to remove any other bacteria or fungi within the sample that might overgrow any Mycobacteria if they are present. It is then used to inoculate the culture media, which are incubated at 35–37 °C for 10–12 weeks and 'read' weekly. At the end of the incubation period, the ZN stain is applied to the colonies to detect the presence of AAFBs.

Blood testing

Two blood-based immunological tests are now commercially available in the United Kingdom – QuantiFERON-TB Gold, and TSPOT-TB Assay. These detect tuberculosis antigens known as 'early secretion antigen target 6' (ESAT-6) and 'culture filtrate protein 10' (CFP-10), interferon gamma produced by T cells in specific response to *M. tuberculosis*, which are not present in the bacillus Calmette–Guérin (BCG) vaccine and are found in only a few strains of environmental mycobacteria. The TSPOT-TB Assay can provide a result within 24 hours.

Clostridium difficile

See Chapter 22 for a more detailed discussion of *C. difficile*.

Historically, the definitive method and 'gold standard' for diagnosing *C. difficile* infection has been the detection of cytotoxin in tissue culture (National *Clostridium difficile* Standards Group, 2003). However, revised guidance on the diagnosing and reporting of *C. difficile* infection was published by the Department of Health on 6 March 2012 (DH, 2012), advising that a two-step approach to testing faecal specimens for *C. difficile* is adopted. The two tests are GDH (glutamate dehydrogenase) EIA (enzyme immunoassays) **or** NAAT (Nucleic Acid Amplification Test) **or** polymerase chain reaction (PCR) **and** a sensitive EIA or cytotoxin assay to detect the presence of toxin gene(s).

GDH is the common antigen seen in all strains of *C. difficile*. If GDH is detected in a faecal specimen from a patient with diarrhoea in the absence of toxin, it indicates carrier status. This means that the patient is carrying *C. difficile*, there is the potential for the patient to develop symptomatic *C. difficile* infection and therefore there is a risk of cross-infection to other patients. If GDH antigen **and** toxin are detected **and** the patient has diarrhoea, then he or she has symptomatic (active) *C. difficile* infection. If neither GDH antigen nor toxin is detected, the patient does not have *C. difficile*, either in a carrier state or as an active infection. See Table 7.1 for a summary of the interpretation of the results arising from GDH antigen and toxin testing.

Table 7.1 Interpretation of *C. difficile* testing

Test	Interpretation	Infection control precautions
GDH antigen negative	*C. difficile* not detected. However, other potential pathogens may need to be excluded.	None, unless there are is a clinical suspicion that there may be another infectious cause for diarrhoea.
GDH antigen positive and toxin negative	Carriage of *C. difficile* detected. Potential risk of cross-infection and/or latent symptomatic infection.	Patient should be isolated if diarrhoea present. Discuss with the Consultant Medical Microbiologist regarding treatment if clinically suspecting *C. difficile* infection.
GDH antigen positive and toxin positive	Toxin-producing strain of *C. difficile*. Risk of cross-infection.	Isolate and treat patient if symptomatic.

Source: Data from DH, 2012.

Other laboratory techniques

There are numerous other investigations undertaken in the laboratory to aid bacterial and viral detection and identification. Some of these techniques, which can be applied to both, are briefly described here. Others are outside of the scope of this book, and the reader is advised to undertake further reading and explore this area further if it is one of particular interest.

Polymerase chain reaction (PCR)

PCR is a relatively new diagnostic technique which has revolutionised the detection of pathogens by amplifying fragments of DNA millions of times to such a degree that specific detection of a pathogen is possible. When DNA replicates, it 'un-zips' into two halves, with each half a template for another one. DNA fragments can be made to 'un-zip' if they are heated, which separates the strands. They are cooled down and then heated again, and this cycle is repeated approximately 10 times, amplifying the DNA logarithmically. It is used in the detection of diseases such as HIV (see Chapter 24) and *Mycobacterium tuberculosis*, and is of particular value in detecting antimicrobial resistance genes.

Reflection point

PCR can also be undertaken for the detection of MRSA, and results can be obtained within a matter of hours. Is PCR available within your laboratory? What might the benefits be for patient care?

Latex agglutination

Antigens or antibodies (see Chapter 8) can be applied to latex particles to detect antibody or antigen reactions. If antigen is added to antibody-coated latex particles, agglutination ('clumping' of particles) will occur and antibody can be detected in the patient's serum.

Immunofluorescence

Antibody specific to the antigen being detected, which may be bacterial or viral, is labelled or 'tagged' with fluorescent dye. If the antibody and the antigen combine, a bright green fluorescent halo will be seen around the antigen in the case of bacteria, or a fluorescent clump if the antigen is a virus.

Serology

During any type of infection, the host response is to form antibodies. Their production and the length of time which they take to form are dependent upon the antigenic stimulation. In the event of a severe infection, antibodies are produced early in the illness and rise sharply over the following 10–21 days. Blood serum samples collected soon after the onset of the illness, and again in the convalescent phase, can be compared for changes in antibody content. Serum dilutions can be made where pathogens are difficult to detect in culture, and serological assays can be performed which focus on the interaction between an antigen and a specific antibody. One of the most commonly used assays is the enzyme-linked immunosorbent assay (ELISA) which was developed in the 1970s for the detection of antibodies (Harwood, 2010). Plastic wells on a microtitre plate are coated with specific antigen, to which a sample from the patient's specimen is added. Any specific antibody within the sample will bind to the antigen, effecting a colour change. Serum antibodies to HIV infection can be detected by an ELISA assay within five to seven weeks of infection.

Typing

A bacterial strain consists of 'the descendants of a single, pure microbial culture' (Willey *et al.*, 2011), and typing is a technique used to identify different bacteria within a species and aid the identification and linkage of cases within an outbreak. For the typing of cases of MRSA in the event of a hospital or community care home outbreak, for example, typing of MRSA-positive isolates from colonised or infected patients would be undertaken to identify the *spa* (staphylococcal protein A) type of each isolate in order to identify the clone that the strain originated from (this could be extended further to include other typing methods – see Chapter 20). There are a number of typing methods that can be used depending on the organism and the facilities available. Typing is also commonly undertaken for *C. difficile* isolates and can be a useful tool in the event of a period of increased incidence or outbreak (see Chapter 4) to help the Infection Prevention and Control Team determine whether cross infection has occurred.

Genome sequencing

DNA contains the cell's genes and its genetic code and is integral to the proper functioning of the cell (Engelkirk and Duben-Engelkirk, 2011). The information that makes up the genetic code consists of four nucleotides, or bases – **A** (adenosine), **T** (thymine), **G** (guanine) and **C** (cytosine) – that are strung together in a long sequence, resembling two entwined ribbons, which is made up of thousands of millions of individual letters. The sequence in which these letters appear is different in all organisms, and because of this it is possible to determine the specific, unique sequence of these four bases in an organism. If the order in which these letters or bases appear within the sequence changes, this indicates that a mutation has occurred.

Fact Box 7.5   Genome Sequencing

In 1999, the Human Genome Sequencing Project began (completed in 2003) in which the sequence of three billion DNA subunits was undertaken and all of the human genes were identified (http://www.genome.gov/10001772; Venter, Adams, Myers et al., 2001). In 2005, genome sequencing enabled the **Spanish flu** virus to be re-created (Taubenberger et al., 2005). In 2001, Parkhill et al. reported that genome sequencing of a strain of *Yersinia pestis*, the organism known to have caused the Black Death (plague), had identified the presence of virulence genes acquired from other bacteria and viruses (Parkhill et al., 2001), and more recently, in 2011, approximately 99% of the genome was recovered from the 600-year-old skeletal remains of plague victims buried in the fourteenth century (Bos et al., 2011). (See Fact Sheet 1.8 on the companion website.)

Chapter summary: key points

- Bacterial growth involves an increase in both the size and number of organisms, resulting in an increase in its total mass.

- An adequate supply of nutrients is essential for bacteria's survival.

- All organisms have an optimum growth temperature, where they will be growing at their optimum rate.

- The majority of bacteria will die without an adequate moisture supply, although some bacteria form spores which protect them when the moisture or nutrient supply is low.

- Some bacteria can grow and replicate only in an environment that is either rich or deficient in oxygen. The ability to grow in both is the most advantageous.

- The amount of time that it takes for one single bacterial cell to divide varies amongst bacterial species.

- Bacteria can be artificially grown in the laboratory using culture media and nutrient broths, and various techniques are employed in order to aid bacterial and viral identification.

Further resources are available for this book, including interactive multiple choice questions. Visit the companion website at:

www.wiley.com/go/fundamentalsofinfectionprevention

References

Barer M. (2007).Bacterial growth, physiology and death. In: Greenwood D., Slack R., Peutherer J., Barer M. (Eds.), *A Guide to Microbial Infections: Pathogenesis, Immunity, Laboratory Diagnosis and Control*. 17th ed. Churchill Livingston Elsevier, London: 38–51.

Bos K.I., Schuenemann V.J., Golding G.B., Burbano H.A., Waglechner N. (2011). A draft genome of *Yersinia pestis* from victims of the Black Death. *Nature*. 478 (27 October): 506–510.

Department of Health (2012). *Updated Guidance on the Diagnosis and Reporting of Clostridium difficile*. Department of Health, London.

Engelkirk P.G., Duben-Engelkirk J. (2011). Biochemistry: the chemistry of life. In: Engelkirk P.G., Duben-Engelkirk J. (Eds.), *Burton's Microbiology for the Health Sciences*. 9th ed. Lippincott Williams and Wilkins, Philadelphia: 84–101.

Fitzgerald D.W., Sterling T.R., Haas D.W. (2010). Mycobacterium tuberculosis. In: Mandell G.L., Bennett J.E., Dolin R.D. (Eds.), *Mandell's Principles and Practices of Infectious Diseases*. 6th ed. Churchill Livingstone Elsevier, London. Expert Consult online: http://expertconsult.com (12 December 2012)

Harwood J. (2010). Serology. In: Ford M. (Ed.), *Medical Microbiology*. Oxford University Press, Oxford: 322–327.

Health Protection Agency (2010). *Coagulase Test*. BSOPTP 10, Issue 4. Health Protection Agency, London.

Health Protection Agency (2011a). *Standards for Microbiological Investigations: Inoculation of Culture Media for Bacteriology*. Health Protection Agency, London.

Health Protection Agency (HPA) (2011b). *UK Standards for Microbiology Investigations: Staining Procedures*. Bacteriology TP39, Issue 1. Health Protection Agency, London.

Health Protection Agency (2012a). *UK Standards for Microbiology Investigations: Investigation of Specimens for Screening for MRSA*. Bacteriology B29, Issue 5.2. Health Protection Agency, London.

Health Protection Agency (2012b). *UK Standards for Microbiology Investigations. Investigation of Specimens for Mycobacterium species*. Bacteriology. B40, Issue 6. Health Protection Agency, London.

Levinson W. (2010). Growth. In: *Review of Medical Microbiology*, 11th ed. McGraw-Hill Lange: New York, 4–13.

National *Clostridium difficile* Standards Group (2003). *Report to the Department of Health*. Department of Health, London.

Parkhill J., Wren B.W., Thomson N.R., Titball R.W., Holden M.T., *et al.* (2001). Genome sequence of *Yersinia pestis*, the causative agent of plague. *Nature*. 413 (68555): 523–527.

Pratt R.J., Grange J.M., Williams V.G. (2005). Diagnosis of tuberculosis and other mycobacterial diseases. In: Pratt R.J., Grange J.M., Williams V.G. (Eds.), *Tuberculosis: A Foundation for Nursing and Healthcare Practice*. Hodder Arnold, London: 95–108.

Strohl W.A., Rouse H., Fisher B.D. (2001). Bacterial growth, structure and metabolism. In: Harvey R.A., Champe P.A. (Eds.), *Lippincott's Illustrated Reviews. Microbiology*. Lippincott, Williams and Wilkins, Philadelphia: 101–114.

Taubenberger J.K., Reid A.H., Laurens R.M., Wang R., Guozhong J., *et al*. (2005). Characterisation of the 1918 Influenza virus polymerase genes. *Nature*. 437 (6 October): 889–893.

Venter J.C., Adams M.D., Myers E.W., Li P.W., Mural R.J., *et al*. (2001). The sequence of the human genome. *Science*. 291 (5507): 1304–1351.

Willey J.M., Sherwood J.M., Woolverton C.J. (2011). The evolution of microorganisms and micro-biology. In: Willey J.M., Sherwood J.M., Woolverton C.J. (Eds.), *Prescott's Microbiology*. 8th ed. McGraw-Hill International Edition, New York: 1–24.

8

Understanding the immune system and the nature and pathogenesis of infection

Contents

Fundamentals of Infection Prevention and Control: Theory and Practice, Second Edition. Debbie Weston.
© 2013 John Wiley & Sons, Ltd. Published 2013 by John Wiley & Sons, Ltd. Companion Website: www.wiley.com/go/fundamentalsofinfectionprevention

Introduction

In order to care for patients with an infection or infectious disease, a basic understanding of the workings of the immune system and the pathogenesis (development) of infection is advantageous. This is particularly important given that many of the clinical features of infection are a result of the defence mechanisms employed by the immune system. In order to destroy invading pathogens and protect the host from infection, the immune system has to be able to differentiate between self and non-self – what is foreign to the body and what is not. There are two branches of the immune system which work both independently of each other and together: the innate or natural immune response, and the adaptive or acquired immune response. Since immunology is a complex subject and requires more than just one chapter to do it justice (which is beyond the scope of this book), this chapter aims to provide a broad and brief overview of the disease process, linking together the immune response, the chain of infection and the pathogenesis of infection – common themes which will tie in with Chapters 20–24 in Section 4 of this book. Sepsis and neutropenic sepsis are covered in Chapter 9.

Learning outcomes

After reading this chapter, the reader will be able to:

- Understand the differences between innate and adaptive immunity, and the role played by specialised components of the immune system in fighting infection.

- Understand the terms 'colonisation' and 'infection'.

- Understand the chain of infection and the importance of breaking the links in the chain in order to reduce the opportunities for infection to occur.

- Understand how the clinical features of infection occur by relating them to the workings of the immune response.

The innate, or natural, immune response

Innate immunity, or natural immunity, is quite simply the body's first line of defence; it is always 'switched on' and leaps into action as soon as a pathogen is detected. It is non-specific, meaning that its actions are directed against any pathogen the first time the pathogen is encountered. If it is breached, it focuses and directs the actions of adaptive immunity, or the acquired immune response (Dieffenbach *et al.*, 2009), but unlike adaptive or acquired immunity the workings of the innate immune system do not confer life-long protection upon the host. It consists of physical barriers, internal and external surface secretions and cells, all of which are present in the individual from birth.

The skin

The tough horny outer layer of the skin, with its generally dry condition (although some areas of the skin such as the axillae and the perineum are naturally moist), resident bacterial population and natural secretion of sweat which contains a high concentration of salt, provides an inhospitable living environment for many microorganisms (Willey *et al.*, 2011a). The shedding or desquamation of skin scales also assists in the elimination of microorganisms (Dieffenbach *et al.*, 2009), although this could also contribute to environmental contamination and cross-infection if an individual were to be heavily colonised with a potential pathogen such as meticillin-resistant *Staphylococcus aureus* (MRSA). In spite of these external defence mechanisms, however, any breach in the skin resulting from a traumatic injury, surgical wound (see Chapter 18) or insertion of an IV cannula (see Chapter 16) will create an immediate gateway into the body through which pathogens can swiftly enter and invade body tissues and the bloodstream.

Resident body flora

In normal 'good' health blood, body fluids and tissues are sterile (Ryan and Ray, 2010). However, microorganisms, the amount and type of which can vary between individuals, are present on and in various body sites, colonising the surface of the skin and the respiratory, gastro-intestinal (GI) and genito-urinary tracts. These are known as resident, or commensal, body flora.

Fact Box 8.1   Resident flora

It is estimated that 'normal' body flora probably consists of more than 1000 different species of microorganisms (Ryan and Ray, 2010), and that the surface area of the skin (approximately 2 m^2) is home to 10^{12} bacteria (Willey *et al.*, 2011b).

Colonisation of these body sites prevents pathogens from taking up residence (known as colonisation resistance), as they have to compete with the commensal flora, which outnumber them, for nutrients. However, although they are not generally pathogenic, resident flora are often opportunists and can cause infections if they are transferred to other body sites. For example, bowel flora such as *Escherichia coli* (see Chapter 10) are a common cause of urinary tract and wound infections, and staphylococci residing on the skin can cause wound, IV site and bloodstream infections. These are known as endogenous infections because they arise from the individual's own commensal flora.

Fact Box 8.2   Endogenous and exogenous infection

Patients can sometimes be the source of endogenous infections themselves through the transfer of bacteria from one body site to another – on their hands if they touch their wounds or urethral catheters, for example – but commensal flora can also be transferred exogenously (cross-infection) to other patients, on the hands of healthcare workers by contact with other patients or with contaminated equipment.

Table 8.1 identifies some of the common commensal flora which colonise the body.

Table 8.1   Common commensal flora

Skin flora	Staphylococci (*S. aureus* and *S. epidermidis*) Micrococci Yeasts (especially *Candida* spp.) Corynebacteria *Propionibacterium*
Respiratory tract (including mouth and teeth)	Staphylococci Actinomycetes *Streptococcus mutans* *Streptococcus pneumoniae* *Streptococcus pyogenes* *Haemophilus influenzae* *Neisseria* *Candida* *Bacteroides* spp.
GI tract	*E. coli* and other *Enterobacteriaceae* Enterococci Yeasts *Clostridium* spp. *Bacteroides* spp. Bifidobacteria
Genito-urinary tract (including the perineum and urethra)	Skin flora colonising the perineum plus *Bacteroides* spp., *Clostridium* spp. and *Bifidiobacterium* Yeasts Lactobacilli Actinomycetes Streptococci

Defence mechanisms of the respiratory, GI and genito-urinary tracts

Intact mucosal surfaces, which are often only one cell thick in places (Bannister *et al.*, 1996), can be invaded by bacteria and viruses, but they have their own defence mechanisms which can ward off the invaders.

Tissue fluids containing enzymes called lysozymes, which are present in the lachrymal secretions of the conjunctivae, are active against the peptidoglycan layer in the bacteria cell wall (see Chapter 5), and naturally have an inhibitory effect on microorganisms (Dieffenbach *et al.*, 2009).

Gastric acid and peptide enzymes in the stomach account for the very few resident organisms found there because of the naturally acidic environment which is not particularly conducive to microbial life.

Within the **large bowel**, the resident bowel flora (10^{10} organisms per gram of faeces) (Ryan and Ray, 2010) compete for nutrients with, and inhibit the growth of, other bacteria that could become pathogenic if the balance of the microbial population is disturbed (see Chapter 22 on *Clostridium difficile*).

The **ciliated epithelium and mucociliary 'blankets'** which line the respiratory tract trap invading microorganisms and waft the bacteria out.

The **cough reflex** helps to expel them, and 90% of inhaled material is cleared from the respiratory tract within one hour (Dieffenbach *et al.*, 2009).

While the **genito-urinary tract** is sterile above the distal 1 cm of the urethra, the perineum is colonised by skin and bowel flora which can gain entry into the normally sterile environment, particularly if the normally closed urethra is open because of the presence of a urethral catheter, which acts as 'the ladder to the bladder' (see Chapter 17). Usually, however, the normal mechanism of emptying the bladder and the flushing effect of the urine will wash away any potential invaders.

White blood cells

White blood cells (WBCs) or leukocytes are important components of the innate immune system. There are 4500–11 000 WBCs per cubic millimetre of blood, and that number increases in the presence of inflammation or infection. The WBC population consists of natural killer (NK) cells; mast cells, basophils, eosinophils and neutrophils (known as polymorphonuclear leukocytes); and the phagocytic cells (macrophages and neutrophils).

Natural killer cells belong to a group of WBCs known as lymphocytes, and they target abnormal cells such as those infected with viruses, bacteria, parasites, fungi and cancer cells (Sompayrac, 2008a). They are also able to kill cells that are coated with IgG antibody (a process known as antibody-dependent cellular cytotoxicity), as they possess IgG receptors, and they primarily play a role in the adaptive immune response (Roitt *et al.*, 2001).

Mast cells line body surfaces, particularly mucosal surfaces. Their primary role is protection against parasitic infections and response to allergens – the allergic immune response (Sompayrac, 2008a).

Basophils are present in the circulation in very low numbers, accounting for less than 0.2% of the total leukocyte count, and along with eosinophils (1–2% of leukocytes) they play a role in the allergic immune response, increasing in numbers and migrating to sites where an allergic reaction has taken place (Dieffenbach *et al.*, 2009).

Neutrophils have been described as 'professional killers', and there are approximately 20 billion of them in circulation (Sompayrac, 2008a). They are the most abundant WBCs in the blood stream, with between 2000 and 7500 neutrophils per cubic mm of blood, and they flood infected tissues within 24–48 hours of infection. Receptors on the surface of neutrophils enable them to attach to bacteria when the organism is coated with antibody and/or complement, and destroy them. They are phagocytic cells, the marauding scavengers of the immune system.

Cytokines, chemotaxis and phagocytosis

Although phagocytic cells are constantly on patrol, they can be attracted to pathogens by **cytokines**, which are small proteins or molecules released by different types of cells, including bacterial cells.

Cytokines bind to cell surface receptors on pathogens and act as chemical messengers, forming part of an 'extracellular signalling network' which controls and regulates every function of the innate and the adaptive immune responses, including inflammation and proliferation (multiplication) of clones of T and B lymphocytes (Roitt *et al.*, 2001). Interleukins (IL), interferons and tumour necrosis factor (TNF) are cytokines. Although they are integral to the functioning of the immune system, over-stimulation of the immune system by cytokines can cause the host to effect what can best be described as an exaggerated, inappropriate, overwhelming and potentially fatal immune response which is, perhaps appropriately, known as a cytokine storm.

Fact Box 8.3   Cytokines

Cytokines have been implicated in infections such as influenza and severe acute respiratory syndrome (SARS) (Osterholm, 2005), and, in the United Kingdom in 2006, following a drug trial involving a single intravenous injection of a novel monoclonal antibody (Suntharalingam et al., 2006; St Clair, 2008).

The phagocytic cells migrate through the capillary walls and through the tissues to the affected area by the process of chemotaxis, which is a directed movement towards chemical attractants such as products of injured tissue, blood products and products produced by mast cells and neutrophils (Staines *et al.*, 1993; Dieffenbach *et al.*, 2009). When the phagocytic cells encounter a pathogen, dead or dying cell debris or any foreign material, they bind to it; it is then engulfed by a pseudopod, which is an extension of the phagocytic cell membrane, and killed through the combined activity of digestive enzymes and a transient increase in oxygen uptake (respiratory burst), which destroys the cell. This process is known as phagocytosis, and it plays an important role in the process of wound healing, ingesting cellular debris.

Macrophages

Macrophages are large phagocytic cells derived from monocytes, which are white blood cells formed from stem cells in the bone marrow. They reside in all body tissues at strategic locations through which blood and lymph pass, and are particularly concentrated in areas such as the lungs (alveolar macrophages have a role to play in trying to ward off infection from *Mycobacterium tuberculosis*), liver, spleen, kidneys and lymph nodes, where their role is to filter out pathogens and remove them from the circulation (Staines *et al.*, 1993).

The adaptive, or acquired, immune response

The adaptive or acquired immune response is uniquely remarkable for its specificity, diversity and immunologic memory (the ability to recognise specific antigens and pathogens when they are next encountered) (Staines *et al.*, 1993), and can be divided into humoral (antibody) and cell-mediated (lymphocyte) responses. Its actions are targeted against specific antigens, which are molecules capable of inducing an immune response and reacting with antibodies and/or T lymphocytes, such as bacterial toxins or bacterial cells. It takes three to five days for the adaptive immune response to be activated, so the innate immune system comes into play initially. The first encounter with the antigen generates a primary response and, following this initial exposure, a more powerful and rapid response is generated on encountering the antigen or pathogen a second time (Roitt *et al.*, 2001).

There are two different types of lymphocytes – T and B. They are produced in the bone marrow and found throughout the body in blood, lymph fluid and lymph tissue, where their role is to recognise and react to antigens (Staines *et al.*, 1993)

T lymphocytes

T lymphocytes enter the peripheral circulation and pass through the thymus gland where they mature and acquire specificity, along with recognition molecules, or T cell receptors (TCRs) on their cell surface, which enable the T lymphocyte to interact with the antigen. Following maturation, they leave the thymus gland and re-enter the peripheral circulation, taking up residence in the lymph nodes and the spleen where they undertake surveillance for antigens, constantly re-circulating through the blood, lymph nodes and lymph fluid (Staines *et al.*, 1993).

Fact Box 8.4   T cells

Two different types of T cells assist in the cellular immune response. T helper cells (TH2 cells) express CD4 molecules on their surface and assist the B lymphocytes in generating antibody responses by secreting cytokines which signal the B lymphocyte to differentiate, or change, into an antibody-secreting B lymphocyte. Unfortunately for CD4 cells, they act as receptors for the HIV virus, which specifically targets T lymphocytes and eventually, over time, succeeds in destroying the immune system and killing the host.

T suppressor cells, which express CD8 molecules on their surface (also known as cytotoxic, or killer, T cells), target cells infected with viruses or other microorganisms, and control the responses of the T helper cells and suppress their actions (Roitt *et al.*, 2001).

B lymphocytes

B lymphocytes do not pass through the thymus. They are descended from stem cells and approximately one billion are produced in the bone marrow every day, where they achieve maturation and specificity (Sompayrac, 2008a), and from there enter the peripheral circulation and migrate directly to the lymph nodes and the spleen. When it is exposed to an antigen, the B cell 'switches on' and differentiates into a plasma cell which secretes antibodies, forming a clone of daughter cells which secrete the same antibody as the parent cell. Plasma cells have a short lifespan of only two to three days, but approximately 10% of them survive to become antigen-specific B memory cells, able to respond immediately to the antigen if they encounter it a second time as they are already primed to secrete antibody.

Antibodies

Also known as immunoglobulins, antibodies are soluble globular Y-shaped proteins, some of which are carried on the surface of B cells where they act as receptors for antigens, while others circulate freely in the peripheral blood or lymph fluid (Staines *et al.*, 1993; Roitt *et al.*, 2001). They also assist in triggering the complement cascade. They are antigen specific, binding to and reacting with the antigen that initiated their formation through sites called paratopes that bind with a specific part of that antigen, called the epitope. This essentially 'labels' the antigen, effectively marking it for destruction by other components of the immune system, such as phagocytic cells which may possess particular receptors for that antibody subtype. There are five antibody classes, or isotypes, and these are described in Table 8.2.

Table 8.2   Classes of antibody

IgM	The first antibody to be produced during the primary immune response, and able to activate complement more effectively than other classes of antibody. Often associated with immune responses to blood-borne organisms.
IgG	Has a long half-life of 23 days (4–10 times longer than other classes of antibody). Found in blood, lymph, peritoneal fluid and cerebral spinal fluid, and is the only antibody carried across the maternal placenta to the foetus. The predominant antibody produced during the secondary immune response.
IgA	Found in mucous, tears, sweat, gastric fluid and colostrum, where it protects mucosal surfaces and prevents colonisation of areas of the body such as the GI, respiratory and genito-urinary tracts.
IgD	Present in low amounts in serum. Plays a role in signalling B cells, but other host defence functions are undetermined.
IgE	Low concentrations in serum but primarily concerned with the allergic immune response, binding to allergens and triggering histamine release from mast cells, causing anaphylactic shock. Has a role in defence against parasitic infections.

Source: Staines *et al.*, 1993; Roitt *et al.*, 2001; Stewart, 2003; Dieffenbach and Tramont, 2004; Sompayrac, 2008b.

Complement

The complement system, so called because it facilitates and complements the actions of antibodies (Staines *et al.*, 1993; Roitt *et al.*, 2001), consists of more than 30 soluble proteins, some of which, when activated by either an innate or an adaptive immune response, interact in a cascade and activate each other sequentially. Complement has three main functions:

- Rupture (lysis) of the bacterial cell membrane, resulting in cell death (this destructive action is also directed against cancerous cells and transplanted tissues and organs, i.e. 'foreign' material) (Levinson, 2010)
- The generation of inflammatory mediators
- The enhancement, or opsonisation, of phagocytosis.

Table 8.3   Actions of some of the key complement components

C1	Binds to antibody (classical pathway) and bacterial cell wall (alternative pathway).
C3	The key component, or linchpin, of the complement system involved in both the classical and alternative pathways. Splits to create C3a and Cb3.
C3a	An inflammatory mediator; increases vascular activity and activates the respiratory burst (in phagocytosis). Effects chemotaxis, attracting leukocytes to the site of tissue inflammation.
C3b	Identifies bacteria for destruction by tagging or coating the organism; C3b is coated onto the surface of the bacteria, enhancing phagocytic activity.
C5a	An inflammatory mediator. Activates polymorphonucleocytes – enhanced phagocytic activity. Causes degranulation of mast cells and basophils, triggering the release of histamine in the allergic response.

Source: Staines *et al.*, 1993; Wilson, 1995; Sompayrac, 2008a; Levinson, 2010.

There are three complement activation pathways: the classical pathway is initiated through the formation of antigen–antibody complexes, the alternative pathway by the presence of microbial pathogens and the lectin activation pathway by a protein formed in the liver called mannose-binding lectin (MBL) which is activated by carbohydrate molecules found on the surface of pathogens (Roitt *et al.*, 2001; Sompayrac, 2008a). Table 8.3 describes the actions of some of the key complement components.

The immune response and allergy

Hypersensitivity reactions

Repeated exposure to a particular antigen or allergen can stimulate the adaptive immune response to initiate an intense reaction each time the antigen or allergen is encountered. Allergens, defined as any foreign substance that causes an immune response (Roitt *et al.*, 2001), can be ingested, inhaled, injected or encountered through direct contact. The extent and severity of the immune response, which can cause local or systemic effects and can be so extreme that it can result in damage to the host's own tissues and even in the death of the host, are results of either excessive amounts of antigen or allergen, or because the quantity of antibody to the antigen or allergen is too high. There are four types of hypersensitivity reaction – types I, II and III are antibody mediated, and type IV reactions are T cell mediated.

Type I hypersensitivity reactions are associated with atopy and anaphylaxis. Atopic disorders such as eczema, asthma and hay fever often occur in individuals where there is a family history. Anaphylaxis (derived from the Greek words 'ana' = non/opposite, and 'phylaxos' = protection) (Roitt *et al.*, 2001; Sompayrac, 2008b) occurs as a response to certain foods such as peanuts, shellfish and drugs (e.g. penicillin) **and is the most extreme allergic reaction of all** (see www.anaphylaxis.com;). IgE antibodies are generated over time in response to repeated low-dose exposure to an allergen, and they bind to IgE receptors on the surface of mast cells and basophils.

Fact Box 8.5   Mast cells and histamine release

When the allergen is encountered, the mast cells and basophils degenerate, releasing hista-mine (which is a potent activator of the immune response) and prostaglandins. As mast cells and basophils are situated under the skin and in the mucous membranes of the eyes, nose, lung and throat, this is where the majority of the clinical signs of an allergic response are seen (Sompayrac, 2008b).

In anaphylaxis, an immediate hypersensitivity reaction occurs as the allergen enters the circula-tion very rapidly. The release of excessive amounts of histamine stimulates an overwhelming and potentially life-threatening immune response, giving rise to the cardinal signs of anaphylaxis which can manifest themselves within seconds or minutes of exposure. **Anaphylaxis constitutes a medical emergency**, and individuals with known allergies to food, drugs, latex rubber and insect stings should carry a pre-loaded injectable adrenaline pen. Box 8.1 describes the cardinal signs of anaphylaxis.

Type II hypersensitivity reactions, involving IgM or IgG, are known as cytotoxic reactions as they damage host cells and tissues (Roitt *et al.*, 2001). Incompatible blood transfusions fall into this class of hypersensitivity reaction, where the recipient has antibodies that react against the donor erythrocytes, hence the need for cross-matching prior to transfusion.

In **type III** hypersensitivity reactions, an immune complex is formed every time the antibody (IgG or IgM) meets the antigen, resulting in reactions in the bloodstream or the tissues. Immune complexes within the tissues give rise to tissue damage caused by an acute inflammatory response from the activation of complement, platelets and phagocytosis (Dieffenbach *et al.*, 2009).

Type IV delayed hypersensitivity reactions are slowly evolving reactions involving T lymphocytes and macrophages that take between 24 and 72 hours to manifest after the allergen has been encountered (Dieffenbach *et al.*, 2009). Contact hypersensitivity reactions occur at the point of contact with the allergen, resulting in an eczema-type reaction on the skin. It takes 10–14 days for the individual to become sensitised to the allergen, and when the allergen is next encountered, an immune response is directed against it. Latex allergy falls into this category (see Chapter 13; and Royal College of Physicians, 2008). Delayed hypersensitivity reactions are also seen following the tuberculin skin test (see Chapter 21). This involves immunologic memory; a previous encoun-ter with purified protein derivative (PPD) which acts as the antigen is remembered, and an immune response involving lymphocytes is generated at the injection site (Staines *et al.*, 1993).

Box 8.1   The cardinal signs of anaphylaxis

Urticaria: 'nettle rash' or 'hives'; palpable raised wheels – can occur anywhere on the skin and may be intensely itchy

Angioedema: swelling of the deeper layers of the skin, commonly affecting the hands, feet, eyes and mouth, and due to build-up of fluid; can be severe

Flushing: of the skin; due to vasodilation (widening of the blood vessels)

Dyspnoea: shortness of breath due to bronchoconstriction (narrowing of the airways); may also be accompanied by coughing and wheezing

Rhinitis: similar to the symptoms of a cold or hay fever.

Understanding the chain of infection

The 'chain of infection' is the phrase used to describe the process by which infection can spread from one susceptible individual to another. It has been criticized for being a biomedical model as opposed to a biosocial model, focusing on the microbiological, physical and environmental aspects of the infection process, and excluding the various social and psychological factors that play a role in cross-infection (Elliott, 2009). However, it has its origins in what is known about the nature of microorganisms and how they are transmitted, and the concept of there being a 'chain' in the infection process is one which has become firmly established and utilised widely within infection prevention and control. For an infection to occur, all of the links in the chain must be intact and in the correct order. In order to break the chain, it is important that healthcare workers understand how the different components of the chain interact and facilitate the spread of infection. Then, the basic principles of infection prevention and control can be applied to clinical practice to break the chain.

Link 1: causative organism

This can be any organism that demonstrates pathogenicity and/or virulence, which are not necessarily one and the same thing. Pathogenicity is the ability of the organism to cause infection. Not all organisms are pathogenic, and those that are may cause infections that range from asymptomatic or mild, to severe. Virulence refers to the organism's ability to cause severe disease, and while all pathogens are able to cause disease, some are more virulent than others. The degree of virulence is dependent on the host's susceptibility and the virulence factors that the organism possesses (see Chapter 5).

Fact Box 8.6   Virulence

An example of virulence can be demonstrated by looking at *Shigella* and *Salmonella*, two medically important bacteria which cause severe diarrhoea. While 10–1000 *Salmonella* cells are required to cause salmonellosis, only 10 *Shigella* cells will cause diarrhoea, making *Shigella* a more virulent organism than *Salmonella* (Engelkirk and Duben-Engelkirk, 2011).

The organism's infectiveness, or ease with which it can spread to other people, its invasiveness, which is related to its ability to spread through the body; and its toxigenicity, or toxin-producing properties, are other important contributing factors (Bannister *et al.*, 1996; Roitt *et al.*, 2001).

Link 2: reservoir or source

The reservoir is the site where the organism usually lives, and where it will find the nutrient and moisture supply necessary for its growth and survival. It may be environmental, human or animal, and in the healthcare setting, environmental and human reservoirs are commonly the most problematic and difficult to control. As discussed in this chapter, the human body is the reservoir for the bacteria that colonise the skin, bowel and respiratory tract. They generally do not harm the host unless the immune system is impaired, when they can cause opportunistic infections in immunocompromised patients. The hospital environment can serve as a reservoir for organisms if standards of cleanliness are not adhered to.

Fact Box 8.7   Reservoirs and sources

Patients can become a source of infection if they have infected skin lesions, skin scales, secretions and excretions which can easily be transferred to other people. Organic material such as dirt, blood and body fluids can harbour bacteria and viruses, and any equipment that has been in contact with the patient can serve as both a reservoir and a source of infection. Bed frames, mattresses and manual handling equipment have all been implicated in the spread of infection (O'Connor, 2002).

Links 3 and 4: portal of exit and portal of entry

There are many different portals of exit, which are the routes by which the organism leaves the reservoir and enters the host. These include the respiratory and gastro-intestinal tracts and the skin and mucosa, with organisms carried in blood and body fluids, in respiratory droplets and on the surface of the skin. In some organisms, the portal of exit can be the same as the portal of entry, such as the respiratory tract in tuberculosis, or it may be different; in *Salmonella* infections, the route of entry is the mouth as *Salmonella* has to be ingested, and the exit route is in the faeces.

Link 5: mode of transmission

This refers to the way in which the organism is spread and acquired.

Direct contact with infected body fluids, secretions and lesions can transmit infections such as HIV, the common cold and impetigo. The hands of healthcare workers are the most important source of cross-infection, transferring resident and transient skin flora (see Chapter 14). Fomites are objects which can become contaminated with organisms from patients or staff, and subsequently become a source of cross-infection. They include IV stands, pumps and monitors, bed linen, computer keyboards and telephones. The risk that these pose depends largely on the degree or extent to which the object or piece of equipment is contaminated, the microbial load and the amount of direct contact that it has with the patient. However, even if it does not come into contact with the patient, the hands of any healthcare workers who may have had contact with it could serve as vehicles for cross-infection.

Airborne transmission of particles such as dust, water and respiratory droplets, which can all contain microorganisms, can result in infection if they are inhaled or if they settle on equipment or wounds. *Legionella* is present in aerosols which can, depending on wind speed, travel up to 500 m and infect large numbers of people. Pathogens may be expelled from the respiratory tract during coughing, sneezing and talking. These droplets partially evaporate to form droplet nuclei, where they remain suspended in the air for long periods of time and can subsequently be inhaled. Other droplets, or large dust particles, may fall rather rapidly and settle on furniture, bedding or equipment, and although they are unlikely to become airborne again, they can still cause infection.

Bacteria may be **ingested** through consuming contaminated food or water (e.g. cholera, *Campylobacter* and *Salmonella*). Patients may also acquire some infections as a result of faecal-oral transmission, whereby their hands have become contaminated and they subsequently move their hands to their mouth (e.g. *C. difficile*). Norovirus can be spread by both the airborne and the faecal-oral routes (Chapter 23).

Transmission of blood-borne viruses such as HIV and hepatitis B and C via **inoculation injury**, either from a contaminated sharp (see Chapters 14 and 24) or a splash of blood or body fluids into the mucosa, can pose a big risk to healthcare workers.

As described in this chapter, some infections may also be spread **endogenously** – they are acquired as the result of the patient's own body flora being transferred from one body site to another.

Link 5: the susceptible patient

Any patient in a hospital bed is potentially at risk of contracting an infection during their in-patient stay, but there are many factors which significantly increase that risk.

Age: With increasing age, the ability of the immune system to fight infection naturally declines. This affects the efficiency of both the innate and the acquired responses, particularly decreased antibody and lymphocyte responses, and lowered response to vaccination. This is a natural decline known as immunosenescence (Dieffenbach *et al.*, 2009).

Fact Box 8.8   Immunosenescence

A weakened immune response means that fever, which is a normal clinical response to infection, may be absent or suppressed, and the first indications of an infection may actually be non-specific signs such as lack of appetite, confusion and malaise (Rajagopalan and Yoshikawa, 2001; Destarac and Ely, 2002). Elderly individuals often have a reduced cough reflex and are more vulnerable to serious respiratory tract infections, particularly pneumonia, as up to 40% of lung function decreases by the age of 70 (Knight and Nigam, 2008a). The skin is more easily damaged and prone to tears due to the weakening of the collagen content of the dermis, which means that the skin loses some of its elasticity or 'bounce-back' (Bianchi and Cameron, 2008). While gastric acid secretion is part of the immune defence, creating an inhospitable, acidic environment for microorganisms, it can cause gastric ulcers by weakening and damaging the protective stomach lining or mucosa (Knight and Nigam, 2008b). To reduce gastric acid secretion and prevent gastric ulcers, proton pump inhibitors such as Omeprazole are prescribed. However, the downside of this is that they can increase the risk of colonisation or infection with *C. difficile* (Dial *et al.*, 2004).

Babies in the uterus are sterile up until the membranes rupture, and then they are exposed to the genital and perineal flora of the mother during childbirth, and to the outside world, and they rapidly become colonised (Ryan and Ray, 2010). Premature infants are particularly susceptible to infection, and have no immunological memory together with a reduced ability to develop specific antibodies against the microorganisms that they are exposed to (Petrova and Mehta, 2007). Their protection against infection is mostly dependent upon innate immune defences. However, due to their prematurity, natural barriers such as the skin and mucosa are weakened. They have an immature and undeveloped population of T lymphocytes, and decreased neutrophil efficiency (although the neutrophil count rises abruptly within the first 24 hours after birth and stabilizes within 72 hours, neutrophil production in response to an infection is underwhelming) (Petrova and Mehta, 2007), and they are deficient in some components of the complement cascade (Petrova and Mehta, 2007; Anderson-Berry and Bellig, 2010).

Nutritional status: Poor nutritional intake compromises the immune system and increases the risk of infection (Cowan *et al.*, 2003; Kenkmann *et al.*, 2010). Malnutrition, which affects 40–60% of older people admitted to hospital (Morse and High, 2004), results in low concentrations of serum albumin (hypoalbuminemia), which can be a poor prognostic indicator when treating serious infections, for example severe *C. difficile* infection (see Chapter 22).

Loss of mobility: This can breach the body's first line of defence, the skin, leading to skin damage and potential pressure sore formation.

Co-existing illness or disease: The presence of a known or undetected underlying illness increases an individual's susceptibility to infection. For example, wound infection is a major complication of diabetes as a result of impaired leukocyte function and delayed migration of neutrophils and macrophages to the wound or site of inflammation (Hirsch *et al.*, 2008), and the risk of surgical wound infection is estimated to be 2–5 times greater in diabetics, as compared to non-diabetics (Golden *et al.*, 1999).

Immunocompromised as a result of underlying illness or treatment: In individuals who are immunocompromised as a result of chemotherapy or radiotherapy, damage occurs to the mucosal barriers in the mouth and GI tract, leading to inflammation, ulceration and diarrhoea. Neutrophils can become severely depleted owing to suppression of the bone marrow, giving rise to a potentially life-threatening condition known as neutropenia, which is a neutrophil count of less than $1000/mm^3$, with the risk of infection increasing substantially if the count drops below $500\ mm^3$ (see Chapter 9).

Medication: The balance of the resident microbial population of the colon can be adversely affected by the administration of antibiotics. While the colonic micro-flora is generally resistant to colonisation by *C. difficile*, which is part of the normal bowel flora in 2–5% of the population and readily acquired in the healthcare setting, with carriage rates reported of approximately 15% (Poutanen and Simor, 2004), *C. difficile* can grow unchecked, proliferating within and colonising the colon, and giving rise to systemic infection (see Chapter 22).

The presence of invasive indwelling devices: The presence of an invasive indwelling device that breaches the skin (e.g. a peripheral intravenous cannula) or a sterile organ (e.g. a urinary catheter inserted into the bladder) significantly increases the risk of infection as critical lines of defence are breached.

Duration of hospital stay: The duration of hospital stay and bed occupancy hospital rates increase the risk of patients becoming colonised with MRSA (see Chapter 20) or *C. difficile*. The average bed occupancy rates in 1996–1997 were 80.8%, increasing to 86.5% in 2002–2003; in 2008/09–2009/10, one-quarter of NHS Trusts had bed occupancy rates exceeding 90%. Trusts with greater than 90% occupancy were found to have MRSA rates that were 10 times greater than those with bed occupancy rates of less than 85% (Department of Health, 2007).

Reflection point

Think of a microorganism, or reflect on a colonised or infected patient care in your care, and then work your way through the chain of infection, considering each of the remaining five links in turn and the infection control precautions and preventions that need to be taken in order to interrupt each link.

Colonisation, infection and the inflammatory response

Not all patients with an 'infection' are genuinely infected, so the isolation of an organism from a body site is not necessarily clinically significant.

Colonisation

Once an organism has made contact with the host and adhered to the skin or mucosal surfaces, it often establishes itself at that site and colonises it, without causing any adverse effects or harm. The length of time in which a site may be colonised is variable and depends on both host factors and the properties of the organism involved. The host may go on to develop immunity to the organism by developing specific T cell or antibody responses (immunity to *Neisseria meningitidis* is acquired this way). The status quo may change, however, if the relationship between the host and the organism alters to the extent that the organism can extend beyond colonisation to local invasion of the tissues, or even the whole body (Bannister *et al.*, 1996).

Infection

Infection is the process of microbial invasion which results in tissue damage at the site of the infection or, in the worst-case scenario, the death of the host. Unlike colonisation, infection manifests itself both physically and physiologically. These signs may be either localised or systemic.

There are several stages in the pathogenesis of infection:

Attachment: The organism needs to attach itself to the tissues so that it can penetrate them. Adherence often occurs at a mucosal surface, enabling the bacteria to establish itself either on or in the host, colonising the site of entry and attachment, and occurs because of interactions between adhesins (molecules which mediate adherence of bacteria to the host) and receptors on the host cell wall (Petri *et al.*, 2009). Hair-like protrusions known as pili (see Chapter 5) enable bacteria to adhere to these receptors.

Entry of the organism: As seen in the chain of infection, there are a number of ways in which the organism can enter the host.

Multiplication, invasion and spread: Once attached, and providing that the environmental conditions required for the organism's growth and survival are right, it will begin to multiply. It can do this locally at the site of attachment, or it may invade the bloodstream and be carried to other body sites. Clinical signs of infection then become apparent.

Evasion of host defences: The organism will try to avoid the effects of the host's immune system. The mechanisms that organisms employ in order to do this are discussed in Chapter 5.

Damage to tissues or the host: In some cases, the damage resulting from the infection may be so severe that it leads to the death of the host. Much of this damage is a result of bacterial toxins produced by Gram-positive and Gram-negative bacteria (Chapter 5).

When the body suffers a traumatic injury, or is invaded by microorganisms, it generates an inflammatory response, which is designed to localise the infection and limit its spread. The success of the inflammatory response, however, depends on the strength of the host's immune system and the pathogenicity, virulence and toxigenicity of the organism involved. The physiological events that subsequently take place give rise to the cardinal signs of infection, or inflammation:

- Redness or erythema (rubour)
- Heat (calour)
- Swelling (tumour)
- Pain (dolour)
- Loss of function.

Vasodilation (widening of the blood vessels) occurs at the site of 'injury', caused by the release of histamines and prostaglandins from damaged cells. This results in an increased blood flow, which contains plasma proteins, neutrophils and phagocytes, to the affected site. The temperature of the skin rises as a result of the increased blood supply and an increase in the metabolic activities in the cells of the tissues at the damaged site.

The capillaries that line the epithelial cells dilate, releasing plasma which causes swelling; depending on the site involved and the severity of the swelling, this may lead to loss of function. The process of phagocytosis begins with the release of chemokines, which attract the phagocytes to the area where they are needed. The phagocyte then attaches itself to the bacteria, surrounds it and ingests it. Some pathogens are able to evade phagocytosis, either by producing a toxin (leukocidin) which destroys the phagocyte, or because the pathogen has the ability to survive within it and multiply, yet remain in a dormant state, resulting in disease months or even years later.

An inflammatory exudate forms at the site of inflammation, consisting of fluid, cells and cellular debris. Purulent discharge or pus, often seen in wound infections or at infected intravascular cannula sites, contains living and dead organisms, phagocytes and cell debris. With some organisms such as staphylococci and streptococci, the inflammatory exudate may be excessive. Once the invading bacteria have been dealt with, the damaged tissues and cells begin the process of repair. However, if the immune response has been weak and/or the infection overwhelming, the host may die.

Fact Box 8.9   Inflammatory markers

Inflammatory markers detect acute inflammation that may indicate infection or disease, and also measure the effectiveness of treatment or resolution of infection. They are measured by blood tests.

C-reactive protein (CRP): CRP is an 'acute phase' protein found in the blood in very low levels (5–10 mg/l). It binds to a molecule called phosphocoline, which is found on the surface of dead or dying cells, including some bacteria, and plays a role in activating the complement system, enhancing phagocytosis. Where there is tissue damage, CRP levels start to increase 4–6 hours after an inflammatory response is generated, generally peaking at 35–50 hours. CRP levels may decrease without intervention due to the effectiveness of the immune response. If they continue to increase, particularly after antibiotic therapy has been initiated, they indicate a worsening infection or treatment failure.

Erythrocyte sedimentation rate (ESR): The ESR is a non-specific marker of infection and inflammation. It is a blood test that measures the rate at which red blood cells separate and fall to the bottom of a test tube of anticoagulated blood in an hour. A raised ESR indicates a 'problem'.

White blood cells (WBCs): The number of white blood cells increases in bacterial infections and inflammation. The normal range is 4 to 11×10^9/L (4000–11 000 per cubic millimetre of blood) and consists of:
- Neutrophils (2–7.5×10^9/L)
- Lymphocytes (1.3–3.5×10^9/L)
- Eosinophils (0.04–0.44×10^9/L)
- Monocytes (0.2–0.8×10^9/L)
- Basophils (up to 0.01×10^9/L)

Chapter summary: key points

- In order to destroy invading pathogens and protect the host from infection, the immune system has to be able to differentiate between what is foreign to the body and what is not.

- The immune system consists of two branches, or arms: innate (or natural) immunity and adaptive (or acquired) immunity. They work both independently of each other and together.

- Innate or natural immunity is the body's first line of defence. Its actions are directed against any pathogen the first time the pathogen is encountered, but they do not confer life-long protection. The innate immune system consists of physical barriers, internal and external surface secretions and cells, all of which are present in the individual from birth.

- The actions of the adaptive or acquired immune response are targeted against specific antigens, which are molecules capable of inducing an immune response and reacting with antibodies and/or T lymphocytes, such as bacterial toxins or bacterial cells. The first encounter with the antigen generates a primary response, and following this initial exposure, a more powerful and rapid response is generated on encountering the antigen or pathogen a second time.

- Repeated exposure to a particular antigen or allergen can stimulate the adaptive immune response to initiate an intense reaction each time the antigen or allergen is encountered.

- Overstimulation of the immune system can result in damage to the host, and possibly death.

- The isolation of an organism from a body site is not necessarily clinically significant unless infection manifests itself both physically and physiologically. These signs may be either localised or systemic. There are five significant stages in the pathogenesis of infection.

- When the body suffers a traumatic injury, or is invaded by microorganisms, it generates an inflammatory response, which is designed to localise the infection and limit its spread. The success of this depends on the strength of the host's immune system and the ability of the organism to cause severe infection or disease.

- The uncontrolled spread of bacteria or their toxins in the bloodstream results in septicaemia and septic shock, which may overwhelm the immune response.

Further resources are available for this book, including interactive multiple choice questions. Visit the companion website at:

www.wiley.com/go/fundamentalsofinfectionprevention

References

Anderson-Berry A.L., Bellig L.L. (2010). *Neonatal Sepsis*. eMedicine. http://emedicine.medscape.com/article/978352-overview (accessed 20 March 2013)

Bannister B.A., Begg N.T. Gillespie S.H. (1996). The nature and pathogenesis of infection. In: *Infectious Diseases*. Blackwell Science Ltd, London: 1–21.

Bianchi J., Cameron J. (2008). Assessment of skin integrity in the elderly. *British Journal of Community Nursing*. 13 (3): S26–S33.

Cowan D.T., Roberts J.D., Fitzpatrick J.M., While A.E., Baldwin J. (2003). Nutritional status of older people in long term care settings: current status and future directions. *International Journal of Nursing Studies*. 41 (3): 225–237.

Department of Health (2007). *Hospital Organisation, Specialty Mix and MRSA*. Department of Health, London.

Destarac L.A., Ely E.W. (2002). Sepsis in older patients: an emerging concern in critical care. *Advances in Sepsis*. 2 (1): 15–22.

Dial S., Airsdsdi K., Manoukian C., Huang A., Menzies D. (2004). Risk of *Clostridium difficile* diarrhoea among hospital patients prescribed proton pump inhibitors: cohort and case control studies. *Canadian Medical Journal Association*. 17 (1): 33–38.

Dieffenbach C.W., Tramont E.D. (2004). Innate (general or non-specific) host defence mechanisms. In: Mandell G., Bennett J., Dolin R. (Eds.), *Mandell's Principles and Practices of Infectious Diseases*. 6th ed. Churchill Livingstone, Edinburgh. PPID Online: www.ppidonline.com (accessed 20 March 2013)

Dieffenbach C.W., Tramont E.C., Plaeger S.F. (2009). Innate (general or nonspecific) host defence mechanisms. In: Mandell G., Bennett J., Dolin R. (Eds.), *Mandell, Douglas and Bennett's Principles and Practice of Infectious Diseases*. 7th ed, Churchill Livingstone Elsevier, London. http://expertconsult.com (accessed 18 December 2012)

Elliott P. (2009). Biomedical versus biopsychosocial perspectives. In: *Infection Control: A Psychosocial Approach to Changing Practice*. Radcliffe Publishing, Oxford: 51–71.

Engelkirk P.G., Duben-Engelkirk J. (2011). Pathogenesis of infectious disease. In: *Microbiology for the Health Sciences*. 9th ed. Lippincott Williams and Wilkins, Philadelphia: 238–250.

Golden S.H., Peart-Vigilance C., Kao W.H., Brancati F.L. (1999). Perioperative glycaemic control and the risk of infection complications in a cohort of adults with diabetes. *Diabetes Care*. 22: 1408–1414.

Hirsch T., Spielmann M., Zuhail B. (2008). *Enhanced susceptibility to infections in a diabetic wound model*. http://www.biomedcentral.com/1471-2482/8/5 (accessed 18 December 2012)

Kenkmann A., Price G.M., Bolton J., Hooper L. (2010). *Health, wellbeing and nutritional status of older people living in UK care homes: an exploratory evaluation of changes in food and drink provision*. http://www.biomedcentral.com/1471-2318/10/28 (accessed 10 January 2012)

Knight J., Nigam Y. (2008a). Exploring the anatomy and physiology of ageing: part 2 – the respiratory system. *Nursing Times*. 104 (32): 24.

Knight J., Nigam Y. (2008b). Exploring the anatomy and physiology of ageing: part 3 – the digestive system. *Nursing Times*. 104 (43): 22–23.

Levinson W. (2010). Complement. In: *Review of Medical Microbiology and Immunology*. 11th edition. McGraw-Hill Lange, New York: 419–421.

Morse C.G., High K.P. (2004). Nutrition, immunity and infection. In: Mandell G. L., Bennett J.E., Dolin R.D. (Eds.), *Mandell, Bennett and Dolin's Principles and Practice of Infectious Disease*. 6th ed. Churchill Livingstone, Edinburgh. PPID Online: www.ppidonline.com (accessed 20 March 2013)

O'Connor H. (2002). Decontaminating beds and mattresses. *Nursing Times*. 96 (Suppl.): 2–5.

Osterholm M.T. (2005). Preparing for the next pandemic. *New England Journal of Medicine*. 352 (18): 1839–1842.

Petri W.A., Mann B.J., Huston C.D. (2009). Microbial adherence. In: Mandell G. L., Bennett J.E., Dolin R.D. (Eds.), *Mandell, Bennett and Dolin's Principles and Practice of Infectious Disease*. 6th ed. Churchill Livingstone, Edinburgh. PPID Online: www.ppidonline.com (accessed 20 March 2013)

Petrova A., Mehta R. (2007). Dysfunction of innate immunity and associated pathology in neonates. *Indian Journal of Paediatrics*. February (74): 185–191.

Poutanen S.M., Simor A.E. (2004). *Clostridium difficile* associated diarrhoea in adults. *Canadian Medical Association Journal*. 171 (1): 51–58

Rajagopalan S., Yoshikawa T.T. (2001). Antimicrobial therapy in the elderly. *Medical Clinics of North America*. 85: 133–147; vii.

Roitt I., Brostoff J., Male D. (2001). *Immunology*. 6th ed. Mosby, London.

Royal College of Physicians (2008). *Latex Allergy: Occupational Aspects of Management. A National Guideline*. Royal College of Physicians, London.

Ryan K.J., Ray C.G. (2010). Infection. In: Ryan K.J., Ray G.C. (Eds.), *Sherris Medical Microbiology*. 5th ed. McGraw Hill Medical, New York: 3–18.

Staines N., Brostoff J., James K. (1993). *Introducing Immunology*. 2nd ed. Mosby, London.

St Clair E.W. (2008). The calm after the cytokine storm: lessons from the TGN1412 trial. *Journal of Clinical Investigation*. 118 (4): 1344–1347.

Stewart J. (2003). Innate and acquired immunity. In: Greenwood D, Slack R.C.B., Peutherer J.F. (Eds.), *Medical Microbiology. A Guide to Microbial Infections: Pathogenesis, Immunity, Laboratory Diagnosis and Control*. 16th ed. Churchill Livingstone, Edinburgh: 121–145.

Sompayrac L. (2008a). Lecture 2: the innate immune system. In: *How the Immune System Works*. 3rd ed. Blackwell Publishing, Oxford: 13–23.

Sompayrac L. (2008b). Lecture 3: B cells and antibodies. In: *How the Immune System Works*. 3rd ed. Blackwell Publishing, Oxford: 24–37.

Suntharalingam G., Perry M.R., Ward S., Brett S.J., Castello-Cortes A., *et al.* (2006). Cytokine storm in a phase 1 trial of the anti-CD28 monoclonal antibody TGN1412. *New England Journal of Medicine*. 355 (September 7): 1018–1028.

Willey J.M., Sherwood L.M., Woolverton C.J. (2011a). Nonspecific (innate) host resistance. In: *Prescott's Microbiology*. 8th ed. McGraw Hill International Edition, New York: 761–788.

Willey J.M., Sherwood L.M., Woolverton C.J. (2011b). Microbial interactions. In: *Prescott's Microbiology*. 8th ed. McGraw Hill International Edition, New York: 713–738.

Wilson J. (1995). *Infection Control in Clinical Practice*. Bailliere Tindall, London, 77–105.

9

Sepsis

Contents

Fundamentals of Infection Prevention and Control: Theory and Practice, Second Edition. Debbie Weston.
© 2013 John Wiley & Sons, Ltd. Published 2013 by John Wiley & Sons, Ltd. Companion Website: www.wiley.com/go/fundamentalsofinfectionprevention

Introduction

At some point, healthcare staff working in community settings such as nursing homes, or healthcare staff working on a general surgical or medical ward, will be involved in the care of a 'septic' patient. This brief chapter aims to provide an overview of the pathogenesis of sepsis and its infection control management, along with the infection control management of neutropenic sepsis.

Learning outcomes

After reading this chapter, the reader will be able to:

- Understand the definitions of sepsis, septicaemia and septic shock.
- Understand the patient risk factors for developing sepsis.
- Understand the pathogenesis of septic shock and the presenting features.
- Understand the early and late signs of neutropenic sepsis.
- Understand the infection control management of neutropenic sepsis.

Sepsis and septicaemia

Fact Box 9.1   Sepsis and septicaemia

Sepsis is the 'umbrella' word frequently used to describe systemic infection; 18 million people die from sepsis worldwide each year (Slade *et al.*, 2003). In the United Kingdom, mortality ranges from 37 000 to 64 000 deaths per year (www.uksepsis.org; and see Daniels, 2011).

Septicaemia is the systemic illness which arises as a result of the uncontrolled spread of bacteria or their toxins through the bloodstream, and is the leading cause of death in intensive care units (Robson and Newell, 2005; Wheeler, 2009).

Sepsis definitions

There has been confusion over the definition of the word sepsis (Bone *et al.*, 1992) which is often used interchangeably with septicaemia and septic shock, and historically there has been a general lack of consensus in actually agreeing these definitions. However, in 1991 clear and concise definitions were agreed (Bone *et al.*, 1992; Vincent, 2002) for the terms sepsis, severe sepsis and septic shock, together with the introduction of a new term known as systemic inflammatory response syndrome (SIRS).

Systemic inflammatory response syndrome

Systemic inflammatory response syndrome (SIRS) is defined as a clinical response arising from a non-specific insult and which includes more than two of the following:

- Temperature greater than 38 °C or less than 36 °C
- Tachycardic, with heart rate > 90 beats/minute
- Tachyapnoeic – respiratory rate > 20 breaths/minute
- White cell count > 12 000 per mm3 or < 4000 per mm3.

Sepsis

Sepsis is defined as SIRS with a presumed or confirmed infection and accompanied by two or more of the SIRS criteria (Bone *et al.*, 1992).

Severe sepsis

Severe sepsis is said to occur if there is a known or suspected infection, along with two or more SIRS criteria *plus* more than one sign of acute organ dysfunction, which can involve any of the major body organs. Signs of organ dysfunction may manifest themselves as:

- altered mental state
- hyperglycaemia (in the absence of diabetes)
- hypoxia (oxygen saturation < 93% or arterial blood gas < 9 kPa)
- urine output < 0.5 ml/kg/hr, and/or raised urea and creatinine
- coagulopathy (INR > 1.5, activated partial thromboplastin time > 60 seconds or platelets < 100).

Box 9.1 summarises the patient risk factors for developing sepsis.

Box 9.1   Patient risk factors for developing sepsis

Age
Obesity
Intensive care unit patients
Patients with invasive indwelling devices
Underlying chronic diseases – chronic obstructive pulmonary disease (COPD), heart failure and chronic renal failure
Immunocompromised – due to drugs or disease
Cellulitis
Urinary tract infections
Meningitis
Abdominal surgery
Infection with an antibiotic-resistant organism.

Reflection point

Consider the patients within your clinical area. How many have two or more sepsis risk factors?

The pathogenesis of septic shock

Septic shock is defined as severe sepsis together with cardiovascular dysfunction, and is characterised by hypotension which does not respond to fluid resuscitation (Vincent 2002; Dellenger et al., 2004). It is commonly seen as a complication of septicaemia caused by Gram-negative endotoxins (or Gram-positive toxins such as staphylococcal enterotoxins), which initiate a cascade of events, leading to hypotension and disseminated intravascular coagulation (DIC), which may be irreversible.

Toxin release

The release of toxins trigger the release of inflammatory mediators into the bloodstream, such as histamine, serotonin, noradrenalin and plasmakinins, along with tumour necrosis factor (TNF) and interleukin 1 (IL1), which are released from macrophages. These inflammatory mediators cause the blood vessels to dilate. TNF and IL1 also cause disturbances in temperature regulation, giving rise to signs of fever.

Activation of the complement system

The macrophages activate the complement system and release other inflammatory cytokines, which have an effect on vascular endothelial cell function and integrity. As the blood capillaries become more permeable and fluid leaks out of the general circulation, the blood pressure falls due to the drop in circulating volume, and the patient becomes hypovolaemic. The coagulation pathway becomes activated, triggering clotting abnormalities, and DIC may develop. As a result of blood-clotting abnormalities, purpuric lesions may develop and manifest as areas of petechiae on the skin, as seen in meningococcal septicaemia. Small blood clots develop in the blood vessels, which result in poor tissue and organ perfusion, and can affect digits or an entire limb. The affected limb will initially appear ice cold, white and bloodless and will eventually become blackened and necrosed as arterial and venous occlusion progresses.

Systemic effects

Multi-organ dysfunction swiftly develops. An increasing respiratory rate heralds the onset of impending respiratory failure; impaired cerebral confusion and metabolism attributed to hypotension, hypoxia and acidosis lead to decreased neurological function and may result in coma; and reduced renal perfusion will contribute to renal failure.

The management of sepsis and septic shock

In 2002 the Surviving Sepsis Campaign, an international campaign with the aim of improving the early identification and management of patients with sepsis and reducing mortality, was launched, incorporating a series of evidence-based outcomes and care bundles (www.survivingsepsis.org). Aggressive treatment influences survival and the severity of the illness (Ahrens and Tuggle, 2004; Dellenger *et al.*, 2004), and should begin immediately after sepsis is recognised. Box 9.2 lists the sepsis six – six tasks which can be initiated and undertaken by any team of healthcare professionals (e.g. nursing and medical staff on a general ward environment), and which should be delivered within **one hour** of recognition of sepsis (www.survivingsepsis.org).

Treatment begins with the establishment of vascular access and aggressive fluid resuscitation as the first priority. Patients will require ventilatory support to reduce the respiratory workload, and are at risk of developing acute respiratory distress syndrome (ARDS) which can arise from pulmonary capillary leak, or pulmonary oedema secondary to left ventricular failure. The administration of inotropes in the form of dopamine and dobutamine are required to help restore renal perfusion and cardiac function, along with adrenaline and noradrenaline to restore blood pressure.

Box 9.3 summarises the infection control investigations that should be carried out to determine the cause of sepsis.

Box 9.2   The sepsis six

Give high-flow oxygen via a non-rebreathe bag.
Take blood cultures.
Give intravenous (IV) antibiotics.
Start IV fluid resuscitation with Hartmann's solution or equivalent.
Check haemoglobin and lactate.
Monitor accurate hourly urine output.

Box 9.3   Investigations to determine the cause of sepsis

Blood culture
Arterial blood gas
Full blood count (FBC)
Urea and electrolytes
Clotting screen
Blood culture
Full blood count
Glucose
Chest X-ray
Electrocardiogram (ECG)
Culture – urine, sputum and cerebral spinal fluid (CSF)
Swabs – wounds, peripheral IV or central venous catheter (CVC) lines, wound drainage sites and pressure sores
Remove invasive indwelling devices.
Surgical debridement or drainage of abscesses, if appropriate.

The choice of antibiotic, which may necessitate combination therapy, should be guided by the susceptible patterns of microorganisms in both the community and the hospital, should have activity against likely bacterial and fungal pathogens and should penetrate to the presumed source of sepsis (Ahrens and Tuggle, 2004; Robson and Newell, 2005). Attempts should also be made to control the source of sepsis, such as removing potentially infected invasive devices, debriding any necrotic tissue and draining any abscesses if present.

Neutropenic sepsis

The management of neutropenic sepsis, which is a recognised complication of treatment for cancer and an acute medical emergency, is a clinical priority in the United Kingdom, and evidence-based best-practice guidance for its prevention and management was published by the National Institute for Clinical Excellence (NICE) in September 2012. **Note**: This section does not cover the prevention and management of neutropenia in general but attempts to give a brief overview of the immediate actions that need to be implemented if a patient is admitted to a general hospital (outside of a specialist oncology unit or ward) with neutropenic sepsis, something that Infection Prevention and Control Specialist Nurses are commonly asked about.

As discussed in Chapter 8, neutrophils (white blood cells) are the 'professional killers' of the innate immune response, whose role is to flood infected tissues within 24–48 hours of infection and attach to microorganisms in order to destroy them.

Fact Box 9.2   Chemotherapy

The administration of highly cytotoxic chemotherapy agents not only causes irreparable damage to the DNA of neoplastic (malignant) stem cells (undifferentiated cells that have the ability to continuously divide and differentiate into other kinds of cells or tissue) but also damages and suppresses the production of other living cells. These include neutrophils, cells lining the mucosa of the mouth and gastro-intestinal tract, and stem cell production within the bone marrow, and can give rise to anaemia, neutropenia and bone marrow suppression (Nikolousis, 2009; NICE, 2012).

When neutrophil production is suppressed and the absolute neutrophil count falls to its lowest level, which is generally 5–7 days after chemotherapy begins, it takes 2–4 weeks for the neutrophil count to recover (NICE, 2012). During this time, patients are extremely susceptible to overwhelming and invasive opportunistic infections, which generally arise from their own resident body flora although they are obviously also at risk of contracting infections from other people.

Confirming a diagnosis of neutropenic sepsis

Neutropenic sepsis should be diagnosed in patients having anticancer treatment whose neutrophil count is 0.5×10^9 per litre or lower **and** who have either a temperature higher than 38 °C **or** other signs or symptoms consistent with clinically significant sepsis (NICE, 2012). The microorganisms commonly implicated in neutropenic sepsis are listed in Box 9.4. The signs of early and late neutropenic sepsis are listed in Boxes 9.5 and 9.6.

Box 9.4   Microorganisms causing neutropenic sepsis

Staphylococcus epidermidis (see Chapter 20)
Staphylococcus aureus (including MRSA) (see Chapter 20)
Pseudomonas aeruginosa (see Chapter 10)
Escherichia coli (see Chapter 10)
Enterobacteriaceae (*Klebsiella*, *Enterobacter* and *Serratia species*) (see Chapter 10, and Fact Sheet 9.3 on the companion website)
Streptococcus pneumoniae
Haemophilus influenzae
Candida species (e.g. *Candida albacans*)
Aspergillus species (see Fact Sheet 9.1 on the companion website)
Cytomegalovirus (CMV) (see Fact Sheet 9.2 on the companion website)
Herpes zoster virus (see Fact Sheet 3.11 on the companion website).

Source: Bannister *et al.*, 1996: Nikolousis, 2009.

Box 9.5   Early signs of neutropenic sepsis

Feeling generally unwell, with or without a temperature
Temperature $\geq$ 38 °C and +/– hypotension or +/– tachycardia
Signs of infection
Shivering, hot and cold, and spontaneous rigor
Diarrhoea.

Note: Patients may not exhibit all of these, and at the early stage the patient will be warm and alert and not look unwell. However, they can deteriorate rapidly and death can follow within hours.

Box 9.6   Late signs of neutropenic sepsis

Cold and clammy
Restless, anxious or confused
Hypothermic or hyperthermic
Hypotensive or tachycardic.

Clinical considerations

Readers are advised to refer to their own local oncology unit or emergency department protocols and pathways for the admission and management of patients with neutropenic sepsis, but generally the following principles should apply regarding the emergency admission of patients with neutropenic sepsis within a general hospital setting:

- Haematology or oncology patients should be aware that they must contact either the chemotherapy unit where they are receiving treatment if they become ill within working hours, **or** an out-of-hours emergency advice line (**not** their GP) **without delay** if they develop signs of neutropenic sepsis.

Blood culture and antibiotics

- As a blood culture needs to be taken (see Chapter 6) **and** IV antibiotics need to be commenced **within one hour** of the patient's arrival either in the Emergency Department or on a ward ('door to needle time'), the patient must be seen **without delay** when he or she arrives at the hospital.

Admission and isolation

- If the patient requires admission and there is no Oncology bed immediately available, the patient should be admitted to an appropriate ward and **not** placed next to patients who are known to be colonised or have infections, and not admitted to a single room on an isolation or infectious diseases ward. **Admission and the commencement of antibiotics must not be delayed because of lack of single-room availability.**
- Admission to a single room is not strictly necessary, and there is limited evidence to support the implementation of 'protective isolation' precautions for neutropenic patients. If there is a room available, the patient can be admitted to it if appropriate, and admission to a single room may help to promote adherence to the application of stringent infection control precautions (Wigglesworth, 2003). However, a risk assessment of the room must be undertaken as it is critical that the patient can be easily observed and monitored, and therefore the room must not be in an isolated area on or off of the main ward.
- The patient must be managed according to the sepsis six pathway and seen by a member of the Oncology Team as soon as possible and within 48 hours of admission (NICE, 2012).

Clinical practice points: infection control precautions

- Hands must be decontaminated with alcohol hand rub directly before and after any episode of direct contact with the patient, and following any contact with the patient's equipment and environment in accordance with the 5 Moments of Hand Hygiene (See Chapter 12).
- Gloves and aprons must be changed in between each task or episode of patient care performed for the patient, and following any contact with the patient's equipment (see Chapter 13).

137

- Neutropenic patients must have their own dedicated patient equipment (e.g. dynamap, blood pressure cuff, tourniquet and commode).
- As previously stated, neutropenic patients must **not** be placed in beds next to patients who are known to be colonised or infected or who have open wounds (including leg ulcers). Additionally, they **must not** be exposed to staff or visitors who may have infections (e.g. coughs, colds or cold sores).

Chapter summary: key points

- Sepsis is the leading cause of death in intensive care units.

- Eighteen million people worldwide die from sepsis each year.

- Septic shock, a complication caused by bacterial toxins, is characterised by hypotension which does not respond to fluid resuscitation.

- The early identification of sepsis and implementation of aggressive treatment are keys to patient survival.

- Neutropenic sepsis is a recognised complication of treatment for cancer and is an acute medical emergency; its management is a clinical priority in the United Kingdom.

- Following chemotherapy or radiotherapy, patients are susceptible to overwhelming opportunistic infections which may be acquired endogenously.

- In patients admitted with neutropenic sepsis, 'door to needle time' is of paramount importance (blood culture to be taken and IV antibiotics to be commenced within one hour of admission).

- Neutropenic patients admitted to a general surgical or medical ward do not necessarily have to be admitted to a single room but must not be exposed to colonised or infected patients or to staff or visitors who may have infections.

Further resources are available for this book, including interactive multiple choice questions. Visit the companion website at:

www.wiley.com/go/fundamentalsofinfectionprevention

References

Ahrens T., Tuggle D. (2004). Surviving sepsis: early recognition and treatment. *Critical Care Nurse*. 24 (5) (Suppl.): 2–13.

Bannister B.A, Begg N.T., Gillespie S.H. (1996). Infections in immunocompromised patients. In: Bannister B.A, Begg N.T., Gillespie S. (Eds.), *Infectious Diseases*. Blackwell Science, Oxford: 403–413.

Bone R.C., Balk R.A., Cerra F.B. (1992). American College of Chest Physicians/Society of Critical Care Medical Consensus Conference. Definitions for sepsis and organ failure and guidelines for the use of innovative therapies in sepsis. *Chest*. 101 (6): 1644–1655.

Daniels R. (2011). Surviving the first hours in sepsis: getting the basics right (an intensivist's approach). *Journal of Antimicrobial Chemotherapy*. 66 (2): 11–23.

Dellenger R.P., Carlet J.M., Masur H., Gerlach H., Calandra T., *et al*. (2004). Surviving Sepsis Campaign guidelines for management of severe sepsis and septic shock. *Critical Care Medicine*. 34 (3): 858–873.

National Institute for Clinical Excellence (NICE) (2012). *Draft Clinical Guideline. Neutropenic Sepsis: Prevention and Management of Neutropenic Sepsis in Cancer Patients*. February. NICE, London.

Nikolousis M. (2009). Special cases: the immunocompromised patient. In: Daniels R. (Ed.), *ABC of Sepsis*. Wiley-Blackwell, Chichester: 62–67.

Robson W., Newell J. (2005). Assessing, treating and managing patients with sepsis. *Nursing Standard*. 19 (50): 56–64.

Slade E., Tamber P.S., Vincent J.L. (2003). The Surviving Sepsis Campaign: raising awareness to reduce mortality. *Critical Care*. 7 (1): 1–2.

Vincent J.L. (2002). Sepsis definition. *Lancet Infectious Diseases*. 2: 135.

Wheeler D.S. (2009). Death to sepsis: targeting apoptosis pathways in sepsis. *Critical Care*. 13: 1000.

Wigglesworth N. (2003). The use of protective isolation. *Nursing Times*. 99 (7): 26.

10

Antibiotics and the problem of resistance

Contents

Introduction

Very few new antimicrobial agents have been developed since the late 1980s and early 1990s, and with the continued rise of multidrug resistance, particularly amongst Gram-negative bacteria, antimicrobial resistance has been acknowledged to be a major public health threat and a global concern since the late 1990s (Department of Health [DH], 2002). Key documents published in the United Kingdom over the last decade by the House of Lords Select Committee on Science and Technology (1998) and the DH (1998) have emphasised the need for the ongoing monitoring and surveillance of antimicrobial resistance, and identified the prudent use of antibiotics as an area requiring intensified control measures. In 2013, the Chief Medical Officer (CMO), principal medical advisor to the UK government, announced that antimicrobial resistance should be placed on the National Security Risk Register, and carry the same level of 'political interest' as MRSA and *C. difficile*.

This chapter is in two parts. **Part A** describes the history of antibiotics and the development of resistance. It goes on to explain how antibiotics work, the problems of antibiotic resistance and the importance of antimicrobial stewardship. **Part B** looks at the problems associated with resistant Gram-negative rods, and the major public health threat posed by carbapenem resistance.

Note: Extensive information on national and global campaigns regarding antibiotic-prescribing policy and antibiotic resistance, including bulletins, reports and guidelines, can be found on the following websites: hpa.org.uk, www.dh.gov, www.cdc.gov, www.who.int, scot.nhs.uk, and www.wales.nhs.uk.

Learning outcomes

After reading this chapter, the reader will be able to:

- Understand the principles of antibiotic therapy.

- Understand why antimicrobial resistance has occurred and how microorganisms become resistant.

- Understand what is meant by 'antimicrobial stewardship'.

- Understand the significance of ESBL and carbapenem resistance, and the infection control management of resistant organisms.

Part A

The discovery of penicillin

The term antibiotic was originally applied to naturally occurring compounds such as penicillin, which attacked bacteria without harming the host. The initial discovery of penicillin was made in 1896 by Ernest Duchesne, a French medical student, and then re-discovered in 1928 by the scientist Alexander Fleming when he noticed that a fungal mould (*Penicillin notatum*), which was growing as a probable contaminant on an agar plate containing *Staphylococcus aureus*, was causing the bacteria to lyse (Willey *et al.*, 2011). Fleming named the substance produced by this mould 'penicillin' but was subsequently unable to demonstrate its effectiveness in practice (Ryan and Drew, 2010a).

Penicillin re-discovered

The first group of broad-spectrum antibacterial agents to be developed were the sulphonamides in 1935, and although they were initially effective and their discovery and introduction marked the beginning of the effective treatment of bacterial infections with antibacterial agents, their usefulness was relatively short-lived and sulphonamide resistance amongst many strains of bacteria soon became common. Then, work undertaken with Fleming's original culture during 1939–1940 by Howard Florey, Ernest Chain and Norman Heatley (which subsequently earned Fleming, Florey and Chain the Nobel Prize in 1945) led to the discovery and production of penicillin (Willey *et al.*, 2011). Its mass production during the 1940s saw it hailed as the 'wonder drug'. It was seen as a 'magic bullet' because of its ability to destroy bacteria without harming the host, and it was perceived that it would completely revolutionise the treatment of infections and infectious diseases. However, the euphoria was short-lived.

The emergence of resistance

Bacteria swiftly gained the upper hand when they started to produce enzymes (penicillinase, or beta-lactamase) that were able to break open the beta-lactam ring, a structural component of penicillin and later cephalosporin. By 1950, penicillinase-producing resistant strains of *S. aureus* began to emerge as a major cause of serious infection in hospital patients (see Chapter 20), and fewer than one-third of all isolates were susceptible to penicillin (Ryan and Drew, 2010a).

The rise of resistant Gram-negative bacteria

During the 1960s and into the 1970s, particularly in response to the emergence of aerobic Gram-negative bacilli as important healthcare pathogens, modified penicillins such as ampicillin and carbenicillin, along with aminoglycosides, glycopeptides, tetracyclines, quinolones and macrolides, were developed, but resistance emerged and the 1970s and 1980s saw significant problems with multidrug-resistant Gram-negative bacteria (French and Phillips, 1997).

Resistance in Gram-positive bacteria

The last 20 years have seen the emergence of opportunistic Gram-positive bacteria, particularly Gram-positive cocci (staphylococci, streptococci and enterococci) that are resistant to some or all of these agents. This is possibly because the widespread use of cephalosporins, aminoglycosides and quinolones for Gram-negative infections has selected Gram-positive species that are inherently resistant to these antibiotics, along with their capacity for acquiring antibiotic-resistant determinants (Gold and Moellering, 1996).

Resistance: a global problem

The Health Protection Agency (HPA, now Public Health England), the World Health Organization (WHO) and the Centers for Disease Control and Prevention (CDC) have all been spearheading the global crusade to halt the global spread of antimicrobial resistance for fear of a return to the pre-antibiotic era of the 1930s and 1940s and a potential 'doomsday' scenario of a world without antibiotics (see www.hpa.org.uk, www.who.int and www.cdc.gov). The emergence and discovery of New Delhi motello (NDM-1), the novel enzyme that confers resistance to the latest antimicrobial agents to be developed, the carbapenems (amikacin, ertapenem, meropenem and doripenem), mean that the feared 'post-antibiotic era' may be fast approaching. Resistance to antiviral agents has also developed markedly, with serious implications for the treatment of patients with HIV or hepatitis B, vulnerable patients at risk from opportunistic infections and influenza (Hayden, 2006; Regoes and Bonhoefter, 2006; WHO, 2008; Ghany and Doo 2009, Hurt *et al.*, 2011). Resistance is also now seen among fungi and protozoa (Bloland, 2001; Hudson, 2001; Sanglard and Odds, 2002).

How antibiotics work

Antibiotics are classified according to their spectrum of activity and mode of action.

Spectrum of activity

This may be narrow or broad. Antibiotics with a **narrow spectrum** have restricted activity and are effective only against certain organisms (i.e. Gram-positives), whereas **broad-spectrum** agents are effective against a wide range of pathogens. Broad-spectrum agents are commonly chosen either where confirmation of the causative organism is unknown (i.e. before laboratory confirmation is received) and/or where the cause of infection may be poly-microbial (more than one organism is implicated). The major disadvantage of using these agents is that they can deplete resident body flora, such as the organisms that reside in the gastro-intestinal tract, leaving a gap in host defences for dominant pathogens (i.e. *Clostridium difficile*) to proliferate.

Mode of action

Antibiotics are generally highly effective at treating infections caused by bacteria because of their selective toxicity. This means that they are able to kill bacteria (**bactericidal**) or prevent their growth and replication (**bacteriostatic**) without actually harming the host (Strohl *et al.*, 2001). The choice of the appropriate antibiotic is multi-factorial and is dependent upon:

- The organism (or likely organism)
- The site of infection (not all antibiotics are able to penetrate bone, joints or cerebral spinal fluid)
- Likely antibiotic susceptibilities
- The severity of the infection
- Whether or not the patient has a past medical history of allergy to any antibiotics (penicillin allergy being the most common).

Interference with bacterial cell wall synthesis

Groups of antibiotics that interfere with bacterial cell wall synthesis, either by preventing the cell wall from forming, or by weakening it so that osmotic pressure exerted outside the cell causes it to swell and burst, include the beta-lactam antibiotics such as the penicillins and the cephalosporins (Strohl *et al.*, 2001). Penicillin, for example, targets the bacterial enzyme transpeptidase, which is necessary for the cross-linking of the peptide–sugar chains which build the peptidoglycan wall.

Disruption of the cell membrane

Polymixins, such as colistin, disrupt the bacterial cell membrane, which causes the cell to break open (Ryan and Drew, 2004).

Inhibition of protein synthesis

Aminoglycosides inhibit protein synthesis in aerobic bacteria (Strohl *et al.*, 2001).

Inhibition of nucleic acid synthesis

Quinolones are among groups of antibiotics that act directly or indirectly on DNA or RNA synthesis, either preventing DNA from being transcribed into RNA, or disrupting the coiling and uncoiling of DNA (Greenwood and Ogilvie, 2003).

Routes of administration

Antibiotics can be administered topically, orally, rectally and by intramuscular (IM) and intravenous (IV) injection.

IM and IV

The IM and IV route is commonly used to treat infections where it is particularly important to ensure that adequate concentrations of the antibiotic have been achieved, or in situations where the oral route cannot be tolerated. In these instances, the concentration of the antibiotic in the bloodstream has to be monitored to ensure that the correct therapeutic dose is being achieved and to detect toxicity. For example, when IV vancomycin is prescribed, blood is taken pre-dose and 1–2 hours post dose every three days, and the dose adjusted where appropriate (either increased or decreased) to ensure that it is within the therapeutic range.

Combination therapy

Antibiotics can also be prescribed in combination, as certain antibiotics have a synergistic effect and work together, with one antibiotic enhancing the effectiveness of the other. Combination therapy can be used in the initial treatment of potentially life-threatening infections before microbiology results are available, if the causative organism cannot be isolated or if the infection is poly-microbial. Combination therapy can also help combat or delay the emergence of antibiotic resistance.

Side effects

All antibiotics have side effects, the most common being gastro-intestinal disturbances following disruption of the normal bowel flora (see Chapter 22 on *C. difficile*). Other side effects include skin rashes, ranging from mild urticaria to Stevens–Johnson syndrome and renal and hepatic toxicity. The most serious allergic reaction is anaphylaxis (see Chapter 8).

144

Antimicrobial resistance

Resistance is acknowledged to be a complex phenomenon, involving the organism, the antimicrobial drug, the environment and the patient, both separately and in their interaction (Cohen and Tartsky, 1997).

Fact Box 10.1   Definition of resistance

An organism can be classed as resistant if it is not inhibited or killed by one or more classes of antibiotic at concentrations achievable after normal dosage. From a microbiology laboratory perspective, this essentially means that a sensitive organism is one that is likely to respond to therapy with the antimicrobial agent tested, and a resistant isolate is one that will not. Resistance gives organisms a distinct competitive advantage, and can be inherent or acquired.

Inherent or acquired resistance

Inherent, or natural resistance, is part of the organism's genetic make-up, and it is encoded on the bacterial chromosome, meaning that the organism is naturally not susceptible to a certain antibiotic. Resistance that is **acquired**, however, is the most worrying, with spontaneous genetic mutations and/or genetic recombinations leading to the emergence of an antibiotic-resistant organism.

Plasmids and transposons

Organisms can acquire resistance through the transfer of genetic material from one organism to another by plasmids or transposons. **Plasmids** are self-replicating circular pieces of DNA which exist outside of the chromosome. They may be transmissible between bacterial species, meaning that other bacteria can readily acquire virulence genes, including those that code for antibiotic resistance (including multidrug resistance) (Nye, 2010), and once it is in possession of a resistance plasmid (R plasmid), either the plasmid or the genes within it can be transferred to other bacteria (Willey *et al.*, 2011).

Fact Box 10.2   Resistance genes and plasmids (staphylococci and enterococci)

The meticillin-resistant *Staphylococcus aureus* (MRSA) resistance gene is known as *mecA* (Que and Moreillon, 2009). In 1992, it was first discovered that the gene that codes for vancomycin resistance, *vanA*, could be transferred from enterococci to MRSA by a plasmid (Moellering, 1992). In 1996, the first strain of *S. aureus* with reduced susceptibility to vancomycin and teicoplanin was isolated in Japan (Hiramatsu *et al.*, 1997) and subsequently in the United States, France, Korea, Africa and Brazil (Hiramatsu, 2001).

Transposons are mobile DNA segments found in Gram-positive and Gram-negative bacteria that often carry genes for resistance and virulence which migrate between unrelated plasmids and/ or the bacterial chromosome (Towner, 2003; Willey et al., 2011). The transfer of plasmids or transposons is acquired through conjugation, transduction or transformation.

Conjugation

Conjugation is the major mechanism for the transfer of antibiotic resistance, and the exchange of genetic material can occur between unrelated species of bacteria (Gladwin and Trattler, 2003). It is the process by which DNA is transferred from a donor cell to a recipient cell, requiring direct cell-to-cell contact (Willey et al., 2011). One cell has to possess a self-transmissible plasmid (F plasmid) which contains a specialised structure known as the sex pilus, which attaches to the recipient cell and penetrates the cell membrane, allowing the transfer of DNA from one cell to another (Neidhardt, 2004).

Transduction and transformation

Transduction involves the transfer of DNA between cells by bacteriophages, viruses which infect bacteria, carrying DNA from one bacterium to another (Ryan and Drew, 2010b). Some bacteria are able to take up DNA from another organism that has been released by lysis of the cell, incorporating it into their own chromosome through recombination. This process is known as transformation, and can occur between closely related species of bacteria (Towner, 2003).

Other mechanisms of resistance

Some bacterial species may produce an enzyme capable of destroying the antibiotic, as seen with S. aureus and penicillin. The bacterial cell wall may be naturally impermeable to certain antibiotics, or the bacteria may acquire an inner membrane protein which acts as an efflux pump and pumps the antibiotic out of the cell (Lee and Lomovskaya, 1998). Bacteria can also alter the target site of the antibiotic; the antibiotic can enter the cell but is unable to inhibit the activity of the cell because of structural changes within it that prevent the antibiotic from binding and attaching to it (Ryan and Drew, 2004). They can also develop an alternative metabolic pathway, so that the antibiotic bypasses the site at which it would normally be effective.

Factors leading to the emergence of resistance and problems within the healthcare setting

Survival of the fittest, or selection

Resistance often occurs among normal bacterial flora in patients receiving antibiotics. If a further infection requiring treatment subsequently develops, that bacterial population is more likely to become resistant than in patients who have not received treatment. Darwin's theory of the 'survival of the fittest' favours selection systems (Turnidge and Christiansen, 2005). Within the microbial population there is variation amongst microorganisms, and selection occurs which favours those organisms with traits that are most advantageous in the prevailing environment.

Fact Box 10.3   Selection pressure

Antibiotics 'select' for resistance by targeting susceptible or antibiotic-sensitive organisms, 'allowing' the resistant ones to survive, so if there is a resistant mutant present, it has a competitive advantage over other bacteria, with natural selection always ensuring that dominant organisms survive. If antibiotic selection pressure is removed (i.e. by temporarily or permanently restricting the use of the antibiotic within a population), mobile resistance genes carried by 'promiscuous' plasmids may be lost, and the 'host' bacterium may revert to being sensitive.

The use of antibiotics in animals

The driving force behind the whole 'resistance problem' has been the widespread use of antibacterial drugs, and the misuse and overuse of antibiotics worldwide in the treatment of humans and animals. Antimicrobial agents are used to treat infections in animals, accounting for in excess of 50% of total antibiotic use (WHO, 2011), but in those animals bred for human consumption they are often administered prophylactically to protect whole herds from disease, and also for growth promotion (Department of Health Standing Medical Advisory Committee Sub-Group on Antimicrobial Resistance, 1998; DH, 2002). They are administered continuously at sub-therapeutic levels, often in feed, and the agents used are either the same, or belong to the same classes, as those used for the treatment of infections in humans (WHO, 2011).

Fact Box 10.4   Transfer of resistant bacteria from animals to humans

Either resistant bacteria are transferred to humans via the food chain (as in the case of glyco-peptide-resistant enterococci [GRE]), or resistant pathogens in animals transfer resistance genes to human pathogens (Witte, 2000).

Antibiotic prescribing in the healthcare setting

Within the United Kingdom, 80% of antibiotics are prescribed in the community, predominantly for the treatment of upper respiratory and urinary tract infections (Department of Health Standing Medical Advisory Committee Sub-Group on Antimicrobial Resistance, 1998). Historically, there has been huge pressure on general practitioners to prescribe antibiotics for the treatment of minor coughs and colds and other illness because of the level of patient expectation and demand for treatment. This has led to the prescription and administration of antibiotics in situations where their use is not justified and the emergence of resistant organisms within the community, partly through poor prescribing, with the dose prescribed at sub-therapeutic levels, and partly due to poor patient compliance. Lack of regulation regarding the sale of over-the-counter antibiotics and antibiotic prescribing generally in developing countries has exacerbated the problem of resistance.

Box 10.1 lists some of the factors in relation to prescribing which have exacerbated the development of resistance.

Pressures on healthcare systems for greater efficiency, with greater bed occupancy rates and stretched nursing and medical care, along with heavy antimicrobial use, increase the risk of infection to patients (Wise *et al.*, 1998). Resistant strains can spread amongst patients, with selection of resistance in infected or colonised patients enhanced by various patient factors. These include immunosuppression, the use of indwelling invasive devices, alteration of the patient's own flora during antibiotic therapy, the length of hospital stay, the intensity and duration of exposure to broad-spectrum antibiotics, severity of the illness and other associated co-morbidities, and contact via the contaminated hands of healthcare staff. The hospital environment can harbour resistant organisms, and healthcare staff need to work together to reduce environmental reservoirs (DH, 2002). Box 10.2 lists some of the factors that have exacerbated the spread of resistant microorganisms.

Box 10.1   Prescribing factors which have exacerbated the development of resistance

- Treatment of conditions where antibiotics are not indicated (e.g. coughs or colds due to viral infections)
- Prophylactic administration where there is no proven value, or duration of prophylaxis is too long
- Inadequate dose or duration
- Monotherapy, when treatment with combination antibiotic therapy would be clinically indicated
- Poor patient compliance – course of antibiotics not completed (e.g. because of lack of understanding, side effects or the patient starts to feel better and so doesn't complete the course).

Antimicrobial stewardship

It is a requirement of the Health and Social Care Act 2008, *Code of Practice on the Prevention of Infections and Related Guidance* (DH, 2010), that 'procedures should be in place to ensure prudent prescribing and antimicrobial stewardship' (Criterion 9). According to Carlet *et al.* (2012), antimicrobial stewardship requires a multi-faceted, multi-disciplinary approach to antimicrobial prescribing that takes into account 'optimal selection, dosage and duration of treatment, resulting in the best clinical outcome of the treatment or prevention of cross infection, with minimal toxicity to the patient and minimal impact on subsequent resistance'. It is central to the control of antimicrobial resistance and the effective treatment of infections, and it is the responsibility of medical, pharmacy and nursing staff. The Department of Health Advisory Committee on Antimicrobial Resistance and Healthcare-associated Infections published national evidence-based best-practice guidance on antimicrobial stewardship in 2011, and the principles are summarised in Box 10.3.

Box 10.2   Factors exacerbating the spread of resistant organisms

- Travel to other countries with higher rates of resistant organisms (resistant organisms can be 'imported')
- Indiscriminate use and prescribing, and over-the-counter availability of antibiotics where there are insufficient control measures
- Overcrowding in hospitals, high bed occupancy rates and mixing of patient populations – increased opportunities for cross-infection
- Poor infection control practice (e.g. poor hand hygiene compliance, inappropriate use and disposal of personal protective equipment [PPE], failure to decontaminate equipment appropriately and poor standards of environmental cleanliness).

149

Box 10.3   The principles of antimicrobial stewardship

- Right drug, right dose, right time, right duration and right patient.
- Antibiotics must not be prescribed in the absence of clinical signs of infection.
- If infection is suspected or there is evidence of infection, antibiotics must be prescribed in accordance with local prescribing guidelines.
- Obtain appropriate cultures (e.g. blood, wound swabs and other clinical specimens) before prescribing, but do not delay commencing treatment in the event of potentially life-threatening illness or infection.
- Single-dose antibiotics should be prescribed for surgical prophylaxis where the use of antibiotics has been shown to be effective.
- The indication for prescribing, duration, route, dose and review date must be recorded on the prescription chart.
- The clinical diagnosis and continuing need for antibiotics must be reviewed within 48 hours, and a clear plan of action recorded in the notes (e.g. stop, switch IV to oral therapy, change, continue or Outpatient Parenteral Antibiotic Therapy).

Source: Department of Health Advisory Committee on Antimicrobial Resistance and Healthcare Associated Infections (ARHAI) (2011).

Reflection point

Look at the antibiotic prescription charts of patients within your clinical area. How many of the principles of antibiotic stewardship can you see evidence of? Do the prescriptions comply with the Antimicrobial Guidelines or Prescribing Policy?

In 2012, the HPA published the preliminary results of the first ever national point prevalence survey of antimicrobial use in England, which had been undertaken as part of a national point prevalence survey on healthcare-associated infections (HCAIs). The key findings are summarised in Box 10.4.

Box 10.4   Key findings regarding antimicrobial prescribing

- The prevalence of antimicrobial prescribing was 34.7% in the NHS and 46.7% in the independent sector. These figures will be used as a baseline for future surveys.
- 25 942 antimicrobial agents were prescribed for 18 219 patients.
- Antimicrobial prescribing was highest in Intensive Care Units (60.8%).
- 53% of antibiotics were prescribed for the treatment of community-acquired infections.
- The majority of the antibiotics prescribed were for the treatment of respiratory tract. infections (30.9%) and skin, soft tissue, bone and joint infections (19%).
- 85% of patients surveyed had the indication for prescribing recorded.

Source: Data from HPA, 2012.

Part B

Specific antibiotic-resistant organisms

Extended-spectrum beta-lactamases (ESBLs)

As described in Part A, beta-lactamases are enzymes capable of breaking open the beta-lactam ring, part of the molecular structure of penicillins and cephalosporins. Extended-spectrum beta-lactamases (ESBLs) are classes of beta-lactamase that render bacteria multidrug resistant, to cephalosporins and penicillins predominantly but also to other antibiotics. They were first reported over 30 years ago but have risen to prominence over the last decade. ESBLs are 'expressed' by Gram-negative bacteria (see Chapter 5), mainly those belonging to the genus of bacteria known as *Enterobacteriaeceae*, in particular *Escherichia coli* and *Klebsiella pneumoniae*, as well as *Pseudomonas aeruginosa* and *Acinetobacter bumanii* (Dhillon and Clark, 2012). The use of cephalosporins in animal food production has been linked to the emergence of ESBLs associated with cattle, poultry and pigs (DH, 2012).

Fact Box 10.5   Enterobacteriaeceae

Enterobacteriaeceae exist as part of the normal bowel flora (coliforms), and they harmlessly colonise the colon and/or the environment. They may be present in the bowel in large numbers, posing a risk to patients undergoing procedures in hospital. They can be transferred to other sites on patients by their own hands or to other patients via the hands of healthcare workers and through contact with contaminated equipment.

Box 10.5 lists some of the risk factors for ESBL acquisition (colonisation and infection).

Box 10.5   Risk factors for ESBL colonisation and infection

Previous treatment with antibiotics
Presence of an invasive indwelling device or open wound
Neonatal Intensive Care Unit or Special Care Baby Unit admission
Intensive Care Unit admission

Klebsiella spp.

Klebsiella are opportunistic pathogens implicated in many healthcare-associated infections, with K. pneumoniae a common cause of pneumonia, urinary tract infections, wound infections, blood-stream infections, biliary tract infections and peritonitis (Donnenberg, 2009). Infection is preceded by colonisation (it can be carried by 10% of the 'healthy' population as part of the respiratory flora but may cause pneumonia if host immune defences are impaired) (Levinson, 2010) and is associated with length of stay, the severity of the patient's illness and the manipulation of any invasive indwelling devices (Lucet et al., 1996). Widespread environmental contamination can occur. It is one of the commonest organisms to carry plasmids encoded for multidrug resistance (Donnenberg, 2009).

Fact Box 10.6   Klebsiella outbreak

One documented outbreak of K. pneumoniae involved nearly 300 patients over a period of three and a half years (Hobson et al., 1996).

E. coli

E. coli is a common cause of community and healthcare-associated urinary tract infections (see Chapter 17) and Gram-negative sepsis, and in neonates it can cause meningitis and septicaemia, acquired from the mother during birth (Levinson, 2010).

Fact Box 10.7   E. coli 0157

Verocytotoxin-producing E. coli 0157 (VTEC) is a pathogenic strain of E. coli acquired through consumption of food or water contaminated with faeces from infected animals, by contact with animals that carry VTEC or by exposure to contaminated environments such as farms. Cases and outbreaks in children have been associated with 'petting farms', and guidance on the prevention of VTEC is available on the HPA website at http://www.hpa.org.uk/Infectious-Diseases/InfectionsAZ/Escherichiacoli0157.

Acinetobacter

Acinetobacter are encapsulated, non-motile, aerobic, Gram-negative coccobacilli, of which there are at least 21 strains (Allen and Hartman, 2009).

Fact Box 10.8   Laboratory identification of *Acinetobacter*

Their ability to retain crystal violet dye on Gram-staining may lead to them inadvertently being identified as Gram-positive cocci (Allen and Hartman, 2009), and on culture they can be confused with *Neisseria* (Ryan and Drew, 2010c).

As well as colonising the bowel and skin of humans and animals, they are also widespread within the environment, occurring naturally within drinking and surface waters, soils and sewage. Compared to many other organisms, they lack the virulence factors that would class them as major pathogens, but they can cause opportunistic infections, particularly in patients who are immunocompromised, and they can affect any body site.

They have been isolated from traumatic wounds of combat soldiers in Iraq and Afghanistan (Peleg *et al.*, 2008) where they have caused serious infections. However, isolation of *Acinetobacter* in a clinical specimen is not always of clinical significance; the patient's general condition and the antibiotic susceptibilities of the organism need to be taken into account in order to determine whether or not the patient is colonised or infected.

A. bumannii is the most commonly reported species of *Acinetobacter*, accounting for approximately 80% of reported infections such as pneumonia, bacteraemia, wound infections and urinary tract infections. These infections tend to occur in already ill hospitalised patients, and they can be spread by direct or indirect contact, contaminated equipment and environmental exposure. They can be multi-antibiotic resistant, which is defined as resistant to any aminoglycoside, such as gentamicin, as well as resistant to any third-generation cephalosporin, such as cefuroxime and cefotaxime. Some isolates are now also resistant to the carbapenems such as imipenem and meropenem, and these are designated as MRAB-C, a clone which is established within hospitals in London and the southeast of England.

Guidelines on the control and management of multidrug-resistant *Acinetobacter* which incorporate recommendations on isolation, antibiotic prescribing, environmental cleanliness and decontamination were published in 2005 and updated in 2006 and 2008 (HPA, 2008).

Pseudomonas

Pseudomonas is both a coloniser, causing a variety of opportunistic infections, and a contaminant, and is environmentally extremely resilient (Ryan and Drew, 2010c). There are over 100 species, of which *P. aeruginosa* is one of the prolific species associated with healthcare infections. It is a common cause of sepsis, pneumonia (including chronic lower respiratory tract infections in patients with cystic fibrosis), wound infections and urinary tract infections. It produces two pigments, a blue pigment (pyocyanin) and a yellow pigment (fluorescin). Combined, these produce a blue-green pigment that is sometimes seen as exudate on wound dressings.

Fact Box 10.9   Contamination by *Pseudomonas*

P. aeruginosa can contaminate water systems, posing a risk in healthcare facilities, in particular to vulnerable and potentially immunocompromised patients in adult and paediatric intensive care units and burns units (augmented care). In 2012, the DH issued national guidance in *Water Sources and Potential Pseudomonas aeruginosa Contamination of Taps and Water Systems. Advice for Augmented Care.*

Box 10.6 summarises DH best-practice advice relating to the use of hand wash stations.

Box 10.6   Best-practice advice for the use of hand wash stations

Only use the hand wash station for handwashing.
Do not dispose of body fluids at the wash hand basin – use the dirty utility area.
Do not wash any patient equipment in wash hand basins.
Do not use wash hand basins for storing used equipment awaiting decontamination.
Taps should be cleaned before the rest of the hand basin.
Wash patients, including neonates, on augmented care units with water from outlets demonstrated by risk assessments (and, if necessary, by water sampling) as safe.
Do not dispose of used environmental cleaning fluids at wash hand basins.

Carbapenem resistance

In January 2009, a National Resistance Alert was published by the Antibiotic Resistance Monitoring and Reference Laboratory (ARMRL) and the Health Protection Agency (HPA, 2009) concerning the growing problem with the emergence of carbapenemase-producing *Enterobacteriaceae*. Carbapenemase is an enzyme that confers resistance to one of the newest, and most medically important, classes of antibiotics known as carbapenems (imipenem, meropenem, ertapenem and doripenem), which are used to treat serious infections, particularly those due to multidrug-resistant Gram-negative bacteria and including those with ESBL resistance.

The emergence of a novel enzyme conferring carbapenem resistance, NDM-1 (New Delhi Metallo Beta-Lactamase), was first reported in 2008, isolated from a patient repatriated to Sweden from New Delhi, India, with a strain of *K. pneumoniae* (Yong *et al.*, 2009). Muir and Weinbren (2010) later reported a case of NDM-1 in Coventry, United Kingdom, in a patient of Indian origin with an *E. coli* infection who had dialysis in India 18 months previously.

The highly transmissible NDM-1 gene is carried on a 'promiscuous' plasmid by *K. pneumoniae*, *E. coli*, *Citrobacter*, *Enterobacter cloace* and *Morganella morganii* (Kumarasamy *et al.*, 2010), and its evolution is very much considered to have been a random event, with unregulated antibiotic use possibly selecting it and facilitating its spread. NDM-1 producing organisms are generally sensitive to only colistin and tigecycline, which have toxic side effects, and this therefore significantly limits treatment options. At least one in 10 NDM-1 producing strains appears to be pan-resistant (i.e. there is no known antibiotic treatment). A study by Walsh *et al.* (2011) detected

NDM-1 in drinking water and water used for food preparation and washing clothes in New Delhi, and the isolation of NDM-1 in the community and in hospitals in India suggests widespread circulation.

Fact Box 10.10   The naming of antibiotic-resistant enzymes

It is common practice to name antibiotic-resistant enzymes after the place where they were first discovered (e.g. Sao Paulo Metallo [SPM], Brazil; and Verona Imipenemase Metallo [VIM], Verona, Italy) (see http://hpa.gov.uk/Topics/InfectiousDiseases/InfectionsAZ/CarbapenemResistance/GeneralInformation). However, the Indian government strongly objected to NDM-1 being named after New Delhi on the grounds that it implied that healthcare in India was substandard and unsafe and would have a detrimental effect on tourism.

NDM-1 is becomingly increasingly dominant and has been monitored in the United Kingdom since 2008. It has become the most frequent carbapenemase in isolates referred to the ARMRL and the most widely scattered.

Fact Box 10.11   Mortality associated with carbapenem-resistant *K. pneumoniae*

A recently published Eurosurveillance Report (Sisto *et al.*, 2012) has highlighted the increasing numbers of carbapenem-resistant *K. pneumoniae* infections, predominately respiratory tract and bloodstream infections (bacteraemia), in Italian hospitals. The Report makes particular reference to an article by Borer *et al.* (2009), in which crude and attributable mortality rates of 71.9% and 50%, respectively, have been reported, and where 65% of patients with a carbapenem-resistant *K. pneumoniae* bacteraemia developed septic shock (see Chapter 9 on sepsis).

Advice on Carbapenemase Producers: Recognition, Infection Control and Treatment was published by the HPA in 2010 and contains a one-page checklist of actions for Trusts to implement in order to minimise the risk of carbapenemase spread. In the United States, the Centers for Disease Control and Prevention (CDC) has published an extensive Tool Kit for the management of these organisms (CDC, 2012). As yet, no further guidance has been issued in England by the HPA or the DH. Risk factors for carbapenemase-producing coliforms are listed in Box 10.7.

Box 10.7   Risk factors for colonisation or infection with carbapenemase-producing coliform

- Travel to or residence in the Indian sub-continent (India and Pakistan)
- Medical treatment or healthcare exposure in India or Pakistan
- Treatment within a hospital (in the United Kingdom or abroad) where there have been cases or clusters

Clinical practice points: the infection control management of patients colonised or infected with an ESBL or carbapenem-resistant organism

Stringent adherence to infection control precautions is critical in the prevention of spread of antibiotic-resistant organisms to other patients, and in the case of carbapenem-resistant organisms in particular, it is essential that staff fully understand the implications of cross-infection. There should be an Infection Control Policy in the Infection Control Manual within all healthcare organisations regarding the management of patients with ESBL or carbapenem-resistant organisms.

Isolation: Patients must be isolated in a single room (preferably en-suite where applicable). The decision to discontinue isolation of the patient should be made by a member of the Infection Prevention and Control Team following a clinical risk assessment, and documented in the medical notes. It may be appropriate in some areas to cohort colonised or infected patients with the same ESBL-resistant organism, such as neonates on an Neonatal Intensive Care Unit or Special Care Baby Unit. (See also Chapter 11.) **Note**: Patients either infected or colonised with a carbapenem-resistant organism must be isolated in a single room for the **duration of their hospital stay, with strict adherence to standard precautions and 1:1 nursing** (this will have resource implications in terms of staffing).

Hand hygiene: In the event of carbapenem resistance, the HPA (2010) recommend that staff wash their hands with liquid soap and water, rather than decontaminate them with alcohol hand rub, after contact with the patient, with equipment and/or with the patient's environment. Otherwise, the use of alcohol hand rub or gel is generally acceptable when caring for patients who have ESBL colonisation or infection as long as the patient does not have diarrhoea. (See also Chapter 12.)

Personal protective equipment (PPE): Disposable gloves or aprons must be worn for direct contact with the patient and contaminated equipment and must be changed in between each patient. Following removal of PPE, hands must be washed with liquid soap and water if the patient has a carbapenem-resistant organism. Otherwise, the use of alcohol hand rub and gel following the removal of PPE is generally acceptable when caring for patients who have ESBL colonisation or infection as long as the patient does not have diarrhoea. (See also Chapter 13.)

Equipment: Equipment (including a single-use blood pressure cuff and tourniquet) should be dedicated for use with the patient and **not** shared with other patients. Only equipment or items essential for the patient's care on a daily basis should be kept in the room.

Management of invasive devices: As discussed in Chapters 16 and 17, IV devices and urinary catheters can significantly increase the risk of patients developing a bacteraemia if they are not managed appropriately.

Environmental cleanliness: The patients' side room must be cleaned daily with a chlorine-based solution. In the event of a carbapenem-resistant organism, the frequency of cleaning on the ward should be reviewed and special attention paid to cleaning frequent 'touch' areas and equipment, such as computer keyboards, monitors, telephones and door handles. (See also Chapter 15.)

Outbreaks: One case of carbapenemase resistance on a ward (i.e. detected on admission screening from a high-risk patient) should initiate a meeting whereby infection control practice can be reviewed. Isolation of carbapenem resistance from a clinical specimen in a patient who did not meet the criteria for screening, or the detection of a second case on a ward, should trigger an urgent Outbreak Meeting (see Chapter 4) and be reported as a Serious Untoward Incident (SUI). Screening of patient contacts (stools specimens, rectal swabs, and swabs from skin breaks and other sites as requested by the Infection Prevention and Control Team) would be indicated in this situation, as would weekly screening on the ward and screening on discharge.

Chapter summary: key points

- Antimicrobial resistance has been acknowledged to be a major public health threat and a global concern since the late 1990s.

- Resistance is a complex phenomenon, involving the organism, the antimicrobial drug, the environment and the patient.

- Resistance can either be part of the organism's genetic make-up or be acquired, with spontaneous genetic mutation and/or genetic recombinations leading to the emergence of an antibiotic-resistant organism.

- Resistance often occurs among normal bacterial flora in patients receiving antibiotics.

- Within the microbial population, there is variation amongst microorganisms and natural selection always ensures that dominant organisms survive.

- Antimicrobial stewardship is central to the control of antimicrobial resistance and the effective treatment of infections, and it is the responsibility of medical, pharmacy and nursing staff.

- Carbapenemase resistance is an increasing public health threat, and at least one in 10 NDM-1 producing strains appears to be pan-resistant.

- Stringent adherence to infection control precautions is critical in the prevention of the spread of antibiotic-resistant organisms to other patients, and it is essential that staff fully understand the implications of cross-infection.

 Further resources are available for this book, including interactive multiple choice questions. Visit the companion website at:

www.wiley.com/go/fundamentalsofinfectionprevention

References

Allen D., Hartman B.J. (2009). Acinetobacter. In: Mandell G., Bennett J., Dolin R. (Eds.), *Mandell, Douglas and Bennett's Principles and Practice of Infectious Diseases*. 7th ed. Churchill Livingstone Elsevier, London. http://expertconsult.com (accessed 18 December 2012)

Bloland P.B. (2001). *Drug Resistance in Malaria*. World Health Organization, Geneva.

Borer A., Saidel-Odes L., Riesenberg K., Eskira S., Peled N. (2009). Attributable mortality rate for carbapenem resistant *Klebsiella pneumoniae* bacteraemia. *Infection Control and Hospital Epidemiology*. 30 (10): 972–976.

Carlet J., Jarlier V., Harbath S., Voss A, Gossens H. *et al*. (2012). Ready for a world without antibiotics? The Pensieres Antibiotic Resistance Call to Action. *Antimicrobial Resistance and Infection Control*. 1: 11. http://www.aricjournal.com/content/1/1/11 (accessed 18 December 2012)

Centers for Disease Control and Prevention (CDC) (2012). *Guidance for Carbapenem-resistant Enterobacteriaceae (CRE): 2012 Toolkit*. Centers for Disease Control and Prevention, Atlanta, GA.

Cohen F.L., Tartsky D. (1997). Microbial resistance to drug therapy. *American Journal Infection Control*. 25 (1): 51–64.

Department of Health (DH) (2002). *Getting Ahead of the Curve. A Strategy for Combating Infectious Diseases (Including Other Aspects of Health Protection)*. Report by the Chief Medical Officer. Department of Health, London.

Department of Health (DH) (2010). *The Health and Social Care Act 2008: Code of Practice on the Prevention of Infections and Related Guidance*. Department of Health, London.

Department of Health (DH) (2012). *ESBLs – A Threat to Human and Animal Health?* Report by the Joint Working Group of the Advisory Committee on Antimicrobial Resistance and Healthcare Associated Infection (ARHAI) and the Defra Antimicrobial Resistance Co-ordination (DARC) Group. Department of Health, London.

Department of Health (DH) 2013. Annual Report of the Chief Medical Office. Volume Two, (2011). *Infections and the rise of antimicrobial resistance*. Department of Health, London.

Department of Health Advisory Committee on Antimicrobial Resistance and Healthcare Associated Infections (ARHAI) (2011). *Antimicrobial Stewardship: 'Start Smart – Then Focus'. Guidance for Antimicrobial Stewardship in Hospitals (England)*. Department of Health, London.

Department of Health Standing Medical Advisory Committee Sub-Group on Antimicrobial Resistance (1998). *The Path of Least Resistance*. Department of Health, London.

Dhillon R.H.P., Clark J. (2012). ESBLs: a clear and present danger? *Critical Care Research and Practice*. http://www.hindawi.com/Journals/ccrp/2012/625170/ (accessed 18 December 2012)

Donnenberg M. (2009). Enterobacteriaeceae: In: Mandell G., Bennett J., Dolin R. (Eds.), *Mandell, Douglas and Bennett's Principles and Practice of Infectious Diseases*. 7th ed. Churchill Livingstone Elsevier, London. http://expertconsult.com (accessed 18 December 2012)

French G.L., Phillips I. (1997). Resistance. In: O'Grady F., Lambert H.P., Finch H.P., Greenwood D. (Eds.), *Antibiotics and Chemotherapy: Anti-infective Agents and Their Use in Therapy*. Churchill-Livingstone, London: 23–43.

Ghany M.G., Doo E.C. (2009). Antiviral resistance and hepatitis B therapy. *Hepatology*. 49 (5 Suppl.): S174–S184.

Gladwin M., Trattler B. (2003). Bacterial genetics. In: *Clinical Microbiology Made Ridiculously Simple*. 3rd ed. MedMaster Inc., Miami, FL: 16–21.

Gold H.S., Moellering R.C. (1996). Antimicrobial drug resistance. *New England Journal of Medicine*. 355 (19): 1443–1445.

Greenwood D., Ogilvie M.M. (2003). Antimicrobial agents. In: Greenwood D., Slack R.C.B., Peutherer J.F. (Eds.), *Medical Microbiology. A Guide to Microbial Infections: Pathogenesis, Immunity, Laboratory Diagnosis and Control*. 16th ed. Churchill Livingstone, London: 46–60.

Hayden G.C. (2006). Antiviral resistance in influenza viruses – implications for management and pandemic response. *New England Journal of Medicine*. 354: 785–788.

Health Protection Agency (HPA) (2008). *Working Party Guidance on the Control of Multi-Resistant Acinetobacter Outbreaks*. Health Protection Agency, London.

Health Protection Agency (HPA) (2009). *Health Protection Report. National Resistance Alert on Carbapenemase-producing Enterobacteriaceae*. Health Protection Agency, London. http://www.hpa.org.uk/HPR/archives/2009/news0409.htm (accessed 18 December 2012)

Health Protection Agency (HPA) (2010). *Advice on Carbapenemase Producers: Recognition, Infection Control and Treatment*. Health Protection Agency, London.

Health Protection Agency (HPA) (2012). *English National Point Prevalence Survey on Healthcare-associated Infections and Antimicrobial Use, 2011*. Preliminary data. Health Protection Agency, London.

Hiramatsu K. (2001). Vancomycin-resistant *Staphylococcus aureus*: a new model of antibiotic resistance. *The Lancet Infectious Diseases*. 1: 147–155.

Hiramatsu K., Hanaki H., Ino T., Yabuta K., Oguri T., *et al*. (1997). Meticillin-resistant *Staphylococcus aureus* in clinical strain with reduced vancomycin susceptibility. *Journal of Antimicrobial Chemotherapy*. 40: 135–136.

Hobson R.P., Mackenzie F.M., Gould I.M. (1996). An outbreak of multiply-resistant *Klebsiella pneumoniae* in the Grampian region of Scotland. *Journal of Hospital Infection*. 33 (4): 249–262.

House of Lords Select Committee on Science and Technology Report (1998). *Resistance to Antibiotics and Other Antimicrobial Agents*. The Stationary Office, London.

Hudson M.T. (2001). Antifungal resistance and over-the-counter-availability in the UK: a current perspective. *Journal of Antimicrobial Chemotherapy*. 48 (3): 345–350.

Hurt A.C., Chotpitayasunodh T., Cox N.J., Daniels R., Fry A.M. (2011). Antiviral resistance during the 2009 Influenza A H1N1 pandemic: public health, laboratory and clinical perspectives. *The Lancet Infectious Diseases*. 12 (3): 240–248.

Kumarasamy K.K., Toleman M.A., Walsh T.R., Bagaria J., Butt F. (2010). Emergence of a new antibiotic resistant mechanism in India, Pakistan and the UK: a molecular, biological and epidemiological study. *The Lancet Infectious Diseases*. 10 (9): 597–602.

Lee V.J., Lomovskaya O. (1998). Efflux mediated resistance to antibiotics in bacteria: challenges and opportunities. *Antibacterial Research*. 1: 39–42.

Levinson W. (2010). Gram-negative rods related to the enteric tract. In: *Review of Medical Microbiology and Immunology*. 11th ed. McGraw-Hill Lange, New York: 122–140.

Lucet J.C., Chevret S., Decre D., Vanjak D., Macrez A., *et al*. (1996). Outbreak of multiply-resistant Enterobacteriaceae in an Intensive Care Unit: epidemiology and risk factors for acquisition. *Clinical Infectious Diseases*. 22 (3): 403–406.

Moellering R.C. (1992). Emergence of Enterococcus as a significant pathogen. *Clinical Infectious Diseases*. 14 (6): 1173–1178.

Muir A., Weinbren M.J. (2010). New-Delhi Metallo-beta-lactamase: a cautionary tale. *Journal of Hospital Infection*. 75 (3): 239–240.

Neidhardt F.G. (2004). Bacterial genetics. In: Sherris J.C., Ryan K.J., Ray G.C. (Eds.), *Medical Microbiology: An Introduction to Infectious Diseases*. 4th ed. McGraw-Hill, London: 53–75.

Nye K. (2010). Investigation of gastrointestinal specimens. In: Ford M. (Ed.), *Fundamentals of Biomedical Science: Medical Microbiology*. Oxford University Press, Oxford: 227–252.

Peleg A.Y., Seifert H., Paterson D.L. (2008). *Acinetobacter baumanii*: emergence of a successful pathogen. *Clinical Microbiology Reviews*. 21 (3): 538–582.

Que Y-A., Moreillon P. (2009). *Staphylococcus aureus* (including staphylococcal toxic shock). In: Mandell G., Bennett J., Dolin R. (Eds.), *Mandell, Douglas and Bennett's Principles and Practice of Infectious Diseases*. 7th ed. Churchill Livingstone Elsevier, London. http://expertconsult.com (accessed 18 December 2012)

Regoes R.R., Bonhoefter S. (2006). Emergence of drug-resistance influenza virus: population dynamical considerations. *Science*. 312 (5772): 389–391.

Ryan K.J., Drew W.L. (2004). Antibacterial and antiviral agents. In: Sherris J.C., Ryan K.J., Ray G.C. (Eds.), *Medical Microbiology: An Introduction to Infectious Diseases*. 4th ed. McGraw-Hill, London: 193–213.

Ryan K.J., Drew W.L. (2010a). Antibacterial agents and resistance. In: Ryan K.J., Drew W.L. (Eds.), *Sherris Medical Microbiology*. 5th ed. McGraw-Hill: 403–427.

Ryan K.J., Drew W.L. (2010b). The nature ofb. In: Ryan K.J., Drew W.L. (Eds.), *Sherris Medical Microbiology*. 5th ed. McGraw-Hill: 347–386

Ryan K.J., Drew W.L. (2010c). Pseudomonas and other opportunistic Gram-negative bacilli. In: Ryan K.J., Drew W.L. (Eds.), *Sherris Medical Microbiology*. 5th ed. McGraw-Hill: 617–628.

Sanglard D., Odds F.C. (2002). Resistance of candida species to antifungal agents: molecular mechanisms and clinical consequences. *The Lancet Infectious Diseases*. 2: 73–85

Sisto A., D'Ancona F., Meledrani M., Pantosti A., Rossaolini G.M. (2012). Carbapenem non-susceptible *Klebsiella pneumoniae* from Micronet network hospitals, Italy, 2009 to 2012. *Eurosurveillance*. 17 (3). http://www.eurosurveillance.org/ViewArticle/aspx?ArticleId=20247 (accessed 18 December 2012)

Strohl W.A., Rouse H., Fisher B.D. (2001). Vaccines and antibiotics. In: Harvey R.A., Champe P.A. (Eds.), *Lippincott's Illustrated Reviews. Microbiology*. Lippincott Williams and Wilkins, Philadelphia, PA: 35–50.

Towner K.J. (2003). Bacterial genetics. In: Greenwood D., Slack R.C.B., Peutherer J.F. (Eds.), *Medical Microbiology. A Guide to Microbial Infections: Pathogenesis, Immunity, Laboratory Diagnosis and Control*. 16th ed.. Churchill Livingstone, London: 61–72.

Turnidge J., Christiansen K. (2005). Antibiotic use and resistance – proving the obvious. *The Lancet*. 365 (9459): 548–549.

Walsh T.R., Week J., Livermore D.M., Toleman M.A. (2011). Dissemination of NDM-1 positive bacteria in the New Delhi environment and its implications for human health: an environmental point prevalence study. *The Lancet Infectious Diseases*. 11 (5): 355–362

Willey J.M., Sherwood L.M., Woolverton C.J. (2011). Antimicrobial chemotherapy. In: *Prescott's Medical Microbiology*. 8th ed. McGraw-Hill, New York: 826–849.

Wise R., Hart T., Cars D., Strenulens M., Helmuth R., *et al.* (1998). Antimicrobial resistance. *British Medical Journal*. 317 (7159): 609–610.

Witte W. (2000). Selective pressure by antibiotic use in livestock. *International Journal Antimicrobial Agents*. 16 (Suppl.): 19–24.

World Health Organization (WHO) (2008). The World Health Organization's Global Strategy for the prevention and assessment of HIV drug-resistance. *Antiviral Therapy*. 13 (Suppl. 2): 1–13.

World Health Organization (WHO) (2011). *The Evolving Threat of Antimicrobial Resistance: Options for Action*. World Health Organization, Geneva.

Yong D., Toleman M.A., Giske G.G., Cho H.S., Lee K., *et al.* (2009). Characterisation of a new metallo-beta-lactamase-gene, bla_{NDM-1}, and a novel erythromycin esterase gene carried on a unique genetic structure in *Klebsiella pneumoniae* sequence type 14 from India. *Antimicrobial Agents Chemotherapy*. 53 (12): 504–505.

Part Two

The principles of infection prevention and control (standard precautions)

11

Isolation and cohort nursing

Contents

Fundamentals of Infection Prevention and Control: Theory and Practice, Second Edition. Debbie Weston.
© 2013 John Wiley & Sons, Ltd. Published 2013 by John Wiley & Sons, Ltd. Companion Website: www.wiley.com/go/fundamentalsofinfectionprevention

Introduction

Ensuring that patients in hospital who are known or suspected to be infected or colonised with potentially pathogenic microorganisms are 'isolated', or barrier nursed, is an important component in preventing and controlling the spread of healthcare-associated infections and communicable diseases. It can, however, be a challenging and sometimes distressing process for patients, their relatives and carers, and healthcare staff, and is not always appropriate, or easily achieved, in other healthcare settings. This chapter looks at implementing patient isolation in the context of infection control standard precautions. Determining the need for isolation and risk assessment is discussed, along with different methods of isolation such as negative-pressure facilities and cohort nursing, and the challenges of isolating patients in different care areas.

Learning outcomes

After reading this chapter, the reader will:

- Understand the significance of patient isolation and cohort nursing as parts of infection control standard precautions.

- Understand the different categories of isolation.

- Understand what needs to be in place when patients are isolated or cohort nursed.

- Understand the importance of undertaking a risk assessment to ensure that the patient is isolated safely.

- Understand how to apply infection control standard precautions in settings where patients cannot be isolated in a single room or cohort area.

Compliance with the Health and Social Care Act 2008

It is a requirement of the Health and Social Care Act 2008, *Code of Practice on the Prevention and Control of Infections and Related Guidance* (criterion 7) (Department of Health, 2010) that registered healthcare providers who deliver in-patient care:

- Are able to provide, or secure the provision of, adequate isolation precautions and facilities, including facilities within a day care setting
- Have policies in place for the allocation of patients to isolation facilities based on a local risk assessment (to include consideration of the need for special ventilated isolation facilities)
- Ensure that they are able to provide or secure facilities that can be physically separated in their service use from other residents in an appropriate manner in order to minimise the spread of infection.

Care homes are not expected to have dedicated isolation facilities but are expected to implement standard and isolation precautions.

Standard precautions

Most healthcare workers are familiar with the phrase 'universal precautions' or 'standard precautions' (also sometimes referred to as 'standard principles') (Box 11.1).

Box 11.1   Standard precautions

Hand hygiene (see Chapter 12)
The use of personal protective equipment (PPE) and clothing (see Chapter 13)
The safe handling and disposal of sharps (see Chapter 14)
Cleaning and decontamination of equipment and the environment (see Chapter 15)
The handling and disposal of healthcare waste
The handling and disposal of linen and laundry
The management of blood and body fluid spillages (see Chapter 15).

Standard precautions must be used for **all** patients in **all** healthcare settings (including out-patient departments, day hospitals, day units and even the patient's own home) **all** of the time on the assumption that **all** contact with blood, body fluids, secretions and excretions (with the exception of sweat), non-intact skin and mucous membranes, along with contact with the healthcare environment, **may** result in the transmission of infectious microorganisms. If standard precautions are applied appropriately, then there should be fewer opportunities for cross-infection to occur.

Fact Box 11.1   Standard precautions and transmission-based precautions

Transmission-based precautions (air-borne, droplet, respiratory, contact and enteric precautions) are essentially isolation of the patient in conjunction with the application of standard precautions, but with **added emphasis** on hand hygiene and the appropriate use of personal protective equipment . Standard precautions may also be referred to as 'infection control precautions' or 'isolation precautions'.

Within the hospital setting (acute or community) in the context of a patient who is isolated, isolation door signs are used to depict the precautions that staff need to take when patients are isolated for infection control purposes. Given that there are no nationally agreed, standardised isolation door signs, there is great variation in terms of the signage used.

Reflection point

How many different types of isolation door signs are used within your place of work? Do they convey a clear message as to the precautions required? Do you think that they convey too much information, or not enough?

EPIC and NICE guidelines

The Department of Health commissioned the development of national evidence-based best-practice (EPIC) guidelines for the prevention of healthcare-associated infections, which were published in 2001 and undated in 2007 (Pratt *et al.*, 2001, 2007). The Department of Health commissioned a further update in 2012, and these were published as a draft document for a consultation period in June 2013 (Loveday *et al.*, 2013). These guidelines incorporate the standard precautions (or standard principles) for preventing HCAIs and aim to inform best practice based on the best evidence currently available. In 2012, the National Clinical Guideline Centre commissioned the National Institute for Clinical Excellence (NICE) to revise and update guidance on the prevention and control of HCAIs in primary and community care (National Clinical Guideline Centre, 2012). Infection control policies in acute, community and primary care settings should be based upon the evidence-based best-practice recommendations within these documents.

The purpose of isolating patients and different categories of isolation

Isolation can be defined as 'causing a person to remain alone or apart from others . . . as quarantine as a precaution against infection or contagious disease' (http://www.oxforddictionaries.com/definition/english/isolation).

Fact Box 11.2   Quarantine

In an attempt to halt the spread of the infamous Black Death (plague) that swept through Europe between 1346 and 1350, attempts were made to isolate affected communities, and the Venetians were the first to introduce the concept of quarantine by making sure that ships coming into Venice waited at an island for 40 days before entering the city.

Source (standard) isolation

The purpose of 'isolating' patients who are known or suspected to be colonised or infected is to isolate the infectious microorganism, and control or limit its route of transmission, reducing the risk of cross-infection to healthcare staff and other patients. This is best achieved by caring for the patient in a single room (which must have a dedicated clinical handwash basin and which preferably should have en-suite facilities), in conjunction with the application of standard precautions. The isolation room, obviously, forms a barrier between the patient and the other patients on the ward (isolation is often referred to as 'barrier nursing'). Some hospitals may have a designated isolation ward consisting solely of single rooms. Only patients suspected or known to be colonised or infected should be admitted to an isolation ward – under no circumstances should vacant rooms be utilised as part of the hospital bed base. Where dedicated isolation wards are not available, 'patient isolation' can take place in a single room (or side room, as they are often called) on a ward.

It is important that all staff understand that it is *not* the patient who is being isolated but the *organism* and its *mode of transmission*, and it is of paramount importance that this is communicated clearly to patients and their relatives and carers. Source isolation covers all organisms and infections with the exception of respiratory isolation for suspected or confirmed tuberculosis, and rare infectious diseases. Certain microorganisms and infectious diseases pose a higher risk of transmission and cross-infection than others (see Box 11.2), and patients who are colonised or infected will require isolation.

Strict isolation is for very rare infectious diseases (e.g. viral haemorrhagic fever [VHF], SARS and H5N1 influenza [see Chapter 5], pulmonary anthrax and rabies) and will be undertaken in a designated high-security Infectious Disease Unit. There are Fact Sheets on VHF (3.12) and anthrax (11.1) on the companion website.

Protective isolation (see Chapter 9)

Cohort nursing

Cohort nursing can be undertaken in instances where the need for isolation exceeds room capacity. Patients with the same organism (e.g. MRSA colonisation) or those displaying similar

Box 11.2   Organisms with a high risk of transmission and potential cross-infection

- Suspected or confirmed respiratory tuberculosis (TB) (see Chapter 21)
- Suspected or confirmed multidrug-resistant TB (MDR-TB)
- Suspected or confirmed meningococcal disease (see Fact Sheet 3.4 on the companion website)
- Confirmed symptomatic *Clostridium difficile* (see Chapter 22)
- Confirmed symptomatic glutamate dehydrogenase (GDH) antigen positive until the patient has been asymptomatic for 48 hours with 'normal' stools
- Diarrhoea and/or vomiting unless a non-infectious cause can be determined
- ESBL-resistant and carbapenem-resistant organisms (see Chapter 10)
- Pandemic influenza (special precautions will apply)
- Chickenpox and shingles (see Fact Sheet 3.11 on the companion website)
- Measles, mumps or rubella (see Chapter 5)
- Fever +/– respiratory symptoms if the patient has recently returned from foreign travel
- MRSA in multiple body sites (e.g. nose, axilla and one or more other sites), deep leaking wounds or sputum; dermatitis or exfoliative skin conditions; urine positive and urinary catheter in situ; and/or mupirocin-resistant MRSA (see Chapter 20).

signs and symptoms (e.g. norovirus) can be nursed together. The cohort may consist of an entire bay of colonised or infected patients, in which case the patients should be cared for by designated staff in a designated area (bay) of the ward, although it is accepted that this cannot always be readily achieved.

See Chapter 9 for more information.

Isolation and risk assessment

There are several factors that need to be taken into consideration before moving a patient into a single room or transferring him or her to an isolation ward, and, increasingly, risk assessments need to be undertaken by the Infection Prevention and Control Team (IP&CT) in conjunction with the Nursing staff and Bed Managers. These take into account:

- The organism
- Its mode of transmission
- The risk of cross-infection to healthcare staff and other patients
- The implications of cross-infection
- Patient safety
- The facilities available.

Sometimes, difficult and unpopular decisions have to be made. Patients who are admitted to a single room for non–infection control purposes (e.g. at their own request or because it is the only available bed) should always be informed on admission that it cannot be guaranteed that they will be able to remain in the room for the duration of their stay, and this should be clearly documented in the nursing notes. In the event of a patient receiving end-of-life care in a single room, it is always extremely distressing for the patient, their family and the nursing staff if the patient has to be moved to an open bay. However, the IP&CT *have* to balance the needs of one patient against the risk of cross-infection to other patients and also healthcare staff. This needs to be handled sensitively, and advice may need to be sought.

In the event of a patient not being safe if he or she is moved to a single room, the IP&CT may have to insist that 1:1 nursing is implemented depending on the organism concerned. This is highly likely to have resource implications and may require escalation to the Matron or Head of Nursing if additional nursing staff are required.

Where a patient cannot be isolated, it may be acceptable for the patient to be nursed on the open ward based on a risk assessment following discussion with the IP&CT as long as standard precautions are stringently applied (e.g. MRSA colonisation or ESBL colonisation depending upon the antibiotic sensitivities) along with any other advice or recommendations from the IP&CT. The nurse looking after the patient is responsible for recording this in the nursing notes and for ensuring that it is reviewed and updated daily. The patient should not be placed next to other patients with open wounds or invasive devices because of the implications of cross-infection.

Infection control precautions within specialist areas

Intensive Care Units (ITUs), Coronary Care Units (CCUs), Neonatal Intensive Care Units (NICUs) and Emergency Departments may have very few single rooms or none at all. Both stringent application of standard precautions and enhanced cleaning are essential in order to reduce the risk of cross-infection. If standard precautions *are* diligently and properly applied by *all* healthcare workers in contact with the patient at *all* times, and compliance is monitored, there should be no cross-infection.

Within ITUs, even if the patient has a respiratory pathogen, it may be possible for them to remain on the open unit if they are ventilated. Special care will need to be taken to ensure that the ventilator circuit does not accidentally become disconnected, and a closed circuit must be maintained.

If the patient has symptomatic *C. difficile* infection, is in a CCU with no single rooms and is not medically fit for transfer to a ward for isolation, there will be no option other than to keep the patient within CCU. Enhanced environmental cleaning and the cleaning of equipment will be required with a sporicidal agent, along with handwashing in place of alcohol hand rub. For patients who are faecally incontinent or who have profuse diarrhoea, a faecal or bowel management system that contains infectious diarrhoea and protects the patient's skin may be an option.

Within NICUs, an incubator serves as a physical barrier, effectively isolating the infected or colonised neonate within a contained area. Stringent attention to hand hygiene in particular is essential given the increased susceptibility to infection amongst this patient group.

Reflection point

Within your ward, are patients isolated appropriately? Are there any patients in single rooms who could be moved out, and are there any patients in the open ward who should be isolated?

Box 11.3 lists the 'precautions' that need to be in place when patients are isolated in a single room.

If the patient cannot be isolated and is in an open bay with patients who are *not* colonised or infected, or is in a cohort bay:

- Alcohol hand rub must be available at the point of care.
- There must be a dedicated clinical hand wash basin within the bay.
- PPE must be available.
- A toilet or bathroom should be dedicated for the patient or cohort bay if possible.
- Equipment should be dedicated to the patient or the cohort bay.
- If the bay has doors, they should be closed.
- Enhanced cleaning will be required because of the increased risk of environmental contamination.

Reflection point

Unless a patient is in a single room with an isolation door sign displayed on the door, staff may not be aware of colonised patients, or patients with an infection, who are nursed on the open ward. How do you ensure that this is communicated to staff, such as medical teams, phlebotomists and therapists?

Box 11.3   What needs to be in place when patients are isolated?

- The appropriate isolation door sign needs to be displayed on the door.
- The door should be kept closed (if this is not possible, e.g. the door must be kept open so that the patient can be readily observed, this must be documented in the nursing notes each shift).
- Alcohol hand rub must be available outside the entrance to the room and inside the room at the point of care.
- A dedicated clinical wash hand basin must be in the room, along with liquid soap and paper hand towels.
- Domestic and clinical waste bins must be available, and waste disposed of according to local policy.
- Linen must be disposed of according to local policy.
- Ideally, the room should have en-suite facilities. If this is not possible, a commode should be dedicated for the patient's use.
- Gloves and aprons must be available at the entrance to the room. **Note**: Visitors do not need to wear PPE (unless they are assisting the patient with hygiene needs, in which case they may wish to wear a disposable plastic apron). They should be asked to decontaminate their hands on entering and leaving the side room or ward (see Chapter 12).
- Equipment should be specifically dedicated to the patient, for example a single-patient-use tourniquet and blood pressure cuff, and a sphygmomanometer.
- Generally, the patient's nursing notes and TPR (temperature, pulse and respirations) and prescription charts are kept outside the room. However, if the patient is having 1:1 nursing, or is in a side room in Intensive Care, the notes can remain in the room with the patient. Bedside folders or clipboards should have a covering that is wipeable.
- Domestic services staff need to be informed of the cleaning requirements.
- The patient and his or her family must be given a patient information leaflet.
- If the patient is on a specific Infection Control Pathway or Patient Management Plan, this must be completed each shift or day as required.

169

General points regarding the infection control management of infected and colonised patients

- Patients who are isolated in a single room should not be moved to another ward unless the move is based on clinical need, such as for specialist medical and nursing care.
- It is not strictly necessary for patients to be last on the theatre list, recovered in the anaesthetic room rather than the recovery suite or seen in clinic at the end of the day. However, this does in part depend on the nature of the infection. Generally speaking, this is why the application of standard precautions is so important, in particular hand hygiene, and cleaning of equipment and the environment, in order to greatly reduce the risk of cross-infection. Advice should be sought from the IP&CT.

- Rehabilitation should not be compromised or delayed because the patient is isolated in a single room. Physiotherapy, occupational therapy and speech therapy may be crucial to the patient's recovery and discharge home, and unless the organism is highly transmissible, there is no reason why most activities and risks cannot be effectively managed. The IP&CT will advise.
- Patients should be discharged home as soon as they are medically fit.

Negative-pressure isolation

Patients with suspected or confirmed MDR-TB require isolation in dedicated negative-pressure isolation facilities which conform to the standards described by the Interdepartmental Working Group on Tuberculosis (1998) (and see Chapter 21).

Air currents can transport bacteria and viruses within buildings and rooms, increasing the risk of infection to staff and other patients, and ventilation in buildings, either natural or mechanically induced, dilutes droplet nuclei by removing contaminated air from within the room and replacing it with 'clean' air.

An ordinary, standard ventilated hospital single room will usually have six air changes an hour. The air changes within the room by passing under the door or, whenever the door or a window in the room is opened, mixing with the air in the corridor or within the room. With MDR-TB, it is important to prevent air contaminated with TB bacilli from mixing with 'clean' air, and so the ventilation system must expel the air away from other areas, venting it to the outside so that it is not sucked back into the building.

Where there is no existing negative-pressure ventilation, a suitable single room can be adapted to negative pressure through the installation of a vent-axia exhaust fan, which will discharge air from the room to the outside. Ideally, negative-pressure rooms should be purpose built, with air pressure that is automatically controlled and monitored so that if the system fails, an alarm sounds, alerting staff when the pressure falls. In order to maintain the negative pressure within the room, there should be no gaps underneath or around the doors through which air can enter the room and escape from it, and it should not be possible to open the windows. Negative-pressure rooms should have an en-suite toilet and bathroom, and also be equipped with a telephone and a television – some patients may require isolation for many months.

Important note: Where negative-pressure isolation rooms are available, it is the responsibility of the Ward Manager to ensure that all staff understand how the negative-pressure room functions, their responsibility for ensuring that the room is achieving negative pressure while it is occupied, and the action to be taken in the event of a failure in the negative pressure. Education or training may be required by the Estates Department.

Practical points regarding the management of negative-pressure rooms are summarised in Box 11.4.

Box 11.4   Management of negative-pressure rooms

- Doors must not be left open or wedged open.
- Walls must not be damaged (this will affect the pressure control).
- Damage to the door seals must be avoided.
- Rooms must be re-validated yearly.
- The pressure should be 10 pascals between the entrance lobby and the corridor; this should be monitored and recorded at least daily.

If the pressure fails, Nursing staff must:

- Check that the doors are shut and/or that they have not been left open for a prolonged period.
- Contact the Estates Department once the above checks have been made, in order that the ventilation plant can be inspected.
- Contact the IP&CT.
- Record the time of alarm, and any instructions given and actions taken.

The psychological effects of isolation

It is well documented in the literature that placement of patients in a single room for infection control purposes can have a negative impact on patients' psychological well-being. Research has shown that patients feel 'violated' and often find the whole experience 'traumatic' (Skyman and Sjostrom, 2009). They may believe that they are 'contagious' and 'contaminated' and that they pose a risk to other patients, and can feel 'stigmatised' and 'downgraded', experiencing feelings of anxiety, anger and guilt (Barrett, 2010). It can also have an adverse effect on patient safety as well as patient satisfaction (Abad et al., 2010) if it is not managed sensitively by healthcare professionals.

Care of deceased patients

As previously discussed, we carry an enormous number of microorganisms on and in our bodies. Add to that the fact that many people with a blood borne virus (BBV) infection are asymptomatic carriers and are unaware of their carrier status/infectivity (see Chapter 24), and it is easy to see how important the application of standard precautions is during everyday patient contact.

When patients who are known to be colonised or infected with microorganisms die, care of the body (last offices) and removal to the mortuary generally only requires the application of standard precautions. This may include the requirement for the patient to be placed into a body bag (i.e. invasive group A streptococcal disease, Norovirus), but body bags are generally not required as a rule. However, there are some microorganisms that may pose significant infection risks to mortuary staff and others who subsequently handle the body. These 'high-risk' microorganisms belong to 'hazard group 3 biological agents' (see Chapter 6, Specimen Collection) and include (amongst others) avian influenza, CJD, dysentery, viral encephalitis, hepatitis B and C, HIV, malaria, leprosy, paratyphoid fever, plague, novel coronavirus and respiratory tuberculosis.

It is a Health and Safety Exceecutive (HSE) requirement that all organisations have a Policy for the management of 'high-risk cadavers', that covers deceased patients who die in hospital and who are brought into the mortuary from the community. Where patients are suspected or known to be 'high risk', a 'danger of infection' label should be attached to the outside of the body bag and any accompanying paperwork completed as per Policy. When 'community death' bodies are brought into hospital premises, for example when a thorough medical assessment of the patient has not been undertaken, the body should be treated as 'high-risk'.

Chapter summary: key points

- Standard precautions must be used for *all* patients in *all* healthcare settings *all* of the time on the assumption that *all* contact with blood, body fluids, secretions and excretions (with the exception of sweat), non-intact skin and mucous membranes, along with contact with the healthcare environment, may result in the transmission of infectious microorganisms.

- The purpose of isolation is to isolate or contain the organism and its mode of transmission, rather than the patient.

- The patient's overall condition and his or her safety have to be taken into consideration when isolation is required – where isolation is not possible, a risk assessment must be made, documented and then reviewed each shift or daily.

- Patient care and rehabilitation must not be compromised.

- If standard precautions are stringently implemented, cross-infection should not occur.

 Further resources are available for this book, including interactive multiple choice questions. Visit the companion website at:

www.wiley.com/go/fundamentalsofinfectionprevention

References

Abad C., Fearday A., Safdar N. (2010). Adverse effects of isolation in hospitalised patients: a systematic review. *Journal of Hospital Infection*. 76 (2): 97–102.

Barrett R. (2010). Behind barriers: patients perceptions of source isolation for meticillin-resistant *Staphylococcus aureus*. *Australian Journal of Advanced Nursing*. 28 (2): 53–59.

Department of Health (2010). *Code of Practice on the Prevention and Control of Infections and Related Guidance*. Department of Health, London.

Interdepartmental Working Group on Tuberculosis (1998). *The Prevention and Control of Tuberculosis in the United Kingdom: UK Guidance on the Prevention and Control of Transmission of HIV-related Tuberculosis and Drug-resistant, including Multiple-drug Resistant, Tuberculosis*. Department of Health, London.

Healing T.D., Hoffman P.N., Young S.E.J. (1995). *The Infection Hazards of Human Cadavers*. CDR Review. Volume 5, review number 5. 28th April 1995.

Health and Safety Executive (HSE) (2003). *Safe Working and the Prevention of Infection in the Mortuary and Post-Mortem Room*. HSE, London.

Health and Safety Executive (HSE) (2004). *Advisory Committee on Dangerous Pathogens*. The approved list of biological agents. HSE, London.

Health and Safety Executive (HSE) (2005). *Controlling the Risks of Infection at Work from Human Remains: A guide for those involved in funeral services (including embalmers) and those involved in exhumation*. HSE, London.

Loveday H.P., Wilson J.A., Pratt R.J., Golsorkhi M., Tingle A. *et al* (2013). EPIC3: *National Evidence-Based Guidelines for Preventing Healthcare-Associated Infections in NHS Hospitals in England*. (Draft). Richard Wells Research Centre, University of West London, 2013.

National Clinical Guideline Centre (2012). *Partial Update of NICE Clinical Guideline 2. Infection: Prevention and Control of Healthcare Associated Infections in Primary and Community Care*. National Clinical Guideline Centre, London.

Pratt R.J., Pellowe C.M., Loveday H.B., Robinson M., Smith G.W. and the EPIC Guidelines Development Team (2001). The EPIC Project: developing national evidence-based guidelines for preventing healthcare associated infections. *Journal of Hospital Infection*. 47 (Suppl.): S1–S82.

Pratt R.J., Pellowe C.M., Wilson J.A., Loveday H.P., Harper P.J., Jones S.R.L.K., McDougall C., Wilcox M.H. (2007). *EPIC2: national evidence-based guidelines for preventing healthcare-associated infections in NHS hospitals in England*. http://www.epic.tvu.ac.uk/Downloads/ (accessed 26 February 2013).

Skyman E., Sjostrom H.T. (2009). Patients experiences of being infected with MRSA at a hospital and subsequently source isolated. *Scandinavian Journal of Caring Sciences*. 24 (1): 101–107.

12

Hand hygiene

Contents

Introduction

In 2005, the World Health Organization (WHO) launched the First Global Patient Safety Challenge, *Clean Care Is Safe Care*, to promote best practice in hand hygiene globally and to emphasise the importance of hand hygiene in reducing healthcare-associated infections. This was followed in 2009 by the publication of new evidence-based best-practice *Guidelines on Hand Hygiene in Health Care* (WHO, 2009a). A recent research study evaluating the success of the national *Cleanyourhands* campaign in England and Wales, which looked at the procurement of soap and alcohol hand rub within NHS Trusts, its usage and rates of *Clostridium difficile* infection and meticillin-resistant *Staphylococcus aureus* (MRSA) bacteraemia found that rates of both infections fell, and although there were other national key drives, a national campaign to raise awareness regarding the importance of hand hygiene was undoubtedly a significant factor (Stone *et al.*, 2012).

This chapter explains the difference between resident and transient microorganisms on the skin and hands; how cross-infection via the hands occurs; when hand washing with soap and water, and hand decontamination with alcohol-based hand rubs or gels, should be undertaken; the advantages and disadvantages of each method, and the importance of undertaking hand hygiene and hand decontamination at the point of care in accordance with the 5 Moments for Hand Hygiene.

Learning outcomes

After reading this chapter, the reader will be able to:

- Understand how cross-infection via the hands occurs and the sequential steps involved.

- Understand the microbial flora of the skin, and the difference between resident and transient microorganisms.

- Understand when hand washing and hand decontamination using alcohol-based hand rubs or gels should be undertaken.

- Understand the importance of undertaking hand hygiene at the point of care (the 5 Moments for Hand Hygiene).

Ignaz Semmelweis

In 1841, a Hungarian obstetrician working in Vienna, Ignaz Semmelweis, observed that women in labour who were attended by doctors and medical students were more likely to die following childbirth, dying from puerperal fever (group A streptococcal infection, caused by *Streptococcus pyogenes*) (see Fact Sheet 3.9 on the companion website), than those who had been attended by midwives. He noticed that the doctors came straight to the delivery ward from conducting post-mortems, often carrying 'a disagreeable odour' on their hands (Pittet and Boyce, 2001) which was not removed through hand washing, and that their clothing 'smelt of the dead' (Newsom, 2009). Over time, he collated a considerable amount of data and undertook some research of his own.

When a colleague died three days after sustaining an injury during a post-mortem, Semmelweis deduced that 'cadaveric particles' carried on the hands were responsible for the deaths of his colleague and the women in the delivery ward (Pittet and Boyce, 2001; Best and Neuhauser, 2004).

In 1847, Semmelweis introduced chlorinated lime as a method for decontaminating the hands prior to examining women in labour (Rotter, 1997), and maternal mortality decreased dramatically from 11.4% to 3% (Newsom, 2009). At the same time, he identified that cross-infection between patients could occur. A woman in labour with a discharging cancer of the leg was examined by staff who washed their hands with only soap and water following contact with the leg wound. Several other women in the ward subsequently died, and it became apparent that it was not only 'cadaveric particles' acquired during post-mortems that were responsible for deaths in hospital (Newsom, 2009).

Fact Box 12.1   Ignaz Semmelweis

Semmelweis went on to identify that 'disease' could be spread by contaminated linen and by air, but unfortunately, he was way ahead of his time. Bacteria had not yet been discovered, and his findings met with considerable opposition from his medical colleagues. He ended his days in a mental asylum, where he died from streptococcal blood poisoning, contracted during an operation (Newsom, 2009).

It is of course now universally acknowledged that the hands are the principle route by which cross-infection occurs, and that hand hygiene is the single most important factor in the control of infection (Gould, 1991; Pratt et al., 2001; Centers for Disease Control and Prevention [CDC], 2002; Pratt et al., 2007; Sax et al., 2007; National Patient Safety Agency, 2008; Allegranzi and Pettit, 2009; Edmond and Wenzel, 2010). It is estimated that 'good' hand hygiene practice could contribute to the reduction of healthcare-associated infections (HCAIs) by 15–30% (Pratt et al., 2001; National Audit Office, 2004). However, although it is accepted throughout the healthcare community as a basic clinical procedure essential for the prevention of infections in patients and healthcare workers alike, the vast amount of literature published on the importance of hand washing over the last 30 to 40 years shows that hands are inadequately, infrequently or inappropriately washed and that compliance is poor (Taylor, 1978; Pittet et al., 1999, 2004; Pittet, 2001; Trampuz and Widmer, 2004; Jenner et al., 2006).

The microbial flora of the skin

Fact Box 12.2   The microbial flora of the skin

80% of microorganisms reside within the first five cell layers of the epidermis (Ostrander et al., 2005), and approximately 10 million aerobic bacteria reside on one single square centimetre of skin (Taylor, 2006).

The microbial flora of the skin consists of both resident and transient microorganisms.

Resident skin flora

Fact Box 12.3   Resident skin flora

Resident skin flora, with a population density of between 10^2 and 10^3 colony-forming units (CFU) of bacteria per cm^2 of skin, are deep seated within skin crevices, sweat glands and hair follicles and beneath the finger nails, and are more resistant to mechanical removal with soap and water than transient organisms (Trampuz and Widmer, 2004). They are generally of lower pathogenicity, they have a role to play in protecting the skin from colonisation by other more potentially pathogenic bacteria (colonisation resistance) and it is unnecessary (and potentially damaging to the skin) to remove them from the hands during routine clinical care. However, they can be pathogenic if they are transferred into susceptible sites during invasive procedures.

Transient skin flora

Transient microorganisms are more of a problem within the healthcare setting, and they are frequently associated with infections in hospital.

Fact Box 12.4   Transient skin flora

Transient microorganisms do not reside on the skin but colonise it and are readily acquired through touch (e.g. through contact with other people, equipment or body sites), and although they do not survive on the skin for more than a few hours due to the skin's inherent antibacterial properties, there is sufficient time for them to be transferred to other patients and equipment. How easily they are transmitted to other patients or objects depends on the organism, the number of organisms and the moisture of the skin (Patrick *et al.*, 1997).

While most transient microorganisms are likely to be acquired from heavily contaminated material such as body fluids, they can also be acquired from contact with apparently 'clean' objects or surfaces such as patients' skin, bed linen and work surfaces. MRSA and *C. difficile* are examples of microorganisms that can be carried on the hands transiently.

How cross-infection via the hands occurs

The transmission of microorganisms from one patient to another via the hands, or from hands that have been contaminated from the environment, can result in cross-infection in the following ways:

Directly:
When microorganisms are introduced directly into susceptible sites, such as surgical wounds and intravenous cannula sites.

Or

Indirectly:
When microorganisms transferred by the hands become established on a patient, subsequently causing infection in susceptible sites.

The transmission of microorganisms on the hands of healthcare workers is the most common mode of transmission within the healthcare setting, and Pittet *et al.* (2006) describe **five sequential steps:**

- Organisms are present on the patient's skin, or are shed onto objects surrounding the patient's environment.
- They are transferred onto the hands of healthcare workers.
- They must be able to survive for a period of time that ranges from mere minutes to as long as 60 minutes.
- Hand washing and hand decontamination must be inadequate or missed entirely, or the wrong agent used.
- Hands must be in direct contact with a patient or objects in the patient's environment.

Hand hygiene

Hand hygiene has a dual role in that it protects both patients and healthcare workers from acquiring microorganisms which may cause them harm, and it results in a significant reduction in the carriage of potential pathogens on the hands. This can be readily achieved by using liquid soap and water with an effective technique, or by using an alcohol hand rub or gel on visibly clean hands.

Hand washing

Hand washing has been defined as 'a vigorous, brief rubbing together of all surfaces of lathered hands followed by rinsing under a stream of water' (Garner and Favero, 1985), and the mechanical action of lathering and rubbing the hands together along with rinsing under running water will remove transient microorganisms from the skin, along with dead epithelial cells. However, while washing hands with liquid soap and water suspends microorganisms in solution, enabling them to be washed off, ordinary soap has minimal or no antimicrobial activity, and does not reduce the microbial load on the skin.

Reflection point

Is it mandatory within your place of work that all healthcare staff have their hand washing and alcohol hand rub or gel application techniques assessed annually? If so, who is responsible for undertaking this, and how is compliance with this recorded?

Hands can become contaminated by bar soap (hence its removal from healthcare settings with the exception of bar soap for individual patient use); taps and sinks (Ehrenkranz and Alfonso, 1991); the removal of contaminated personal protective equipment such as gloves, aprons and masks; and the presence of rings, which can cause the skin underneath the ring to become colonised by Gram-negative bacteria, which would normally be found as transient skin flora (Hoffman *et al.*, 1985). Therefore, hand washing renders hands only socially clean, and will not remove deep-seated skin flora.

Surgical hand antisepsis

The purpose of surgical hand antisepsis is to:

- substantially reduce resident microorganisms
- remove or destroy transient microorganisms
- prevent the re-growth of microorganisms on the hands, wrists and forearms from contaminating the wound and/or from being introduced into tissues in the event of gloves becoming damaged (e.g. split or punctured).

Evidence-based best-practice guidance published by the National Collaborative Centre for Women's and Children's Health in 2008 for the prevention of surgical site infection (NICE Guidance) recommends that:

- The operating team should wash their hands prior to the first operation on the list using an aqueous antiseptic surgical solution, with a single-use brush or pick for the nails, and ensure that hands and nails are visibly clean (3 minutes).
- Before subsequent operations, hands should be washed using either an alcoholic hand rub or an antiseptic surgical solution. If hands are soiled, then they should be washed again with an antiseptic surgical solution (2 minutes).

This is supported by WHO (2009a) and the Association for Perioperative Practice (2011).

Alcohol hand rubs

In 2002, the CDC released guidelines for hand hygiene in healthcare institutions that supported the use of alcohol-based 'sanitisers'. The recommendation to use alcohol hand rubs for routine hand decontamination had previously been made in England within the EPIC guidelines (Pratt *et al.*, 2001), and the recommendation made by the CDC provided added weight to the argument of promoting alcohol-based hand rub as the primary method for hand decontamination.

The use of alcohol hand rubs have now become the 'gold standard' for routine hand decontamination (Pratt *et al.*, 2001, 2007), and they should be used routinely when hands are not visibly soiled (i.e. most of the time).

The rapid efficacy of alcohol-based solutions and their availability at the patient's bedside and point of use have made these products an ideal substitute for conventional hand washing, addressing the real and perceived constraints associated with hand washing, and substantially increasing hand hygiene compliance rates (Bischoff *et al.*, 2000; Maury *et al.*, 2000). They remove microorganisms more effectively, take less time to apply and are less likely to lead to skin irritation (Picheansathian, 2004).

Fact Box 12.5   Alcohol hand rubs or gels

While they are active immediately against a wide range of organisms and are approximately 100 times more effective against viruses than any other form of hand-washing product (Rotter, 1999), there are some disadvantages to alcohol hand rubs or gels. They are *not* cleansing agents, they *do not* work in the presence of organic material such as dirt or blood and they are ineffective against *C. difficile* spores (see Chapter 22), so hand washing with liquid soap and water is absolutely essential in these situations.

It is important that healthcare staff understand that hand washing and the use of alcohol hand rubs and gels are equally important and that there is a place for both within the patient care arena.

Boxes 12.1 and 12.2 highlight the advantages and disadvantages of hand washing and alcohol hand rubs or gels (Pratt *et al.* 2001, 2007; CDC, 2002; NPSA, 2008; WHO, 2009a)

Hand decontamination at the point of care – the 5 Moments for Hand Hygiene

In 2005, WHO launched the First Global Patient Safety Challenge as part of its World Alliance for Patient Safety Initiative, of which one challenge was for participants to develop campaigns specifically to promote and improve both practice and compliance with hand hygiene amongst healthcare workers (Allegranzi *et al.*, 2007).

In September 2004, the National Patient Safety Agency (NPSA) had issued a Patient Safety Alert announcing the phased rollout of the Cleanyourhands campaign during 2004–2005 (National Patient Safety Agency, 2004). The aim of the campaign was to minimise the risk to patient safety posed by poor hand hygiene, and it was implemented in all Acute and Primary Care, Ambulance and Mental Health NHS Trusts in England and Wales, and launched in Ireland in 2008. Scotland's hand hygiene campaign, 'Germs. Wash your hands of them', was successfully launched in 2007.

Box 12.1   Advantages and disadvantages of hand washing (soap and water)

Advantages of soap and water

- Cheap and readily available
- Effectively removes transient microorganisms.

Disadvantages of soap and water

- Requires facilities for washing and drying
- Requires space and plumbing
- Requires time
- Can damage the skin.

Source: Pratt *et al.*, 2001; CDC, 2002; Pratt *et al.*, 2007; NPSA, 2008; WHO, 2009a

Box 12.2   Advantages and disadvantages of alcohol hand rubs or gels

Advantages of alcohol hand rubs or gels

- Requires no additional facilities
- Useful for community-based healthcare workers where access to hand-washing facilities may be lacking
- Active immediately against a wide range of microorganisms
- More effective in destroying transient microorganisms
- Kinder to the skin due to added emollients
- Useful for rapid bedside or point-of-care hand decontamination between patients
- Can be used for surgical hand decontamination.

Disadvantages of alcohol hand rubs or gels

- Not a cleansing agent – not effective in the presence of dirt, blood or body fluids
- Ineffective against bacterial spores
- Astringent – makes the skin sting if it comes into contact with skin breaks or minor abrasions
- Can be highly irritant if exposure to the eyes occurs
- Can be harmful if accidentally or deliberately ingested
- Flammable – restrictions on storage.

Source: Pratt *et al.*, 2001; CDC, 2002; Pratt *et al.*, 2007; NPSA, 2008; WHO, 2009a.

The aim of the campaign overall was to increase hand hygiene compliance amongst healthcare professionals through a national strategy of improvement. This involved the placement of alcohol hand rubs or gels at the patient's bedside, the use of posters and other promotional material to inform and influence healthcare staff and patients (see Figures 12.1 and 12.2), and the involvement of patients and the public, encouraging them to ask healthcare workers if they had cleaned their hands.

Fact Box 12.6   The placement of alcohol hand rub or gel dispensers

Soon after the launch of the Cleanyourhands campaign, in addition to being placed at the bedside, hand rubs and gels started appearing at hospital entrances, in ward corridors and in areas where their use could not be adequately supervised. Slips, trips and falls as a result of product spillage, accidental and/or deliberate ingestion, and incidences whereby hand rub or gel had been splashed into the eyes prompted the NPSA to issue a second Patient Safety Alert, re-directing the attention of healthcare staff and the public to hand hygiene at the point of care and requiring hospitals and other organisations to undertake audits and risk assessments in relation to product placement. It was apparent that although the profile of hand hygiene had been raised, it still was not being undertaken at the most appropriate opportunity, and attention had to be focused on improving compliance with hand hygiene at the point of care, leading to the national adoption of the 5 Moments approach.

182

Your 5 Moments
for Hand Hygiene

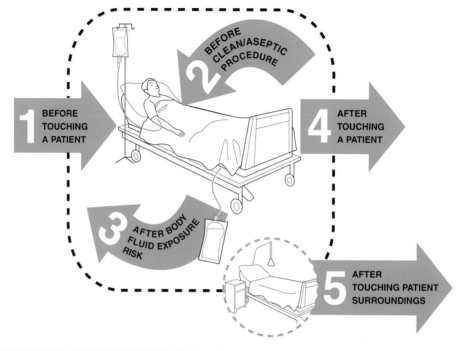

1	BEFORE TOUCHING A PATIENT	WHEN?	Clean your hands before touching a patient when approaching him/her.
		WHY?	To protect the patient against harmful germs carried on your hands.
2	BEFORE CLEAN/ ASEPTIC PROCEDURE	WHEN?	Clean your hands immediately before performing a clean/aseptic procedure.
		WHY?	To protect the patient against harmful germs, including the patient's own, from entering his/her body.
3	AFTER BODY FLUID EXPOSURE RISK	WHEN?	Clean your hands immediately after an exposure risk to body fluids (and after glove removal).
		WHY?	To protect yourself and the health-care environment from harmful patient germs.
4	AFTER TOUCHING A PATIENT	WHEN?	Clean your hands after touching a patient and her/his immediate surroundings, when leaving the patient's side.
		WHY?	To protect yourself and the health-care environment from harmful patient germs.
5	AFTER TOUCHING PATIENT SURROUNDINGS	WHEN?	Clean your hands after touching any object or furniture in the patient's immediate surroundings, when leaving – even if the patient has not been touched.
		WHY?	To protect yourself and the health-care environment from harmful patient germs.

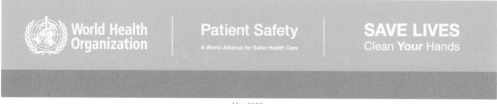

May 2009

Figure 12.1   '5 Moments for Hand Hygiene' poster (bed) (WHO, 2009).

Your 5 Moments
for Hand Hygiene

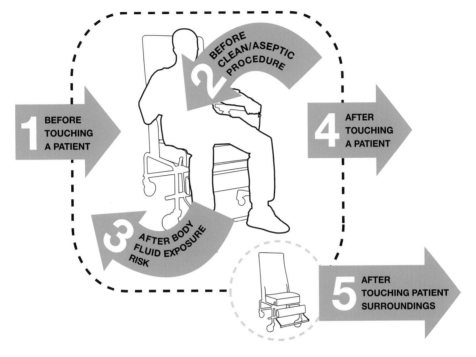

		WHEN?	Clean your hands before touching a patient when approaching him/her.
1	BEFORE TOUCHING A PATIENT	WHY?	To protect the patient against harmful germs carried on your hands.
2	BEFORE CLEAN/ ASEPTIC PROCEDURE	WHEN?	Clean your hands immediately before performing a clean/aseptic procedure.
		WHY?	To protect the patient against harmful germs, including the patient's own, from entering his/her body.
3	AFTER BODY FLUID EXPOSURE RISK	WHEN?	Clean your hands immediately after an exposure risk to body fluids (and after glove removal).
		WHY?	To protect yourself and the health-care environment from harmful patient germs.
4	AFTER TOUCHING A PATIENT	WHEN?	Clean your hands after touching a patient and her/his immediate surroundings, when leaving the patient's side.
		WHY?	To protect yourself and the health-care environment from harmful patient germs.
5	AFTER TOUCHING PATIENT SURROUNDINGS	WHEN?	Clean your hands after touching any object or furniture in the patient's immediate surroundings, when leaving – even if the patient has not been touched.
		WHY?	To protect yourself and the health-care environment from harmful patient germs.

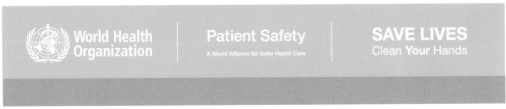

World Health Organization | Patient Safety — A World Alliance for Safer Health Care | SAVE LIVES Clean **Your** Hands

May 2009

Figure 12.2   '5 Moments for Hand Hygiene' poster (chair). (WHO, 2009)

My 5 Moments for Hand Hygiene

The 5 Moments for Hand Hygiene approach to hand hygiene, which was developed as part of the Swiss National Hand Hygiene Campaign and integrated into WHO's Multimodal Hand Hygiene Strategy, recognises three important factors that significantly increase the risk of cross-infection within the healthcare environment (Sax *et al.*, 2007):

- Colonised or infected patients are the main reservoir for many of the microorganisms that are responsible for HCAIs.
- Transmission of infection from the environment can occur because of the variety of microorganisms that can be found there (environmental microorganisms and those shed from patients).
- The immediate patient environment (known in the 5 Moments as the patient zone) will be heavily contaminated with microorganisms from the patient.

The patient's environment is separated into two distinct geographical zones: the patient zone and the healthcare zone.

The patient zone

This is the area immediately 'surrounding' the patient and encompasses the patient and 'touch surfaces' (see Chapter 15) such as the bed, bed linen, bedside furnishings (e.g. table, chair and locker), personal belongings and equipment. In other words, it comprises all surfaces and items that are either temporarily or permanently dedicated to the patient. The patient zone also encompasses 'critical sites', such as body sites, where there may be blood or body fluid exposure, or sites of invasive devices. The patient zone will be heavily contaminated or colonised by the patient's own body flora.

Fact Box 12.7   The patient zone

The patient zone is not static; it moves with the patient, so in an operating theatre, outpatient clinic or health centre, for example, it would include the theatre trolley, examination couch or wheelchair, all equipment used on the patient and all surfaces immediately around the patient. Although cleaning will take place within the patient zone every day and in between patient episodes, it is impossible to keep the area completely free from contamination by the patient's own flora in between cleaning.

The healthcare zone

This encompasses the zones of other patients and the wider environment where other patient contacts and healthcare activities take place, and will be heavily contaminated with microorganisms from patients and healthcare staff. These microorganisms will be varied and may even include those that are multidrug resistant. As the hands of healthcare workers will be exposed to, and in contact with, microorganisms on intact and non-intact skin, mucous membranes, blood and body fluids, inanimate objects, waste and food up to tens of thousands of times a day (Sax *et al.*, 2007), hand hygiene **has** to take place at the right time in order to prevent or reduce contamination of objects within the environment, and colonisation and infection of patients.

The indications for hand hygiene are whenever healthcare workers' hands move (WHO, 2009b):

- from the healthcare zone to the patient zone
- from the patient zone to the healthcare zone
- from one critical site to another body site on the same patient
- away from the patient.

The aims of effective hand hygiene are therefore (WHO, 2009b):

1. To interrupt the transmission of microorganisms, and therefore potential cross-infection on the hands:
   - between the healthcare zone and the patient zone
   - between the patient zone and the healthcare zone
   - at a critical risk site on the patient (e.g. mucous membranes, non-intact skin or an invasive device)
   - from blood and body fluids.
2. To prevent colonisation of the patient from:
   - potential pathogens
   - dissemination of potential pathogens in the healthcare area, infections caused by endogenous microorganisms.
3. To prevent the colonisation and infection of healthcare workers.

It is therefore essential that hand hygiene occurs at the right time, **at the point of care**, in order to interrupt the potential transmission of microorganisms during critical moments in patient care.

Fact Box 12.8   The point of care

The 'point of care' is where patient contact and patient care take place, and is defined by WHO (2009b) as 'the place where three elements come together: the patient, the HCW [healthcare worker] and care or treatment involving contact with the patient'.

The 5 Moments can be applied in any patient care setting, and in 2012, WHO published guidance specifically to the application of the 5 Moments in a variety of out-patient, home-based care and long-term care facilities (WHO, 2012).

Moment 1. Before patient contact: Hands must be decontaminated prior to contact with the patient (whether direct skin contact or contact with the patient's clothing or bed clothes) because the healthcare worker is moving from the healthcare zone to the patient zone. Examples of application of Moment 1 include before helping a patient to stand or mobilise, undertaking observations (recording vital signs) or applying an oxygen mask. The application of alcohol hand rub at this point will destroy the transient flora that the staff member is carrying. Healthcare workers can apply alcohol hand rub to their hands when entering a bay, side room or examination room and approaching the patient, or immediately at the bedside or chair side, as long as they are not going to have any contact with equipment or the environment. However, if a healthcare worker then draws the curtains around the bed or has to move the patient's bedside table, he or she will need to decontaminate his or her hands again (see Moment 5).

Moment 2. Before a clean or aseptic task: Moment 2 takes place before any clean or aseptic procedure in order to prevent the transfer of microorganisms from the environment, and also to prevent transfer of the patient's own flora into susceptible sites on the patient. This moment for hand hygiene is important in preventing colonisation and subsequent infection. Examples include before helping to feed a patient, cleaning a patient's teeth or giving mouth care.

Moment 3. After blood or body fluid exposure: Moment 3, which includes hand decontamination following the removal of gloves, takes place immediately following contact with blood or body fluids, to reduce the risk of transmission of microorganisms from a colonised site to a clean site and to protect the healthcare worker. Examples include following clinical specimen collection (see Chapter 6), after cleaning any contaminated surface, after removing soiled or contaminated linen, and after removing a commode or bedpan. **Note**: Non-sterile examination gloves should be worn for procedures involving exposure to blood and body fluids (see Chapter 13). However, this does not negate the need for hand decontamination.

Moment 4. After touching a patient: Hand decontamination following patient contact protects the healthcare worker, prevents contamination with the patient's flora and prevents dissemination to, and contamination of, the healthcare zone. Examples include after helping a patient to stand, sit or mobilise; after feeding a patient; after handling bed linen and after accessing the patient's urinary catheter.

Moment 5. After touching patient surroundings: Hands must be decontaminated following contact with any surface within the patient zone as it will be contaminated with the patient's flora. This includes curtains, the bedside locker or table, equipment attached to the patient and any equipment within the patient zone that has been removed from the bedside for cleaning. Examples include after looking at the patient's end-of-bed notes, moving the patient's bedside furniture or adjusting the patient's bed.

Note: Obviously, not all of the 5 Moments will apply in every patient care situation, and in some situations moments can be combined. The companion website has some scenarios that can be worked through and discussed.

Fact Box 12.9   Bare Below the Elbows (BBE) and hand hygiene

In 2007, the Department of Health introduced a new dress code policy of Bare Below the Elbows for medical staff – no wristwatches, bracelets, long sleeves and white coats (or ties) – as part of the drive to reduce HCAIs, in particular MRSA and *C. difficile*. The public's perception was that uniforms and work wear contributed to the problem of HCAIs, although there was very little evidence to suggest that this was actually the case. Medical staff were therefore required to remove their white coats, jackets and cardigans; roll up their sleeves; remove their wristwatches and remove or tuck in their ties when entering clinical areas. This caused outrage amongst medical staff up and down the country, primarily because the scientific evidence base for this was rather weak but also because they were concerned that their professional image would be compromised (it led to the rather rapid demise of the white coat). From the perspective of IP&CTs, however, it made perfect sense as effective hand hygiene is hampered by the presence of wristwatches and long sleeves. The concept of Bare Below the Elbows is now well embedded in the NHS, and has naturally extended to include all uniformed and non-uniform-wearing staff groups who have patient contact and led Trusts to extensively revise their Uniform and Dress Code policy for all staff groups. Compliance with BBE is audited as part of hand hygiene compliance.

Reflection point

Observational audits of compliance with hand hygiene, the 5 Moments and BBE should take place in all healthcare settings.

Who undertakes these audits within your place of work?
What is the average percentage of compliance for your workplace:
  A. Overall?
  B. Amongst specific staff groups?
How is this acted upon?

Hand hygiene: patients and the public

While much of the focus is, quite rightly, on compliance with hand washing and hand decontamination amongst healthcare workers in preventing the spread of infection, the role of the patient's hands in the spread of endogenous infection should not be ignored (Banfield and Kerr, 2005). They can acquire microorganisms on their hands from the environment, and they can also 'auto-infect' themselves, moving commensal flora from one body site to another (endogenous infection – see Chapter 8). Patients should be encouraged to wash their hands or use alcohol hand rub or gel before eating and obviously after using the toilet or commode. Where this is not possible, they should be provided with disposable hand wipes.

Reflection point

What opportunities for hand hygiene are provided for patients and clients within your place of work?
How well do staff actively encourage hand hygiene amongst patients?

Although visitors will carry their own resident flora on their hands, and will acquire transient organisms from contact with the healthcare environment, the risks and implications are not the same as for patients. However, visitors should be advised and encouraged to use alcohol hand rub or gel on leaving the ward (or hand wash with liquid soap and water if the patient has diarrhoea).

Reflection point

What advice is given to visitors regarding hand hygiene within your place of work?
Are there posters and notices at the hospital entrances, along with alcohol hand rub or gel stations, requesting that everyone decontaminate their hands on entering the ward? How is this monitored?
Are there posters and notices at ward and department entrances requesting that visitors decontaminate their hands on leaving?

Care of the hands

Taking care of the hands is just as important as ensuring that they are washed and decontaminated appropriately, and Box 12.3 summarises the key points for staff relating to hand care.

Box 12.3   Hand care

- Rinse hands thoroughly after applying soap – soap residue may cause skin irritation.
- Dry hands thoroughly with paper towels in order to prevent sore, cracked skin. Also, transient microorganisms are more readily acquired on wet hands.
- Do not hand wash *and* apply alcohol hand rub or gel afterwards.
- Rub alcohol hand rubs or gels into the skin thoroughly until dry. Certain products also contain emollients, so there are added benefits for the skin as long as the product is applied properly.
- Apply hand cream or moisturiser regularly (even if the alcohol hand rub or gel contains emollients).
- Skin irritation is commonly due to poor hand-washing technique, inadequate hand drying, or over-use of hand washing or application of alcohol hand rub or gel. Staff experiencing problems with their hands should arrange to have their hand-washing and alcohol hand rub techniques re-assessed by the Infection Control Link Practitioner, the Occupational Health Department or one of the Infection Control Nurse Specialists. **However**, it may be caused by irritant or allergic **dermatitis** and staff should self-refer to the Occupational Health Department if they have **any** 'hand concerns'. Signs of dermatitis are:
  - Dry, red and itchy skin
  - Flaking, blistering and cracking of the skin (in severe cases, the skin may 'weep')
  - Pain.

Information on contact dermatitis can be found at http://www.hse.gov.uk/skin/employ/dermatitis.htm. All staff should be provided with written advice on the prevention of contact dermatitis by the Occupational Health Department.

Chapter summary: key points

- Hand hygiene is the single most important intervention that healthcare workers can undertake to prevent HCAIs.

- Microorganisms on the hands can be transferred by direct or indirect contact, and hands are frequently implicated in cross-infection.

- Hand hygiene has a dual role, protecting both patients and healthcare staff (and also visitors) from acquiring potentially pathogenic microorganisms.

- Hand washing with liquid soap and water renders only socially clean hands.

- Alcohol hand rubs or gels, which decontaminate (disinfect) the hands, have been the 'gold standard' for routine hand hygiene for over a decade.

- While hand washing and hand decontamination with alcohol hand rubs or gels have their advantages and disadvantages, they are both equally important.

- For hand hygiene to be really effective, it has to take place at the point of care in accordance with the 5 Moments.

- Patients should also be informed about hand hygiene and encouraged or assisted to clean their hands at appropriate moments.

- Staff must be provided with written information from the Occupational Health Department on the prevention of contact dermatitis, and must self-refer to the Occupational Health Department if they have any concerns about their hands.

Further resources are available for this book, including interactive multiple choice questions. Visit the companion website at:

www.wiley.com/go/fundamentalsofinfectionprevention

References

Allegranzi B., Pettit D. (2009). Role of hand hygiene in healthcare associated infection prevention. *Journal of Hospital Infection*. 73: 305–311.

Allegranzi B., Storr J., Dziekan G., Leotsakos A., Donaldson L. *et al*. (2007). The First Global Patient Safety Challenge, 'Clean Care Is Safer Care': from launch to current progress for achievement. *Journal of Hospital Infection*. 65 (Suppl. 2): 115–123.

Association for Perioperative Practice (2011). *Standards and Recommendations for Safe Perioperative Practice*. Association for Perioperative Practice, Harrowgate.

Banfield K.R., Kerr K.G. (2005). Could hospital patients' hands constitute a missing link? *Journal of Hospital Infection*. 61(3): 183–188.

Best M., Neuhauser D. (2004). Ignaz Semmelweis and the birth of infection control. *British Medical Journal Quality & Safety in Health Care*. 13: 233–234.

Bischoff W.E., Reynolds T., Sessler C., Edmond M., Wenzel R.P. (2000). Handwashing compliance by healthcare workers; the impact of introducing an accessible alcohol based hand antiseptic. *Archives of Internal Medicine*. 160 (7): 1017–1012.

Centers for Disease Control and Prevention (CDC) (2002). Guideline for hand hygiene in health-care settings: recommendations of the Healthcare Infection Control Practices Advisory Committee and the HICPAC/SHEA/APIC/IDSA Hand Hygiene Task Force. Society for Healthcare Epidemiology of America/Association for Professionals in Infection Control/Infectious Diseases Society of America. *Morbidity Mortality Weekly Review*. 51 (RR–16): 1–45.

Edmond M.N., Wenzel R.B. (2010). Isolation: In: Mandell G.L., Bennett J.E., Dolin R.D. (Eds.), *Mandell's Principles and Practices of Infectious Diseases*. 6th ed. Churchill Livingstone Elsevier, London. Expert Consult online: http://expertconsult.com (accessed 19 December 2012)

Ehrenkranz N.J., Alfonso B.C. (1991). Failure of bland soap handwash to prevent hand transfer of patient bacteria to urethral catheters. *Infection Control Hospital Epidemiology*. 12 (11): 654–662.

Garner J.S., Favero M.S. (1985). *Guidelines for Hand Washing and Hospital Environmental Control*. Hospital Infections Program Center for Infectious Diseases, Centers for Disease Control and Prevention, Atlanta, GA.

Gould D. (1991). Nurses' hands as vectors of hospital-acquired infection: a review. *Journal of Advanced Nursing*. 16 (10): 1216–1225.

Hoffman P.N., Cooke P.M., McCarville E., Emmerson A.M. (1985). Microorganisms isolated from the skin under wedding rings worn by hospital staff. *British Medical Journal*. 290 (6463): 206–207.

Jenner E.A., Fletcher B., Watson P., Jones F.A., Miller L., *et al.* (2006). Discrepancy between self-reported and observed hand hygiene behaviour in healthcare professionals. *Journal Hospital Infection*. 63 (4): 418–422.

Maury E., Alzieu M., Baudel J.L., Haram N. (2000). Availability of an alcohol solution can improve hand disinfection compliance in an intensive care unit. *American Journal Respiratory Medicine*. 162 (1): 324–327.

National Audit Office (2004). *Improving patient care by reducing the risk of hospital acquired infection: a progress report*. Report by the Comptroller and Auditor General. HC 876 Session 2003–2004, 14 July. National Audit Office, London.

National Patient Safety Agency (2004). *Patient Safety Alert: Clean Hands Help to Save Lives*. 2 September. National Patient Safety Agency, London.

National Patient Safety Agency (2008). *Patient Safety Alert: Clean Hands Save Lives*. 2nd ed., 2 September. National Patient Safety Agency, London.

Newsom S.W.B. (2009). Semmelweis and handwashing. In: *Infections and Their Control: A Historical Perspective*. Infection Prevention Society and SAGE Publications Ltd, London: 7–12.

National Collaborative Centre for Women's and Children's Health (2008). *Surgical Site Infection: Prevention and Treatment of Surgical Site Infection*. NICE Clinical Guideline 74. NICE, London.

Ostrander R.V., Botte M.J., Brage, M.E. (2005). Efficacy of surgical preparation solutions in foot and ankle surgery. *Journal of Bone and Joint Surgery, American Volume*. 87: 980–985.

Patrick D.R., Findon G., Miller T.E. (1997). Residual moisture determines the level of touch-contact-associated bacteria transferred following handwashing. *Epidemiology and Infection*. 119: 319–325.

Picheansathian W. (2004). A systematic review on the effectiveness of alcohol-based solutions for hand hygiene. *International Journal of Nursing Practice*. 10: 3–9.

Pittet D. (2001). Improving adherence to hand hygiene practice: a multi-disciplinary approach. *Emerging Infectious Diseases*. 7 (2): 234–240.

190

Pittet D., Allegranzi B., Sax H., Dharan S., Pessoa-Silva C.L. *et al.* (2006). Evidence based model for hand transmission during patient care and the role of the hands. *Lancet Infectious Diseases*. 6: 641–652.

Pittet D., Boyce J.M. (2001). Hand hygiene and patient care: pursuing the Semmelweis legacy. *The Lancet Infectious Diseases*. 1: 9–20.

Pittet D., Mourouga P., Perneger T.V. (1999). Compliance with hand washing in a teaching hospital; infection control programme. *Annals of Internal Medicine*. 130 (2): 126–130.

Pittet D., Simon A., Hugonnet S., Pessoa-Silva C.L., Sauvoan V., *et al.* (2004). Hand hygiene among physicians: performance, beliefs and perceptions. *Annals of Internal Medicine*. 141: 1–8.

Pratt R.J., Pellowe C.M., Loveday H.B., Robinson M., Smith G.W. and the EPIC Guidelines Development Team (2001). The EPIC Project: developing national evidence-based guidelines for preventing healthcare associated infections. *Journal Hospital Infection*. 47 (Suppl.): S1–S82.

Pratt R.J., Pellowe C.M., Wilson J.A., Loveday H.P., Harper P.J., *et al.* (2007). EPIC2: national evidence-based guidelines for preventing healthcare-associated infections in NHS hospitals in England. *Journal of Hospital Infection*. 65 (Suppl. 1): S1–S64.

Rotter M.L. (1997). 150 years of hand disinfection: Semmelweis' heritage. *Hygiene and Medicine*. 22: 332–339.

Rotter M.L. (1999). Handwashing and hand disinfection. In: Mayhill C.G. (Ed.), *Hospital Epidemiology and Infection Control*. 2nd ed. Lippincott Williams and Wilkins, Philadelphia: 1339–1355.

Sax H., Allegranzi B., Uckay I., Larson E., Boyce J., *et al.* (2007). 'My Five Moments for Hand Hygiene': a user centred design approach to understand, train, monitor and report hand hygiene. *Journal of Hospital Infection*. 67: 9–21.

Stone S., Fuller C., Savage J., Cookson B., Hayward A. *et al.* (2012). Evaluation of the national Cleanyourhands campaign to reduce *Staphylococcus aureus* bacteraemia and *Clostridium difficile* infection in hospitals in England and Wales by improved hand hygiene: four year, prospective, ecological, interrupted time series study. *British Medical Journal*. 2012; 344: e3005. doi:10.1136/bmj.e3005

Taylor B.Z. (2006). Cutting surgical site infection rates for pacemakers and implantable cardioverter defibrillators. *Nursing*. 36: 18–19.

Taylor L. (1978). An evaluation of handwashing techniques – 1. *Nursing Times*. 74 (2): 54–55.

Trampuz A., Widmer A.F. (2004). Hand hygiene: a frequently missed lifesaving opportunity during patient care. *Mayo Clinic Proceedings*. 79 (1): 109–116.

World Health Organization (WHO) (2009a). *WHO Guidelines on Hand Hygiene in Health Care: First Global Patient Safety Challenge, Clean Care Is Safe Care*. World Health Organization, Geneva.

World Health Organization (WHO) (2009b). *Hand Hygiene Technical Reference Manual*. World Health Organization, Geneva.

World Health Organization (WHO) (2012). *Hand Hygiene in Outpatient and Home-based Care and Long-term Care Facilities*. World Health Organization, Geneva.

13

Personal protective equipment

Contents

Fundamentals of Infection Prevention and Control: Theory and Practice, Second Edition. Debbie Weston.
© 2013 John Wiley & Sons, Ltd. Published 2013 by John Wiley & Sons, Ltd. Companion Website: www.wiley.com/go/fundamentalsofinfectionprevention

Introduction

Personal protective equipment (PPE) is defined as 'all equipment that is intended to be worn or held by a person at work and which protects them against one or more risks to health or safety' (Royal College of Nursing, 2012). With regard to infection prevention and control, the main purpose of wearing PPE (gloves, aprons, masks and eye protection) is to protect healthcare workers from blood-borne pathogens and prevent the transmission of microorganisms to both patients and staff. Unfortunately, the wheres and wherefores of PPE cause great confusion amongst healthcare staff, who are often discovered by Infection Prevention and Control Specialist Nurses to be wearing it inappropriately. This chapter aims to clarify when and how PPE should be worn and disposed of.

Learning outcomes

After reading this chapter, the reader will be able to:

- Understand when gloves, aprons and respiratory and facial protection should be worn.

- Understand the implications of not wearing or disposing of PPE correctly.

Personal protective equipment: risk assessment

The EPIC and NICE guidelines (Pratt *et al.*, 2001, 2007; National Clinical Guideline Centre, 2012) clearly state that the selection of personal protective equipment (PPE) must be based on a risk assessment of the risk of transmission of microorganisms to the patient or healthcare worker, and the risk of contamination with blood, body fluids, secretions and excretions or exposure to chemicals. Therefore, two simple questions need to be asked:

- What is the task that the healthcare worker is about to undertake?
- What is the risk of exposure to blood, body fluids, chemicals (e.g. when making up solutions) and infection?

PPE: common mistakes and important points

- The incorrect use of gloves and disposable plastic aprons (both under-use and over-use) can increase the risk of cross-infection to patients, and contaminate equipment and the environment.
- Putting on a disposable apron or a pair of gloves is often one of the first things that healthcare workers do in preparation for a task or patient care activity. It should actually **be the last thing that the healthcare worker does** before he or she attends to the task or patient.
- Disposable plastic aprons are obviously not sterile, but they are **clean** at the point at which they are put on. Healthcare workers will often put on a disposable apron; go to the patient's bedside (disappearing behind the curtains or into a side room) and then re-emerge wearing the apron; leave the bay or side room to go to the linen cupboard, store room or clean utility

room; then make a telephone call or use the computer, and then go back to the patient. The perception of the Infection Prevention and Control Nurse Specialist who happens to be passing by is that the healthcare worker has been undertaking some kind of intervention or interaction that necessitated the wearing of an apron, and is now walking around the ward in PPE that is contaminated. Even if the healthcare worker has not actually had any interaction with the patient, the fact that he or she has worn it to go to the linen cupboard or store room or to sit at the desk means that it is **no longer clean**; it should not have been worn outside of the patient's bed area, and it must be changed.

- Healthcare workers must not leave a bay or a side room wearing an apron and/or a pair of gloves **unless** there is an emergency **or** they are removing a bedpan or commode or carrying a urinal (PPE will provide protection from body fluid contact, and the wearing of PPE on leaving the patient's bedside in this instance is a continuation of that patient's care), or transporting dirty equipment to the sluice, in which case as soon as the task has been completed in the sluice, the PPE must be removed and hands decontaminated or washed.
- PPE dispensers must be located appropriately (e.g. outside bays and side rooms). Gloves and aprons should be available in the sluice for cleaning commodes and attending to 'dirty' tasks in the sluice, but not put on in the sluice and then worn to give direct patient care. Gloves should not be kept in bathrooms – they will become easily contaminated with faecal organisms such as *Clostridium difficile* spores (see Chapter 22) and norovirus (see Chapter 23).
- The wearing of gloves does not replace the need for hand hygiene, and wearing gloves inappropriately means that opportunities for hand decontamination are missed and the risk of cross-infection to patients is increased.

Fact Box 13.1   Gloves, universal (standard) precautions and latex allergy (see Chapter 8)

The introduction of standard precautions, or universal precautions, for healthcare workers in the 1980s for protection against blood-borne viruses (see Chapter 24) led to what the Health and Safety Executive (HSE) called an 'unprecedented demand' for the use of sterile and non-sterile latex examination gloves, and a significant increase in the number of healthcare workers with natural rubber latex (NRL) allergy (http://www.hse.gov.uk/skin/employ/latex.htm). Fifty percent of all cases of latex allergy are now reported in healthcare professionals (http://www.worldallergy.org/public/allergic_diseases_centre/latexallery/latexallery.php).

Disposable gloves are manufactured from both natural and synthetic materials, such as NRL, vinyl (polyvinyl chloride) and nitrile (acrylonite). While the protection offered by all gloves has the potential to fail if they are damaged or torn during use, polythene gloves can leak, and for this reason they are no longer used in healthcare (Pratt *et al.*, 2001).

Latex gloves have been popular because of their durability, their elasticity and the dexterity that this affords, and their low microbial and fluid penetration rate which offers all-important protection against blood-borne viruses (Pratt *et al.*, 2007; NHS Plus, Royal College of Physicians, and Faculty of Occupational Medicine, 2008). However, healthcare workers are at risk of developing contact dermatitis from prolonged glove use and/or over-use (see also Chapter 12). Powdered latex gloves are no longer used as part of PPE. Corn starch powder was traditionally introduced as a lubricant to facilitate the donning and removal of gloves, but the corn starch acts as a vector for the NRL proteins which leach into it, and when the gloves are removed the powder becomes airborne, increasing the level of latex powder and, if inhaled, triggering respiratory sensitisation (NHS Plus, Royal College of Physicians, and Faculty of Occupational Medicine, 2008; Royal College of Nursing, 2012). The National Patient Safety Agency (NPSA) and the HSE require Trusts to protect the health of their staff and patients with respect to exposure to latex and, consequently, to safeguard the safety of staff and patients; the use of latex gloves is now reduced to a minimum, used by those staff who are designated 'essential users', where fit and dexterity cannot be equalled by an alternative product.

Box 13.1 and Table 13.1 provide examples of when sterile and non-sterile gloves should be worn.

Figure 13.1 illustrates the correct procedure for donning (putting on) and removing non-sterile gloves.

Box 13.1   Indications for the use of sterile or non-sterile gloves

Healthcare workers wear gloves to protect themselves **and/or** to protect the patient. Gloves:

- Provide a physical, protective barrier, protecting the healthcare worker's hands (skin) from coming into direct contact with blood, body fluids (e.g. urine, faeces or vomit) and microorganisms.
- Provide protection for healthcare workers' hands when they come into contact with chemicals (e.g. when making up cleaning solutions, decontaminating endoscopes, or preparing cytotoxic drugs).
- Prevent the transmission of microorganisms from healthcare workers to patients during invasive procedures.
- Protect the healthcare worker from injury resulting from exposure to chemicals as part of Control of Substances Hazardous to Health (COSHH) measures.

This means that they must be worn (either on their own or in conjunction with other PPE):

- for invasive procedures
- for contact with sterile body sites
- for contact with non-intact skin
- for contact with mucous membranes
- where there is a risk of exposure to or contact with blood and/or body fluids
- where there is a risk of exposure to or contact with microorganisms
- when handling sharp or contaminated instruments
- when handling chemicals or drugs where the COSHH certificate states that gloves must be worn.

See also: WHO, 2009.

Table 13.1   When sterile or non-sterile gloves are required

When to wear sterile gloves	Any type of surgical procedure, including taking biopsies, lumbar puncture, insertion of central lines, urinary catheterisation, vaginal examination in obstetric patients and vaginal delivery
When to wear non-sterile gloves	**Contact with blood, body fluids, chemicals or infection**: For example, with patients known or suspected to be colonised or infected (e.g. in a cohort bay or isolation side room); for cannulation, venepuncture, removal of vascular access devices, vaginal examination in non-obstetric patients, rectal examinations, urinary catheter removal, taking a catheter specimen of urine (CSU), obtaining a clinical specimen or IV drug administration; as part of wound care procedures or endotracheal suctioning; during insertion, aspiration or removal of a naso-gastric tube; when administering suppositories and enemas; when emptying urinals, bed pans and vomit bowls; when changing incontinence pads and nappies, emptying or changing stoma bags, handling or cleaning instruments, handling clinical waste bags, cleaning up blood or body fluid spills and handling soiled bed linen or clothing; and during eye care (if infection present)

Gloves are not routinely required for: contact with patients **unless** in a cohort bay or isolation side room; washing or bathing patients (**unless** there is contact with blood or body fluids); bed making; removal of bed linen (**unless** visibly soiled); assisting patients with mobility; entering an isolation side room **unless** patient contact is anticipated; moving patient equipment and furniture (**unless** it is visibly soiled); pushing theatre trolleys, mortuary trolleys and wheelchairs; taking or recording vital signs; placing patients on oxygen or non-invasive ventilation, or inserting nasal cannula; and giving injections.
Note: The reason that gloves are not **routinely** required for the above tasks and activities is because hands are less likely to become heavily contaminated, and the microorganisms that **do** get picked up on the hands are easily removed through the use of alcohol hand rub, or washing with liquid soap and water if they are visibly soiled.

Aprons and gowns

Uniforms can become heavily contaminated during direct contact, and although there is little evidence to suggest that uniforms play a role in the spread of infection and contribute to HCAIs (Department of Health [DH], 2010), disposable plastic aprons protect the part of the healthcare workers uniform or clothing that is most in contact with the patient. Full-length fluid-repellent gowns offer a greater degree of protection against contamination from blood and body fluids. Box 13.2 and Table 13.2 list the indications for wearing aprons and gowns.

- Aprons must not be worn folded down at the waist.
- They must be worn as single-use items for one procedure or one episode of care. Therefore, they may need to be changed in between interventions on the same patient.

When the hand hygiene indication occurs before a contact requiring glove use, perform hand hygiene by rubbing with an alcohol-based handrub or by washing with soap and water.

I. HOW TO DON GLOVES:

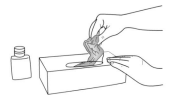

1. Take out a glove from its original box.

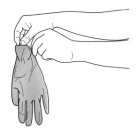

2. Touch only a restricted surface of the glove corresponding to the wrist (at the top edge of the cuff).

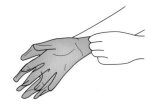

3. Don the first glove.

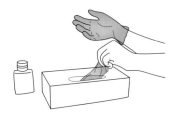

4. Take the second glove with the bare hand and touch only a restricted surface of glove corresponding to the wrist.

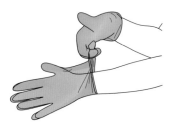

5. To avoid touching the skin of the foream with the gloved hand, turn the external surface of the glove to be donned on the folded fingers of the gloved hand, thus permitting to glove the second hand.

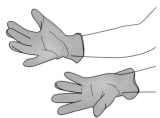

6. Once gloved, hands should not touch anything else that is not defined by indications and conditions for glove use.

II. HOW TO REMOVW GLOVES:

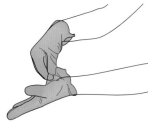

1. Pinch one glove at the wrist level to remove it, without touching the skin of the foream, and peel away from the hand, thus allowing the glove to turn inside out.

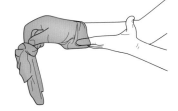

2. Hold the removed glove in the gloved hand and slide the fingers of the ungloved hand inside between the glove and the wrist. Remove the second glove by rolling it down the hand and fold into the first glove.

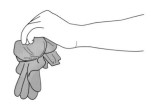

3. Discard the removed gloves.

4. Then, perform hand hygiene by rubbing with an alcohol-based handrub or by washing with soap and water.

Figure 13.1   How to don and remove non-sterile gloves (WHO, 2009).

Box 13.2   Indications for wearing aprons and gowns

Disposable plastic aprons must be worn when close contact with the patient, materials or equipment is anticipated and when there is a risk that clothing may become contaminated with pathogenic microorganisms or blood, body fluids, secretions or excretions (with the exception of perspiration) during healthcare interventions. They may be worn on their own or in conjunction with other PPE.

Full-body fluid-repellent gowns must be worn when there is a risk of extensive splashing of blood, body fluids, secretions or excretions onto the skin or clothing of healthcare personnel.

Table 13.2   When wearing aprons or gowns is required

When to wear disposable plastic aprons	Contact with patients in isolation side rooms or cohort bays (yellow, white or clear apron); venepuncture or cannulation; assisting with washing or bathing; changing dressings; assisting patients with using commodes or bed pans; cleaning commodes; emptying catheter drainage bags; cleaning or decontaminating equipment; changing soiled or contaminated linen; cleaning bathrooms or toilets, or general ward areas; and working in ward kitchens or serving patient food (according to NPSA colour coding – see Chapter 15)
When to wear full-length fluid-repellent gowns	Any situation or intervention where there is a risk of extensive contamination of the arms and uniform from blood and/or body fluids, such as surgery or invasive procedures, and childbirth

Disposable plastic aprons are not required for: routine contact with patients, such as when taking vital signs, assisting with mobility or giving oral medication or injections.

- They must be removed as soon as the patient care or intervention has been completed and **before** leaving the side room or bay **unless** the healthcare worker is taking a commode, a bedpan, a urinal or dirty equipment to the sluice.
- They must be disposed of as clinical waste.

Figure 13.2 illustrates the correct procedure for donning and removing a plastic apron.

Respiratory and facial protection: masks, goggles and visors (face shields)

While masks, goggles and visors are the less commonly used components of PPE, they are just as important in certain situations as aprons and gloves but they are not always worn appropriately.

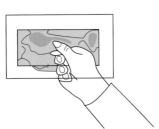

1. Remove a plastic apron from the dispenser.

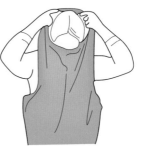

2. Put the apron on by slipping the neck end over the head.

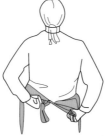

3. Secure the apron to the body by tying the waist ties.

Howe to safely remove a plastic apron

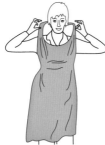

1. Grasp the sides of the apron at the top and pull to break the neck end gently and roll inwards.

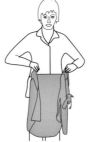

2. Grasp the sides of the apron (at waist level) and pull to break the waist ties, and gently roll plastic apron inwards.

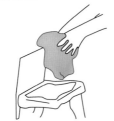

3. Remove from the body and discard into the waste bin.

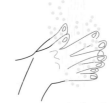

4. Decontaminate the hands.

Figure 13.2 How to wear and remove a plastic apron (Damani, 2012).

Box 13.3   Aerosol-generating procedures

Cardiopulmonary resuscitation (CPR)
Intubation or extubation
Non-invasive or continuous positive airway pressure ventilation (BIPAP/CPAP)
Sputum induction or chest physiotherapy
Suctioning
Bronchoscopy
Certain procedures within surgery or post-mortem where high-speed devices are used.

Source: Data from HPA, 2012a.

The mucous membranes of the eyes, nose and mouth are susceptible portals of entry for micro-organisms (Seigel *et al.*, 2007), and during certain patient care activities and interventions, they will be exposed to splashes or sprays of blood, body fluids and/or respiratory secretions or excretions.

Respiratory and facial protection offers the wearer protection against potentially infectious microorganisms in the air which may be in the form of:

- **Aerosols**: small suspensions of solid or liquid particles in air or gas that can travel short or long distances depending on their size, the speed with which they are generated (e.g. a cough versus a sneeze) and the environmental conditions (e.g. ventilation and air currents). Certain procedures within healthcare settings can generate aerosols (see Box 13.3).
- **Droplets**: larger than aerosols. They can remain suspended in the air for several minutes, and although large droplets will fall out of suspension within a few seconds, smaller droplets can evaporate to form droplet nuclei (see Chapter 21).
- **Splash particles**: larger than droplets. Blood and body fluids can be splashed or sprayed as an airborne mist during surgical procedures, or expelled violently if the patient experiences a sudden hematemesis (vomits blood), or if they hit a surface with any force.

Masks

Surgical face masks

Surgical face masks protect the healthcare worker by providing a barrier to splashes and droplets of blood and body fluids that may enter the nose, mouth and respiratory tract. They are not classed as respiratory PPE, but their use is recommended when caring for patients with confirmed or suspected seasonal influenza (not pandemic influenza) or other respiratory tract infections if the healthcare worker is in close contact with the patient (defined as within three feet or one meter) (HPA, 2012a). They must also be worn when dealing with spillages of faeces or vomit during norovirus outbreaks if there is a risk of splashing (HPA, 2012b). They should be fluid repellent, are single-use items, are not designed to be worn for prolonged periods and must be changed when they become damaged or wet (DH, 2009; HPA, 2012a). Although there is a metal strip that is flexed so that a mask fits across the bridge of the wearer's nose, surgical face masks are not tight-fitting and they do not mould to the face. They need to be secured tightly around the back of the head to ensure that the fit is as close as possible.

Respiratory protection

Masks worn to protect the respiratory tract have to conform to European Standard EN149:2001, which is the European Respiratory Protection Standard for disposable filtering respirators which are worn as face masks covering the nose, mouth and chin and filter particles, including bacteria and viruses.

Filtering face piece (FFP) class 3 disposable respirators (FFP3 masks) offer healthcare workers the highest level of respiratory protection (HPA, 2012a; National Clinical Guideline Centre, 2012), reducing exposure to infectious particles by at least a factor of 20 if the respirator is fitted properly, and should be worn when undertaking aerosol-generating procedures or caring for patients with multidrug-resistant tuberculosis (see Chapter 21), pandemic or avian influenza, severe acute respiratory syndrome (SARS) or novel coronaviruses (see Chapter 5).

Fact Box 13.2   Fit testing

Healthcare workers have to undergo fit testing for FFP3 masks, to ensure that the respirator is a suitable and close fit for the shape of their face and that there are no gaps under or around the mask for unfiltered air to pass through. Fit testing is a trained procedure, and it is the responsibility of the Occupational Health Department to ensure that it is undertaken. The respirator will need fit checking each time one is worn to ensure that it is providing an effective seal and that there are no leaks under or around the mask. Guidance on fit testing and fit checking is available on the DH website at:

http://www.dh.gov.uk/PublicationsandStatistics/Publications/PublicationsPolicyAnd Guidance/DH_110792.

Table 13.3 lists 'do's and don'ts' with regard to the wearing of masks and respirators.

Table 13.3   Masks and respirators: do's and don'ts

Masks and respirators must	Masks and respirators must not
• Be put on immediately before they are required. • Be disposed of as clinical waste in the side room, bay or procedure room **unless** the patient has a respiratory infection, in which case they must be removed **after** leaving the room and disposed of in the nearest clinical waste bin. • Be securely tied in the case of **surgical masks**, using the head straps, and the metal strip must be firmly moulded to the bridge of the nose. • Be fit-checked in the case of FFP3 respirators (having had an initial fit test). • Be changed as required. Surgical face masks will lose any protection when they become wet. FFP3 masks can be worn for up to eight hours of continuous care.	• Be re-used. • Be worn outside of the side room, procedure room or bay **unless** the patient has a respiratory infection, in which case they must be removed after leaving the room. • Be worn dangling around the healthcare worker's neck.

Fact Box 13.3   A cautionary note: The SARS outbreak and the implications of the incorrect use of respiratory PPE and compliance with standard precautions

In March 2003, staff at all hospitals in Ontario, Canada, had been instructed to implement SARS-specific infection control precautions, which included the wearing of personal protective equipment and clothing, using dedicated or disposable equipment, and hand washing in between patient contacts, to halt the progression of SARS among healthcare workers. However, between 28 March when these precautions were implemented and 24 April, 17 cases of probable SARS were seen among healthcare workers at six different hospitals in Toronto. The affected staff were interviewed, and it became apparent that there had been breaches in infection control practice and that compliance was inconsistent. Examples included failure to wear personal protective clothing and equipment, including respiratory protection, some of which was not fit-tested, and failure to dispose of contaminated respiratory equipment and protective clothing appropriately or change it in between patients; failure to decontaminate hands in between patient contacts, after removing gloves and aprons or after handling contaminated equipment; re-using items of equipment that should have been either disposed of after use or decontaminated; and having direct contact with respiratory secretions from SARS patients while failing to wear protection against respiratory droplets. There were other contributing factors. Staff were exhausted from caring for so many patients with SARS, and they took shortcuts. They were confused about the use and removal of personal protective clothing and equipment, which some staff found time-consuming. Staff working in dedicated SARS units, emergency departments and intensive care units were expected to wear protective clothing and respirators throughout their shift, and many reported experiencing nausea, dizziness and shortness of breath when wearing respirators for long hours. Infection control training was felt to have been inadequate.

Source: Data from Ofner-Agnostini *et al.*, 2006.

Goggles and visors

Facial protection in the form of wrap-around goggles and visors or face shields protects the conjunctiva (the thin mucous membrane which covers the white part of the eye [the sclera] and the inside of the eyelid) from splashes and droplets of blood, body fluids and chemicals. They should be worn when any splashing of blood or body fluids is anticipated (e.g. taking patients on and off haemodialysis, or manually cleaning endoscopes prior to placing them in the automated washer disinfector). Ordinary glasses, safety glasses or contact lenses are not suitable substitutes for proper facial protection.

The order of donning and removing PPE

The correct order of donning and removing PPE can be just as important as wearing PPE in the first place, particularly removing it in order to avoid contamination (see Box 13.4).

Box 13.4   The order of donning and removing full PPE

Donning full PPE
Apron
Mask
Eye protection
Gloves

Removing full PPE
Gloves
Apron
Eye protection
Mask

Reflection point

Look at PPE use within your clinical area. What examples of poor PPE use can you see? Is it all staff groups? How is inappropriate PPE use dealt with?

Chapter summary: key points

- PPE is an integral component of standard precautions, but it is often used inappropriately.

- The incorrect use of gloves and disposable plastic aprons (both under-use and over-use) can increase the risk of cross-infection to patients, and contaminate equipment and the environment.

- The selection of protective equipment must be based on a risk assessment of the risk of transmission of microorganisms to the patient or healthcare worker, and the risk of contamination with blood, body fluids, secretions and excretions or exposure to chemicals.

- Staff have a responsibility to ensure that they wear and dispose of PPE appropriately.

- Gloves and aprons must be worn as single use items.

Continued

- Hands must be decontaminated before putting on and after removing gloves.

- The wearing of gloves is not a substitute for handwashing.

- Gloves must not be worn all of the time or for routine activities.

- Gloves and disposable aprons must be changed in between patients, and in between care activities on the same patients.

Further resources are available for this book, including interactive multiple choice questions. Visit the companion website at:

www.wiley.com/go/fundamentalsofinfectionprevention

References

Department of Health (2009). *Pandemic (H1N1) 2009 Influenza. A Summary of Guidance for Infection Control in Healthcare Settings*. Department of Health, London.

Department of Health (2010). *Uniforms and Workwear: Guidance on Uniforms and Workwear Policies for NHS Employers*. Department of Health, London.

Health Protection Agency (2012a). *Infection Control Precautions to Minimise Transmission of Respiratory Tract Infections (RTIs) in the Healthcare Setting*. Health Protection Agency, London.

Health Protection Agency (2012b). *Guidelines for the Management of Norovirus Outbreaks in Acute and Community Health and Social Care Settings*. Health Protection Agency, London.

National Clinical Guideline Centre (2012). *Infection: Prevention and Control of Healthcare-Associated Infections in Primary and Community Care*. National Institute for Health and Clinical Excellence, London.

NHS Plus, Royal College of Physicians and Faculty of Occupational Health Medicine (2008). *Latex Allergy: Occupational Aspects of Management: A National Guideline*. Royal College of Physicians, London.

Ofner-Agnostini M., Gravel D., McDonald C., Lem M., Sarwal S. *et al*. (2006). Cluster of cases of severe acute respiratory syndrome among Toronto healthcare workers after implementation of infection control precautions: a case series. *Infection Control Hospital Epidemiology*. 27 (5): 473–483.

Pratt R.J., Pellowe C.M., Loveday H.B., Robinson M., Smith G.W. and the EPIC Guidelines Development Team (2001). The EPIC Project: developing national evidence-based guidelines for preventing healthcare associated infections. *Journal of Hospital Infection*. 47 (Suppl.): S1–S82.

Pratt R.J., Pellowe C.M., Wilson J.A., Loveday H.P., Harper P.J., *et al*. (2007). *EPIC2: national evidence-based guidelines for preventing healthcare-associated infections in NHS hospitals in England*. http://www.epic.tvu.ac.uk/Downloads/ (accessed 26 February 2013)

Royal College of Nursing (2012). *Tools of the Trade: RCN Guidance for Health Care Staff on Glove Use and the Prevention of Contact Dermatitis*. Royal College of Nursing, London.

Seigel J.D., Rhinehart E., Jackson M., Chiarello L. and the Healthcare Infection Control Practices Advisory Committee (HIPAC) (2007). *2007 Guidelines for Isolation Precautions: Preventing Transmission of Infectious Agents in Healthcare Settings*. http://www.cdc.gov/ncidod/dhqp/pdf/isolation2007.pdf (accessed 26 February 2013)

World Health Organization (2009). *Glove Use Information Leaflet*. World Health Organization, Geneva.

14

The safe handling and disposal of sharps

Contents

Introduction

Healthcare workers are exposed to blood-borne viruses (see Chapter 24) every day through the handling of clinical waste, contact with blood and other high-risk bodily fluids, procedures such as cannulation and venepuncture, and surgery. Sharps or needlestick injuries (also known as inoculation injuries) are the most frequent occupational hazard faced by healthcare workers in hospital and community settings, as well as other individuals. This chapter examines the causes of sharps injuries. Best-practice recommendations for preventing sharps injuries are described, including the use of safety devices in accordance with the European Directive.

Learning outcomes

After reading this chapter, the reader will be able to:

- Understand the different devices that constitute 'sharps'.

- Be able to identify the four key moments during clinical activity when sharps injuries are likely to occur.

- Understand the implications of sharps injuries for healthcare workers and the organisation.

- Understand best-practice recommendations for the prevention of sharps injuries in clinical practice.

The incidence of sharps injuries

Sharps injuries, or needlestick injuries, are one of the most serious health and safety threats in European workplaces, estimated to cause one million injuries each year, and in a National Audit Office (NAO) Report published in 2003, sharps injuries ranked second (behind manual handling) in the list of accidents to healthcare workers (NAO, 2003). Over 20 infectious diseases, including blood-borne viruses (BBVs), can be transmitted via contaminated sharps (http://www.hse.gov.uk/healthservices/needlesticks/index.htm), and between January 1997 and December 2007, the Health Protection Agency (HPA) reported 3773 blood-borne virus exposures in England, Wales and Northern Ireland, with sharps accounting for the most commonly reported exposure (Health and Safety Executive [HSE], 2012). The HPA (2008) reported that over one-third of all sharps injuries reported between 2000 and 2007 were preventable through adherence to standard precautions and the safe disposal of clinical waste. Box 14.1 lists the various devices and implements that constitute 'sharps', Box 14.2 lists the occasions when sharps injuries most commonly occur, and Box 14.3 lists the staff groups most at risk of sharps injuries in hospital, primary care and community care settings.

If the needle or sharp instrument is contaminated with blood or another body fluid, there is the potential for transmission of infection with blood-borne pathogens such as hepatitis B virus (HBV), hepatitis C virus (HCV) and human immunodeficiency virus (HIV).

Box 14.1   Sharps

Intravenous (IV) cannulae
Butterfly needles
Hypodermic needles
Phlebotomy needles
Lancets
Scalpels
Suture needles
Razors
Scissors
Tissues
Fragments of bone.

Source: Data from RCN, 2011.

Box 14.2   When sharps injuries occur

Sharps injuries occur when a needle or other sharp instrument accidentally penetrates the skin:

- During use
- After use and before disposal
- Between steps in procedures
- During disposal
- While re-sheathing or recapping a needle.

Source: Data from HPA, 2008.

Box 14.3   Staff at risk of sustaining sharps injuries

Hospital settings

- Nursing staff
- Medical staff
- Laboratory staff
- Mortuary staff
- Portering staff
- Cleaning staff
- Staff working within laundry services
- Other contracted staff.

Primary care and community care settings

- Nursing and medical staff attached to GP surgeries or health clinics
- Dentists
- District or community nursing staff
- Staff working in nursing or residential homes
- Police and security staff
- Prison officers and probation officers
- Youth workers
- Social workers
- Cleaning staff (within community care settings and the public sector)
- Refuse collectors
- Funeral directors
- Workers in body-piercing and body art (tattoo) shops.

Fact Box 14.1   Factors influencing the risk of infection following a percutaneous injury

- The depth of the injury
- The type of sharp (hollow-bore needles present the greatest risk)
- Whether the needle was in a vein or an artery
- The infectivity of the patient at the time of the injury.

The risk of BBV infection has been estimated at:

- 1 in 3 for HBV
- 1 in 30 for HCV
- 1 in 300 for HIV.

Source: UK Health Departments, 1998; RCN, 2011.

Exposure to blood-borne viruses through sharps-related injuries is largely preventable, and while healthcare workers have to accept responsibility for the sharps that they use, there is an extensive legal framework governing their safe use and disposal. Box 14.4 summarises the legal framework regarding the prevention of sharps injuries and inoculation injuries.

A significant exposure is classed as a percutaneous exposure to blood and body fluids from a source that is known to be, or as a result of the incident is found to be, HBV surface antigen (HBsAg), HCV or HIV positive (HPA, 2008) (see Chapter 24). Not only are healthcare workers at risk from injury from sharps, particularly needles and scalpel blades, but so too are patients if

Box 14.4   Preventing sharps injuries – the legal framework

The Health and Safety at Work Act 1974

Health and Safety (First Aid) Regulations 1981

The Health and Safety at Work Regulations 1991

Personal Protective Equipment Regulations 1992

The Provision and Use of Work Equipment Regulations 1992

Reporting of Injuries and Dangerous Diseases Regulations (RIDDOR) 1999

The Control of Substances Hazardous to Health (COSHH) Regulations 2002

The Health and Social Care Act 2008, *Code of Practice on the Prevention and Control of Infections and Related Guidance* (Department of Health, 2010) – relevant considerations from this Act regarding the safe handling and disposal of sharps include:

- Risk management and training in the management of mucous membrane exposure and sharps injuries and incidents
- Provision of medical devices that incorporate sharps protection mechanisms where there are clear indications that they will provide safe systems of working for staff
- A policy that is easily accessible and understood by all groups of staff
- Safe use, and secure storage and disposal, of sharps
- Auditing of compliance with policy.

sharps are inappropriately used and carelessly discarded (e.g. used needles left amongst the bedclothes, on bedside lockers or in sharps bins are easily accessible) (Medical Devices Agency, 2001).

In the United Kingdom, the Health Protection Agency Centre for Infections monitors significant occupational exposures and potential transmission of HIV, HCV and HBV from patients to healthcare workers through a national surveillance scheme (EPINet). Data are reported in the *Eye of the Needle* report, which is regularly updated and can be accessed at www.hpa.org.uk/Publications/InfectiousDiseases/BloodBorneInfections/EyeoftheNeedle.

Safety devices

In the United States in 2000, the Needlestick Safety and Prevention Act was introduced, requiring employers to implement safety devices as part of an ongoing strategy to reduce sharps injuries and promote safer working practices (http://www.osha.gov/needlesticks/needlefaq.htm).

In May 2010, the European Union (EU) Council in Brussels adopted a new EU directive (transposed into national law in each member state by May 2013) specifically designed to help prevent injuries and infections to healthcare staff from sharps such as needles and intravenous cannulae through the use of 'safety-engineered protection mechanisms', since numerous studies have demonstrated their key role in reducing needlestick injuries. The Directive confirms employers' responsibilities to protect their employees from sharps injuries, and compliance is mandatory.

Safety devices fall into two categories: those with a safety mechanism that the user is required to activate after use (active safety devices), and passive safety devices in which the safety mechanism automatically engages once the device has been used (e.g. self-retracting needles). As with all devices, there are numerous products available but not one that is recommended over all others. Determining which safety device(s) to implement requires the organisation of a comprehensive trial and evaluation involving key staff groups in order to determine user acceptability; failure to organise a trail increases the likelihood of the implementation being doomed to failure, making staff non-compliant with policy and at continued risk of sharps injuries, and the organisation non-compliant with the EU Directive and national guidance.

Reflection point

Have safety devices been implemented within your place of work? How was this achieved (e.g. did a Business Case need to be developed for funding, or was a product trial or user acceptability study undertaken)?

The Safer Needles Network and the Partnership for Occupational Safety and Health in Healthcare (POSHH) have agreed advice for the NHS on preparing for implementation of the sharps Directive (see www.saferneedles.org.uk), and the National Institute of Clinical Excellence (NICE) states that 'needle safety devices must be used where there are clear indications that they will provide safer systems of working for healthcare personnel' (National Clinical Guideline Centre, 2012). The *Code of Practice for the Prevention and Control of Healthcare Associated Infections* (Department of Health, 2010) and related guidance require NHS bodies to implement policies that encompass 'the provision of medical devices incorporating sharps protection mechanisms where there are clear indications that they will provide safe systems of working for healthcare workers'. A Report published by the RCN (2011) also concluded that safety-engineered devices are an effective means of reducing needlestick injuries. Their use is also supported by the HSE (www.hse.gov.uk), who have undertaken inspections of sharps safety and management in NHS Trusts in England, Scotland and Wales, and published an evaluation report on the efficacy of safety devices (HSE, 2012).

Boxes 14.5 and 14.6 summarise the best-practice recommendations for the prevention of sharps and inoculation injuries within the operating theatre environment and in general.

Box 14.5   Best practice recommendations: the prevention of sharps injuries in the theatre environment

- Eliminate any unnecessary use of sharp instruments and needles; use blunt-tipped needles and stapling devices where possible.
- Have no more than one person working in an open wound or body cavity at any time (unless it is essential to the safe and successful outcome of an operation).
- Use a 'hands-free' technique where the same sharp instrument is not touched by more than one person at the same time, and avoid hand-to-hand passing of sharp instruments during an operation.

Continued

- Use scalpels which are disposable, have retractable blades or incorporate a blade release device.
- Assure a safer passage of necessary sharp needles and instruments via a 'neutral zone', and announce when a sharp instrument or needle is placed there. The 'neutral zone' may be a tray, a kidney basin or an identified area in the operative field.
- Consider double gloving when the healthcare worker undertakes either an exposure-prone procedure (see Chapter 24) or one where glove punctures are likely.
- Ensure that scalpels and sharp needles are not left exposed in the operative field, but are always removed promptly by the scrub nurse, having been deposited in the neutral zone by the operator or assistant.
- Use instruments rather than fingers for retraction, and for holding tissues while suturing.
- Use instruments to handle needles and to remove scalpel blades.
- Direct sharp needles and instruments away from own non-dominant, or assistant's, hand.
- Remove sharp suture needles before tying suture; tie suture with instruments rather than fingers.
- Ensure that appropriately sized sharps containers are appropriately sited, for example in the anaesthetic room, on the anaesthetic trolley and in recovery.
- Ensure that there is a theatre rectangular container for the disposal of disposable instruments.

Source: UK Health Departments, 1998; Association of Surgical Technologists, 2006.

Box 14.6   General best-practice recommendations for the safe handling and disposal of sharps and the prevention of sharps injuries

- All clinical staff must receive education regarding sharps handling and disposal and the management and reporting of sharps injuries and BBV exposures on induction, and as part of mandatory infection control training thereafter.
- Compliance with the 'Sharps Policy' must be audited annually, and the results fed back to wards and departments. When standards are non-compliant, the Ward or Department Manager or other individual (e.g. the GP Practice Manager) must devise an action plan for implementation, and then practice and compliance must be re-audited against the action plan.
- Staff's understanding of the action to be taken in the event of a sharps injury or BBV exposure should be audited randomly by the Occupational Health Department and Infection

Prevention and Control Team, and educational campaigns held to raise awareness and promote safe practice.

- Staff working in primary and community care settings, and their Managers, must ensure that they are aware of their local 'Sharps Policy' and the action to be taken in the event of a sharps injury or BBV exposure. Unlike hospital-based staff, they may not have rapid and easy access to an Occupational Health or Emergency Department.
- Clear signage regarding sharps safety and the management of sharps injuries and BBV exposures should be displayed in clinical areas for easy reference and as a supplement to a more detailed 'Sharps Policy'.
- Sharps containers must be properly assembled; do not mix and match bases and lids from different makes or types of container. The date and time that the container was assembled must be recorded on the label, along with the name of the healthcare worker who assembled it. Once in use, the container has an expiry date of three months – if not two-thirds full by then, it must be sealed and discarded and a new container assembled.
- Sharps containers must never be filled above the fill line.
- Healthcare workers must never insert their hand into a container to retrieve a sharp, use the flat of their hand to forcefully close a container that is over-filled or attempt to force sharps into a container.
- Sharps must not be carried in the hands. Sharps containers with integral trays that can be taken to the patient at the point of care must be used in order that sharps can be disposed of by the user immediately following use.
- Where sharps containers are being transported by community staff (e.g. District Nurses), they must be sited safely and closure mechanisms used.
- Where sharps are used at the bedside, the healthcare worker using the sharp is responsible for ensuring that the sharp is properly disposed of and not left on the patient's bed, bedside table or locker or discarded into the domestic or clinical waste bin.
- Sharps must never be passed by hand.
- Needles and syringes must not be disassembled after use.
- Needles must not be re-sheathed after use.
- Do not dismantle infusion bags prior to disposal – wrap the giving set into the bag, and dispose of it as clinical waste.
- Containers must be stored away from the public, especially confused patients and small children. Where this is not practical and containers need to be accessible in clinical areas (e.g. wall mounted in Emergency or Minor Injuries Departments), the temporary closure mechanism must be used.
- Containers must not be stored on radiators, window sills or other areas where they can fall or be knocked off, or on the floor where they can be knocked over. Sharps brackets, clips and container stands should be used to secure them.
- Compliance with the use of safety devices must be monitored and audited, and additional staff training organised where appropriate.
- When sharps containers are being transported (e.g. taken for disposal), they must be held by the handle.

213

Reflection point

How compliant are staff with safe sharps practice within your place of work?

Chapter summary: key points

- Healthcare workers are exposed to blood-borne viruses every day through the handling of clinical waste, contact with blood and high-risk body fluids, procedures such as cannulation and venepuncture, and surgery.

- Sharps injuries are the most frequent occupational hazard faced by nurses, phlebotomists, doctors and other healthcare workers such as housekeeping, portering, laboratory and mortuary staff. Other individuals working in community settings are also at risk of injury or BBV exposure.

- Sharps present as one of the most serious health and safety threats in European workplaces, and are estimated to cause one million injuries each year.

- Sharps injuries have potentially serious implications for the individual affected and the employer or organisation.

- The person using the sharp is responsible for its safe disposal.

- The use of safety devices to prevent sharps injuries will be mandatory in 2013.

- Sharps injuries can be prevented if staff adhere to best-practice principles regarding the handling and disposal of sharps.

214

 Further resources are available for this book, including interactive multiple choice questions. Visit the companion website at:

www.wiley.com/go/fundamentalsofinfectionprevention

References

Association of Surgical Technologists (2006). *Recommended Standards of Practice for Sharps Safety and the Neutral Zone*. http://www.ast.org/pdf/Standards_of_Practice/RSOP_Sharps_Safety_Neutral_Zone.pdf (accessed 21 March 2013)

Department of Health (DH) (2010). *Code of Practice on the Prevention and Control of Infections and Related Guidance*. Department of Health, London.

Health Protection Agency (HPA) (2008). *Eye of the Needle: UK Surveillance of Significant Exposure to Bloodborne Viruses in Healthcare Workers*. Health Protection Agency, London.

Health and Safety Executive (HSE) (2012). *An Evaluation of the Efficacy of Safer Sharps Devices: Systematic Review*. Health and Safety Executive, London.

Medical Devices Agency (2001). *Safe Use and Disposal of Sharps*. SN 200 (19). Medical Devices Agency, London.

National Audit Office (2003). *A Safer Place to Work. Improving the Management of Health and Safety Risks to Staff in NHS Trusts*. Report by the Comptroller and Auditor General. HC 623 Session 2002–2003, 30 April. National Audit Office, London.

National Clinical Guideline Centre (2012). *Partial Update of NICE Clinical Guideline 2. Infection: Prevention and Control of Healthcare Associated Infections in Primary and Community Care*. National Institute for Health and Clinical Excellence, London.

Royal College of Nursing (RCN) (2011). *Sharps Safety: RCN Guidelines to Support Implementation of the EU Directive 2010/32/EU on the Prevention of Sharps Injuries in the Healthcare Sector*. Royal College of Nursing, London.

UK Health Departments (1998). *Guidance for Clinical Health Care Workers: Protection against Infection with Blood-borne Viruses. Recommendations of the Expert Advisory Group on AIDS and the Advisory Group on Hepatitis*. UK Health Departments, London.

15

Cleaning

Contents

Fundamentals of Infection Prevention and Control: Theory and Practice, Second Edition. Debbie Weston.
© 2013 John Wiley & Sons, Ltd. Published 2013 by John Wiley & Sons, Ltd. Companion Website: www.wiley.com/go/fundamentalsofinfectionprevention

Introduction

Concerns regarding hospital cleanliness have frequently hit the headlines over the last decade, with a general lack of public confidence that hospitals are clean and with healthcare-associated infections such as MRSA and *Clostridium difficile* largely, although not solely, attributed to dirty hospital wards. Cleaning is one of the most important tasks in any healthcare setting, and keeping the environment clean is a challenge for cleaning staff. However, the responsibility does not rest solely with them; all healthcare staff have a role to play in keeping the environment and equipment clean.

This chapter does not discuss the different methods of cleaning, although it does refer to new cleaning technology. Instead, its intention is to provide an overview of the importance of environmental cleanliness, including the cleaning of patient equipment, and encourage healthcare staff to consider their role in it. It begins by setting out the responsibilities of staff for ensuring that patients are cared for in a clean environment, as stipulated in the *Code of Practice on the Prevention and Care of Infections and Related Guidance* (Department of Health, 2010), and looking at the factors that can impede effective cleaning. Examples of environmental contamination with specific pathogens are given, along with the importance of cleaning frequent 'hand-touch' surfaces. Reference is made to the NHS Cleaning Standards and colour coding, and the cleaning of beds, commodes, mattresses and patient equipment, along with the cleaning of isolation side rooms, bays and wards.

217

Learning outcomes

After reading this chapter, the reader will:

- Understand their role and responsibilities with regard to environmental cleanliness and the cleaning of equipment.

- Understand the role that contamination of the environment and equipment can play in the spread of HCAIs.

- Know what 'hand-touch' surfaces are and why it is important that they are cleaned frequently.

- Understand the importance of cleaning items such as beds, mattresses and commodes.

Cleaning and the Health and Social Care Act 2008

The *Code of Practice for the Prevention and Control of Infections and Related Guidance* (Department of Health [DH], 2010) makes the following statements regarding cleanliness within the healthcare environment, and compliance is assessed by the Care Quality Commission:

- Registered providers must provide and maintain a clean and appropriate environment in managed premises that facilitates the control of infections.
- Matrons or persons of similar standing have personal responsibility for delivering a safe and clean care environment.
- The nurse or other person in charge of any patient or resident area has direct responsibility for ensuring that cleanliness standards are maintained throughout that shift.
- The cleaning arrangements detail the standards of cleanliness required in each part of its premises and that a schedule of cleaning frequency is available on request.
- There are effective arrangements for the appropriate cleaning of equipment that is used at the point of care, for example hoists, beds and commodes; these should be incorporated within appropriate cleaning, disinfection and decontamination policies.

Reflection point

Within your workplace

Who monitors cleaning standards on a daily basis?
What is the local escalation procedure in the event of any problems with cleaning?
Is a cleaning schedule on display?
Are there defined responsibilities for the cleaning of equipment amongst nursing and domestic services staff?

Cleaning is the process that physically removes contamination, which is the soiling of inanimate objects with organic material such as blood and body fluids, along with dirt and dust.

Fact Box 15.1   Skin squames and dust

We shed approximately 300 million flakes of dead skin, known as skin squames, into the air each day, and during periods of activity, we may shed 10 000 per minute (Noble, 1975: Wilson, 2006); 10% of these skin squames may contain viable microorganisms which can settle onto equipment and potentially contaminate the environment. Human skin cells (which are grey in colour when shed) are one of the major components of dust, along with human and animal hair, pollen and fibres from textiles and paper. Lots of grey dust in the environment = lots of skin squames!

Cleaning reduces the bacterial bio-burden (the number of bacteria residing on an item) by removing, but not destroying, up to 80% of microorganisms from the surface of the item that is being cleaned. Cleaning is not the sole responsibility of domestic services staff – **all** healthcare staff have an equally important role to play in making sure that the patient environment and patient equipment are kept clean. Box 15.1 identifies some of the factors that can impede effective cleaning.

Box 15.1   Factors that can impede effective cleaning

Poor cleaning technique, which will distribute dirt rather than remove it
Dirty cleaning equipment that is not cleaned after use and stored appropriately
Cluttered work surfaces and other surfaces such as window sills and ledges
Untidy store rooms and items not stored above floor level
Insufficient storage
Healthcare staff not taking responsibility for cleaning
Walls that are not intact (holes, gouges etc.) or not washable
Flooring that is not washable, not intact, and not impervious
Poor-quality finishes to floors, work surfaces and cupboards
Pipes and cable work that are not boxed in
Bedside furniture that is not intact (e.g. chipped bedside tables and lockers, worn wooden arms on bedside chairs, and chair seats or foot stools where covers are not intact and/or are not impervious)

Whether or not environmental contamination can contribute to the transmission of micro-organisms and healthcare-associated infections is dependent upon the ability of the organism to survive on surfaces (hard surfaces, soft surfaces, materials and textiles), the frequency with which surfaces become contaminated (how often they are used or touched) and the extent of contamination (Boyce, 2007).

- It has been demonstrated that the area around the bed space of an MRSA-positive patient will be heavily contaminated with his or her own strain of MRSA (see Chapter 20), which can be acquired on the hands of healthcare staff from direct contact with the patient or the patient's environment, and then transferred to other patients and to equipment (Boyce et al., 1997; Boyce, 2007).
- Norovirus (see Chapter 23) can remain viable within the environment for up to 12 days (Cheesbrough et al. 1997), and contaminated fingers (hands of healthcare staff and patients) can transfer norovirus onto as many as seven clean surfaces (Baker et al., 2004).
- Given the explosive nature of diarrhoea, and the fact that patients with C. difficile (see Chapter 22) may secrete up to 10^9 organisms per gram of faeces (Johnson et al. 1990), there is a real risk of patient-to-patient transmission via the faecal-oral route if the environment becomes heavily contaminated.
- Multidrug-resistant organisms such as Acinetobacter spp. (see Chapter 10) and glycopeptide-resistant enterococci (GRE) can persist in the environment for days, and contaminate surfaces and medical equipment (Seigel et al., 2006) (see Fact Sheet 3.2 on the companion website).

Hand-touch surfaces (see Box 15.2) can present a particular challenge, as these are the surfaces with which both patients and healthcare staff have frequent contact and therefore are likely to become heavily contaminated with pathogens (Dancer, 2009). In outbreak situations, enhanced cleaning of these surfaces should be undertaken, but attention should be paid to them routinely, particularly where patients are nursed in isolation side rooms (Kundrapu et al., 2012). If healthcare

Box 15.2   Examples of hand-touch surfaces

Within the 'patient zone' (see Chapter 12)

- Call bells
- Bed controls
- Bed rails and cot sides
- Bedside chairs, tables and lockers
- Bedside patient equipment (intravenous [IV] stand, infusion pumps and monitoring equipment)
- Bedside curtains (these require changing following the transfer or discharge of a colonised or infected patient; staff should decontaminate their hands following contact with curtains).

Within the 'healthcare zone'

- Commode seats and arms
- Toilet seats and raised toilet seats
- Toilet hand rails
- Toilet flush handles
- Taps
- Door handles and push plates
- Telephones
- PC keyboards.

staff decontaminate their hands strictly in accordance with the 5 Moments for Hand Hygiene at moments 1 and 4 (before patient contact and after contact with the environment; see Chapter 12), then the risk of their hands being vectors for the carriage and transmission of microorganisms should be greatly reduced.

Cleaning standards

The *National Specifications for Cleanliness in the NHS*, which can be accessed at http://www.nrls.npsa.nhs.uk/resources, provide a framework for the cleaning standards and the delivery of cleaning services. There are 49 element standards, covering **all**:

- Walls
- Flooring
- Patient equipment
- Furnishings, fixtures and fittings (including appliances)
- Fixed assets (e.g. sockets, light switches and mirrors)
- Fixtures and appliances in kitchens and bathrooms.

The standard statement for all elements is essentially the same: '**all parts** . . . should be visibly clean, with no blood and body substances, dust, dirt, debris or spillages'. This includes the removal of residue such as adhesive tape and limescale. 'All parts' includes the underside of items.

Reflection point

Select some of the items listed here that are applicable to your workplace. Are they clean to the standard described in this chapter? Who is responsible for cleaning each of these items?

- Bed frames, couches, trolleys and incubators
- Wheelchairs
- Bedside tables, lockers, chairs and footstools
- Bedside lights
- Controls for the bed
- IV stands and infusion pumps
- Monitors
- Ventilators, haemodialysis machines and anaesthetic machines
- Telephones
- PCs (monitor, screen, keyboard, mouse and mobile stand for computers on wheels)
- Electric fans
- Stethoscopes
- Alcohol hand rub and soap dispensers
- Personal protective equipment (PPE) and paper towel dispensers
- Notes trolley
- Linbins in store rooms and shelving
- Sharps trays
- Aseptic non-touch technique (ANTT) trays and dressing trolleys
- Equipment trolleys
- Glucometers and blood gas analysis machines
- Macerator and bedpan washer
- Wash hand basins and taps.

Fact Box 15.2   Cleaning and colour coding

In 2007, the National Patient Safety Agency issued a Safer Practice Notice announcing the development of a national colour-coding scheme for hospital cleaning materials and equipment (National Patient Safety Agency, 2007), whereby differently coloured disposable plastic aprons, cloths, buckets and mop handles are worn or used by cleaning staff depending on which area is being cleaned.

Red: bathrooms, washrooms, showers, sinks, toilets and floors
Blue: general areas within wards and departments, including offices and sinks
Green: catering departments, ward kitchens and when serving patient food in wards
Yellow: isolation areas.

Reflection point

Is a poster depicting the National Colour Coding Scheme clearly displayed within your place of work? Do staff adhere to it?

Decontaminating beds and commodes

Beds

Hospital beds, which have evolved over the years to become rather complex items with undercarriages, hydraulics and various attachments, are classed as medical devices and are the most frequently used pieces of equipment in hospitals. Not surprisingly, given the constant pressure on their use, they are often inadequately decontaminated in between patients (Patel, 2005; Creamer and Humphreys, 2008). Thoroughly decontaminating a bed in the middle of a busy ward with a bucket of Chlor-Clean or other disinfectant is not particularly easy to do to a high standard, and although wiping the frame and other components with a disinfectant wipe will remove surface dirt and is quick and easy to do in between patients, neither method is particularly satisfactory. Many hospitals have made considerable investment in purchasing dedicated bed decontamination units, where beds are taken off of the ward and put through an automated bed washer. Where money and space are issues, dedicated bed-cleaning teams have been implemented; beds are taken off the ward and replaced with an already clean bed, and the 'dirty' bed is then steam-cleaned.

Fact Box 15.3   Mattresses

The Medicines and Healthcare Products Regulator Agency (MHRA) issued a Medical Device Alert (MDA) in 2010, warning of the risk of cross-infection from contaminated mattresses. The Alert and its accompanying poster can be viewed at http://www/mhra.gov.uk/Publications/Safetywarnings/MedicalDeviceAlerts/CON065783.

Systems should be in place to ensure that mattresses are checked (audited) frequently, and that there is documentary evidence that this has been undertaken. The MDA and poster detail how the integrity of mattress covers and their foam cores must be checked.

Commodes

Commodes have been implicated as vehicles of cross-infection in *C. difficile* outbreaks, as they will become heavily contaminated with spores, and one study states that a single commode contaminated with *C. difficile* was the source of cross-infection to eight patients in the space of one week (Cohen *et al.*, 2000). Commodes must be thoroughly decontaminated in between each episode of patient use by the healthcare worker who has removed it from the patient, using either a sporicidal wipe or a sporicidal solution. All areas of the commode must be thoroughly cleaned each time (lid, seat, bedpan rack, arms and arm rests, back rest, commode legs, wheels and foot plate), and this obviously involves turning the commode upside down in order to clean the underneath of the frame and the foot plate. If the commode has detachable arms, the 'arm housing' should also be cleaned. The commode should then be labelled as clean (with date, time and signature given). Commode cleanliness should be audited at least weekly on all wards.

Disinfectant wipes

Disinfectant wipes, which combine dirt removal with disinfection, have become increasingly common in recent years for the decontamination of hard surfaces and equipment. The mechanical action of wiping a surface removes surface dirt, by trapping it within the wipe and at the same time releasing disinfectant. The presence of dirt would otherwise form a barrier preventing the disinfectant from effectively coming into contact with the surface that is being cleaned. They are a boon for busy ward staff, making the cleaning of equipment such as infusion stands, infusion pumps, dynamaps, monitors and hoists quick and easy, and therefore staff are more likely to clean equipment in between patient use when the process is relatively effortless. Sporicidal wipes are also available for the routine cleaning of commodes, surfaces and equipment in isolation side rooms where patients have *C. difficile* infection.

An enormous array of wipes are available on the market, and it is important that the correct decision is made regarding the most suitable product and ensuring that it is fit for purpose; ideally, organisations should restrict themselves to using as few different makes as possible, as healthcare staff can all too easily become confused and mistakenly think that cleaning a piece of equipment with any wipe that is available will suffice (even confusing wipes that are used for patient skin cleansing with wipes for environmental cleaning). It is important that any decision to purchase wipes for the purposes of decontaminating equipment and surfaces involves the Infection Prevention and Control Team, as the efficacy of the wipe and its disinfectant and antimicrobial properties will need to be verified and the literature reviewed. Useful guidance on the selection and use of disinfectant wipes was published by the Royal College of Nursing in 2011.

The cleaning of equipment

The majority of equipment that is frequently used in wards and departments (e.g. dynamaps, infusion pumps and stands, pulse oximeters, electrocardiogram [ECG] machines, cardiac monitors, hoists and patslides) can be easily cleaned in between use with detergent or disinfecting wipes. Glucometers and sharps trays should also be cleaned in between use (blood spillages must be removed appropriately). More specialised equipment will need to be cleaned according to manufacturer's instructions or locally agreed protocols. Box 15.3 summarises some best-practice recommendations for the cleaning of equipment.

How clean is clean?

Determining whether something is clean or not can be difficult. Surfaces that have been cleaned should not feel gritty or grainy; there should not be a high dust burden (although fine dust particles will lightly accumulate within hours of cleaning taking place) and certainly no thick, grey dust; there should be no visible soiling or staining of surfaces, and no dirt or dust lurking in corners of

Box 15.3   Best practice: the cleaning of equipment

- Staff are responsible for cleaning patient equipment after it has been used and in between each patient use.
- Equipment that is connected to a patient or connected to an electrical socket must not be cleaned by cleaning staff.
- All equipment should be labelled after cleaning.
- Equipment that is not in use and that is kept in a store room or equipment cupboard can be cleaned once a week as long as it is covered with a plastic bag or sack and labelled. **Note**: If the item is connected to an electrical socket for charging, it should not be covered.
- Equipment that is used for storage (e.g. trollies and linbins) must be emptied regularly in order that they can be cleaned.

the floors, behind floors, underneath beds, on high surfaces or behind lockers. However, even if an area or an item of equipment looks to be visibly clean (and a visibly clean environment is important for patient perception), it is important to remember that for the most part, contamination will be invisible. This is why ensuring that cleaning standards are being adhered to is so important, and that the monitoring or auditing of cleaning is undertaken frequently.

Fact Box 15.4   New technology – adenosine triphosphate

New technologies such as the 3M Clean-Trace system, which received a level 1 recommendation from the Department of Health Rapid Review Panel in 2008, can be used to determine the effectiveness of cleaning. This system measures levels of adenosine triphosphate (ATP), a molecular compound common to all living things, from organic material through the process of bioluminescence. It does not differentiate between living and dead microorganisms, or between microorganisms and soiling, but it does highlight inadequate cleaning and can be a useful aid when teaching staff or auditing the effectiveness of cleaning.

Cleaning isolation side rooms, and deep cleaning bays and wards

Isolation side rooms and bed spaces in the open bay have to be cleaned following the discharge or transfer of colonised or infected patients (often referred to as an 'infection clean'). However, bays and entire wards also require a thorough clean, referred to as **deep cleaning**, for example following a case of suspected norovirus or *C. difficile* in an open bay, following a period of ward closure or periodically as part of the Trust's cleaning programme. This may involve the use of chemicals or cleaning solutions such as Chlor-Clean or chlorine dioxide, and/or steam cleaning. Some organisations have embraced new technology and decontaminate side rooms, bays or entire wards with hydrogen peroxide vapour (HPV).

Fact Box 15.5   New technology – hydrogen peroxide vapour

The use of HPV for cleaning in hospitals was given a level 1 recommendation by the Department of Health Rapid Review Panel. A mobile vapour generator fills the room or bay with HPV (often referred to as **fogging**), disseminating a layer of HPV over all exposed surfaces. When the HPV comes into contact with microorganisms, it oxidises bacterial cells and spores, inactivating them. It does not work in the presence of dust and organic matter, and all surfaces in the room need to be exposed. The area needs to be completely emptied of patients and staff and sealed off for the duration of the process, which can take up to 90 minutes for a single room, although Boyce *et al.* (2008) report that the process can take from 3 to 12 hours depending on the size of the area being decontaminated.

Box 15.4 lists the 'order of cleaning' within an isolation side room, with cleaning staff working from the top of the room down to the floor.

When the IP&CT request that a ward is to be deep-cleaned, it is important that there is co-operation between nursing and cleaning staff. Deep cleans are disruptive and if it is not possible to decant patients into an empty bay a bay at a time, or decant the entire ward, the clean needs to be planned. Boxes 15.5, 15.6 and 15.7 list the considerations that need to be taken into account when planning and carrying out a deep clean, and the order of cleaning.

Box 15.4   'Order of cleaning' of an isolation side room post patient discharge

- Curtains at the windows and around the bed must be removed before cleaning begins. (**Note**: where blinds are in situ at windows, they must be wiped over.)
- Clean air vents and lights.
- Clean walls to maximum hand reach height.
- Clean clinical wash hand basin, including towels and soap dispensers.
- Clean high and low surfaces (e.g. curtain rails, window sills, bumper rails, radiators, wall-mounted oxygen and suction, bedside lights, bedside entertainment system and patient call bell).
- Clean bedside locker and table.
- Clean bed frame and mattresses.
- Clean bedside alcohol hand rub dispensers, and dispensers outside the bay or single room.
- Clean hard furnishings (e.g. chairs and foot stools).
- Clean and label patient equipment.
- Clean the floor.
- Remake the bed.
- Hang clean curtains.

Box 15.5   Things to consider when planning a deep clean

- Patients who cannot be moved out of bed have to be identified before the clean starts.
- Any activities on the ward that might impede the progress of the deep clean should be identified before starting.
- Empty beds will need to be stripped of linen, and patient belongings bagged up to enable the bedside table and locker to be cleaned.
- Where patients cannot be moved out of bed, they will need to be transferred onto a clean bed so that both the bed frame and the base mattress can be cleaned, unless it is unsafe to do so (e.g. the patient is too ill).
- Isolation single rooms and cohort bays will have to be cleaned after other patient areas.
- Air vents and radiators must be cleaned. (**Note**: This may require the involvement of the Estates Department.)
- Electric fans must be cleaned, and may require dismantling.
- Bedside oxygen tubing and masks, suction tubing and suction catheters will need to be disposed of and replaced (this should be undertaken by Nursing staff).
- Extraneous items within the room or bay will need to be discarded (e.g. dressings and dressing packs).
- Bowls of fruit and opened packets of food (e.g. biscuits) should be discarded.
- Hoist slings must be sent for laundering if not single-patient use or disposable.
- All parts of bed frames must be thoroughly cleaned plus the base mattresses.
- Dynamic mattress systems must be cleaned according to local policy.
- PC monitors, screens, keyboards, stands and handheld mice must be cleaned according to local policy.
- All equipment that is connected to patients must be cleaned by Nursing staff; all other equipment should be cleaned by Cleaning staff according to local policy.
- Laminated posters and signs, including isolation door signs, must be wiped clean.

Box 15.6   Procedure for deep cleaning a ward

In each bay and single room

- Curtains at the windows and around the beds must be removed before cleaning begins. (**Note**: Where blinds are in situ at windows, they can be wiped over.)
- Clean air vents and lights.
- Clean walls and laminated notices.
- Clean high and low surfaces (e.g. curtain rails, window sills, bumper rails, radiators and pipe work, wall-mounted oxygen and suction, bedside lights, bedside entertainment system and patient call bell).
- Clean clinical wash hand basins, including towels and soap dispensers.
- Clean PPE dispensers (internal and external surfaces).
- Clean clinical and domestic waste bins (internally and externally).
- Clean bedside lockers and tables.

- Clean all parts of the bed frames and mattresses.
- Clean bedside alcohol hand rub dispensers, and dispensers outside the bay or single room.
- Clean soft furnishings (e.g. chairs and foot stools).
- Clean and label patient equipment.
- Clean the floor.
- Hang clean curtains.
- Remake the beds.

Box 15.7 Other areas of the ward to be included in a deep clean

- Nurses' station: desktops, telephones, work surfaces, computers, computer keyboards and computers on wheels (COWs)
- Utility and store room: cupboard tops, work surfaces, door frames, storage and linbins, and floor (**Note**: Any equipment in the store room must be cleaned and then labelled.)
- Linen room: shelves and flooring
- Sluice and dirty utility: macerator, commodes, cupboard tops, work surfaces, sink and sluice hopper, wall-mounted soap, towels and alcohol hand rub dispensers, and laminated signs and posters
- Toilets and bathrooms: all fixtures, fittings and floors
- Main ward thoroughfare, including any equipment listed here as well as visitor chairs, display racks and flooring.

227

Chapter summary: key points

- The *Code of Practice* (DH, 2010) clearly states that the nurse in charge of a patient area is responsible for ensuring that cleaning standards are maintained.

- All healthcare staff have an equally important role to play in making sure that the patient environment and patient equipment are kept clean.

- Contamination is often invisible, so it is important to ensure that cleaning standards are being adhered and that the monitoring or auditing of cleaning is undertaken frequently.

- Clutter impedes cleaning.

- Hand-touch surfaces are likely to become heavily contaminated with pathogens and require particular attention.

- Equipment must be cleaned after or in between use.

Further resources are available for this book, including interactive multiple choice questions. Visit the companion website at:

www.wiley.com/go/fundamentalsofinfectionprevention

References

Baker J., Vipond I.B., Bloomfield S.F. (2004). Effects of cleaning and disinfection in reducing the spread of norovirus contamination via environmental surfaces. *Journal of Hospital Infection*. 58 (1): 42–49.

Boyce J.M. (2007). Environmental contamination makes an important contribution to hospital infection. *Journal of Hospital Infection*. 65 (S2): 50–54.

Boyce J.M., Havill M.T., Otter J.A., McDonald C., Adams N.M. *et al*. (2008). Impact of hydrogen peroxide vapor room decontamination on *Clostridium difficile* environmental contamination and transmission in a healthcare setting. *Infection Control and Hospital Epidemiology*. 29 (8): 723–729.

Boyce JM., Potter-Bynoe G., Chenevert C., King T. (1997). Environmental contamination due to meticillin-resistant *Staphylococcus aureus*: possible infection control implications. *Infection Control and Hospital Epidemiology*. 18: 622–627.

Cheesbrough J.S., Barkess-Jones L., Brown D.W. (1997). Possible prolonged environmental contamination survival of small round structured viruses. *Journal of Hospital Infection*. 35 (4): 325–326.

Cohen S.H., Tang Y.J., Rahman D., Silva J. (2000). Persistence of an endemic (toxigenic) isolate of *Clostridium difficile* in the environment of a general medical ward. *Clinical Infectious Diseases*. 30: 952–954.

Creamer E., Humphreys H. (2008). The contribution of beds to healthcare-associated infection: the importance of adequate decontamination. *Journal of Hospital Infection*. 69 (1): 8–23.

Dancer S.J. (2009). The role of environmental cleaning in the control of hospital-acquired infection. *Journal of Hospital Infection*. 73: 378–385.

Department of Health (DH) (2010). *Code of Practice on the Prevention and Control of Infections and Related Guidance*. Department of Health, London.

Johnson S., Clabots C.R., Linn F.V., Olson M.M., Peterson L.R., Gerding D.N. (1990). Nosocomial *Clostridium difficile* colonisation and disease. *The Lancet*. 336 (8707): 97–100.

Kundrapu S., Sunkesula V., Jury L.A., Sitzlar B.M., Donskey C.J. (2012). Daily disinfection of high-touch surfaces in isolation rooms to reduce contamination of healthcare workers hands. *Infection Control and Hospital Epidemiology*. 33 (10): 1039–1042.

National Patient Safety Agency (2007). *Safer Practice Notice: Colour Coding Hospital Cleaning Materials and Equipment. January*. National Patient Safety Agency, London.

Noble W.C. (1975). Dispersal of skin microorganisms. *British Journal of Dermatology*. 93: 477–485.

Patel S. (2005). Minimising cross-infection and risks associated with beds and mattresses. *Nursing Times*. 101 (Suppl.): 52–53.

Royal College of Nursing (2011). *The Selection and Use of Disinfectant Wipes*. RCN guidance. Royal College of Nursing, London.

Seigel J.D., Rhinehart E., Jackson M., Chiarella L. and the Healthcare Infection Control Practices Advisory Committee (HICPAC) (2006). *Management of Multidrug-Resistant Organisms in Healthcare Settings*. Centers for Disease Prevention and Control, Atlanta, GA.

Wilson J. (2006). The epidemiology of infection and strategies for prevention. In: *Infection Control in Clinical Practice*. 3rd ed. Bailliere Tindall, London: 33–63.

Part Three

Clinical practice

16

The management of vascular access devices and the prevention of bloodstream infections

Contents

Fundamentals of Infection Prevention and Control: Theory and Practice, Second Edition. Debbie Weston.
© 2013 John Wiley & Sons, Ltd. Published 2013 by John Wiley & Sons, Ltd. Companion Website: www.wiley.com/go/fundamentalsofinfectionprevention

Introduction

'Vascular access devices' (VADs) is the broad term for the various indwelling devices that are inserted into the peripheral or central veins for the administration of intravenous (IV– i.e. within vein) therapy for therapeutic or diagnostic purposes (Cowley, 2004; Kelly, 2009). The management of VADs in general, from choosing the most appropriate device, to its placement, ongoing care and maintenance through to its removal, is extremely complex, and in hospital and community settings, patients with a variety of devices are sometimes cared for by nursing and medical staff with limited experience, skills and competency to manage them. However, VADs are associated with serious and potentially life-threatening complications, including infection, and the most severe of these is the acquisition of a bloodstream infection (BSI), which is acknowledged to be one of the most dangerous complications of healthcare that can occur (Pratt *et al.*, 2007).

Device-related infections are strongly associated with poor management of the device and are largely avoidable. The Department of Health (DH) (Pratt *et al.*, 2007), the Royal College of Nursing (RCN, 2010), the National Institute for Clinical Excellence (NICE) (National Clinical Guideline Centre, 2012) and the Centers for Disease Control and Prevention's Healthcare Infection Control Practices Advisory Committee (O'Grady *et al.*, 2011) have published extensive evidence-based best-practice guidance on the prevention of VAD-related infection in the United Kingdom and the United States, with the emphasis on the management of peripheral IV cannulae and central venous catheters (CVCs) in particular as these are the devices associated with the greatest risk of infection. The DH have published care bundles as part of the Saving Lives High Impact Interventions initiative to reduce the incidence of peripheral IV cannula infections, and central venous catheter and renal dialysis catheter–related BSIs (DH, 2007a,b,c). Participation in the Matching Michigan project, which was developed in the United States to reduce the incidence of central venous catheter bloodstream infections, and saved approximately 1500 lives in just 18 months, was lead in England by the National Patient Safety Agency between 2009–2011, and demonstrated a 60% reduction in CVC associated blood stream infections in adult Intensive Care Units (Bion *et al.*, 2012).

To cover the management of all VADs is beyond the scope of this book and therefore, although the different types of VADs are briefly covered and referred to within this chapter, the main focus is the infection control management of peripheral IV cannulae. **Note**: It is essential that healthcare workers understand that only staff who have been assessed as competent in the insertion and management of VADs should have contact with them. All healthcare organisations will have evidence-based best-practice guidelines for these devices, and in the majority of healthcare settings, both in acute care and within the community, there are now specialist Vascular Access Teams.

Learning outcomes

After reading this chapter, the reader will:

- Have a basic understanding of the different types of vascular access devices and the indications for their use.

- Understand the pathogenesis of cannula and catheter-related BSI (bacteraemia) and its significance.

- Understand the significance of phlebitis.

- Understand the best-practice principles for management of peripheral intravenous cannulae.

Table 16.1   Different types of vascular access devices

Peripheral venous cannulae	IV lines
Midlines	IV lines
Peripherally inserted central catheters	PICC lines
Skin-tunnelled valved central catheters	Groshong® lines
Skin-tunnelled non-valved central catheters	Hickman® lines
Acute central venous catheters	CVC lines
Implanted ports	Ports
Arterial lines	Arterial lines
Intra-osseous access	EZ-IO

Vascular access devices

It has been estimated that between 27% and 70% of patients require intravenous (IV) therapy (Macklin, 2003), and millions of peripheral IV catheters and central venous catheters (CVCs) are inserted annually in the United Kingdom and the United States (O'Grady *et al.*, 2011; Hadaway, 2012; National Clinical Guideline Centre, 2012). There are various types of vascular access devices (VADs) available (see Table 16.1).

The choice of VAD is dependent upon:

- the indication for insertion, for example the administration of antibiotics (intermittent infusion or bolus), drugs (e.g. insulin, heparin or inotropes), fluids (e.g. crystalloids or colloids), cytotoxic agents (chemotherapy) or nutrition (total parenteral nutrition [TPN])
- the type of blood vessel that it occupies (peripheral venous, central venous or arterial)
- whether short and temporary, long-term or permanent access is anticipated or required.

There are various factors or characteristics that are exclusive to VADs, and these include:

- The site of insertion (peripheral venous, peripheral central, subclavian, femoral or internal jugular)
- Whether the device is tunnelled or non-tunnelled. Tunnelled devices are tunnelled via an incision in order to distance the entry site into the blood vessel from the exit site on the skin, which provides a barrier to infection. They have a cuff partway along their length which is positioned inside the subcutaneous tunnel; tissue granulates around the cuff and has the dual role of reinforcing the barrier to infection and stabilising the catheter.
- Whether the device is cuffed or non-cuffed
- Whether the device is valved or non-valved (the valve opens inwards for blood aspiration and outwards for fluid administration, and remains closed when not in use)
- The number of lumens.

Box 16.1   Complications associated with vascular access devices

Mechanical phlebitis
Infective phlebitis
Thrombophlebitis
Thrombosis
Air embolism
Arterial puncture
Pain
Bleeding
Extravasation
Cardiac arrhythmia
Catheter malposition or migration
Venous spasm
Occlusion
Damage or fracture of the line.

The **right** VAD has to be placed at the **right** time in the **right** environment (for vessel health preservation; see www.vesselhealth.org). VADs are associated with numerous complications (see Box 16.2), some of which are potentially life-threatening, and it is essential that healthcare workers inserting and managing these devices are also competent in recognising and dealing with complications should they arise.

Peripheral venous cannulae

Peripheral cannulation is the most commonly performed invasive procedure in hospitals (Webster et al., 2007; Saini et al., 2011) and is a skilled procedure requiring a high level of competence, yet it is one of the most common procedures undertaken by junior doctors (Sado and Deakin, 2005). Peripheral venous cannulae are the most commonly inserted VAD (Kelly, 2009), and are suitable for short-term venous access of 1–6 days' duration.

Indications for use

- For emergency access
- The administration of IV fluids to prevent or correct dehydration
- The administration of blood and blood products
- The administration of antibiotics as a bolus injection or intermittent infusion
- Infusions of medication such as insulin, heparin and analgesia.

Given the risk of bacteraemia associated with peripheral venous cannulation, unnecessary cannulation should be avoided.

Reflection point

How many patients in your ward have a peripheral cannula in situ? Is the indication for cannula insertion clearly documented in the medical or nursing notes?

Midline catheter (IV line)

A midline is an open-ended line which is placed into a vein at the antecubital fossa or just above. It is approximately 20 cm long, can stay in for up to six weeks and can be shortened to suit the size of the patient. Midlines should be considered where IV therapy is likely to continue for in excess of six days, and they have the potential to provide continuous venous access for patients throughout the duration of the treatment episode, avoiding delays in both recovery and discharge from hospital. Where possible, patients should be considered and assessed for midline suitability at the earliest opportunity when optimum peripheral vein integrity is available. Midlines are also suitable for outpatient and home IV therapy services.

234 Indications for use

Placement of a midline should be considered for patients with difficult venous access and/or who:

- Require delivery of IV therapy (medication, fluids or blood products) with duration of more than six days
- Require regular blood samples
- Require IV therapy in the community.

Peripherally inserted central catheter (PICC line)

The peripherally inserted central catheter (PICC line) is a central vascular access device (CVAD) which is placed via the antecubital fossa using either the basilic or cephalic vein; the tip of the catheter is advanced into the central veins, and resides in the lower one-third of the superior vena cava. PICCs are rapidly becoming an acceptable alternative to traditional CVCs and tunnelled catheters, with the advantages of patient comfort, reduced insertion complications, reduced associated infection risks and ease of placement. PICCs have the potential to provide continuous venous access for patients throughout the duration of the treatment episode, avoiding delays in both recovery and discharge from hospital, and PICCs are also suitable for out-patient and home IV therapy services. However, although they are inserted peripherally, they should not be regarded as conventional peripheral cannulae (Pikwer et al., 2011).

Indications for use

- Where duration of IV therapy is likely to exceed six days, in either the hospital or the community setting.

Skin-tunnelled valved central catheter (Groshong® line)

A tunnelled CVC is an indwelling catheter residing within the superior vena cava. These catheters are tunnelled subcutaneously via an incision to distance the entry site into the vein from the exit site on the skin, providing a barrier to infection. They have a cuff partway along their length which is positioned inside the subcutaneous tunnel and within three to four weeks following insertion, tissue granulates around the cuff, reinforcing the barrier to infection and stabilising the catheter. The Groshong has a patented valve which opens inwards for blood aspiration and outwards for infusion, but remains closed when not in use, sealing the fluid inside the catheter and preventing it from coming in contact with the patient's blood. Weekly flushing with saline keeps the catheter patent.

Indications for use

- The delivery of TPN and chemotherapy.

Skin-tunnelled non-valved central catheter (Hickman®)

Like Groshong lines, a Hickman line is an indwelling catheter within the superior vena cava, tunnelled via an incision to distance the entry site into the vein from the exit site on the skin. Hickman lines also have a cuff partway along their length. Non-valved Hickman lines are used primarily within the haematology setting.

Indications for use

- Double-lumen lines are used for general haematology.
- Triple-lumen lines are required for patients undergoing a stem cell or bone marrow transplant at a specialist hospital.

Central venous catheters

CVCs are inserted into the central veins, with the distal tip residing in the lower thirds of either the superior vena cava or the right atrium. Insertion into the subclavian vein is preferable to the internal jugular or the femoral vein due to the risk of contamination of the entry site. The internal jugular site is susceptible to potential contamination from oral-pharyngeal secretions and is difficult to access, and the femoral area carries an increased risk of contamination from genital or bowel flora.

Indications for use

Short-term CVCs are suitable for therapy or treatment of between one and three weeks' duration and for the measurement of central venous pressure in acutely ill patients.

Implanted ports

Implanted ports are totally implantable venous access devices designed to provide repeated access to the venous system. They consist of a reservoir attached to a catheter and are designed to deliver IV therapy centrally, with the tip residing in the lower third of the superior vena cava.

The port is accessed by puncturing the skin covering the reservoir with a huber, or gripper, needle, through which treatment is delivered (Kelly, 2009). Using correct management techniques, the port can remain in situ indefinitely and the reservoir can be punctured up to 2000 times (Kelly, 2009).

Indications for use

- For the delivery of IV therapy and blood sampling.

Arterial lines

Arterial lines are generally inserted in patients requiring intensive or cardiac care. The radial artery is the preferred site for placement as it is associated with fewer complications.

Indications for use

- Invasive arterial blood pressure recording and frequent arterial blood sampling in critical care patients.

Intra-osseous (IO) access

IO devices should be used only in an emergency, such as life-threatening trauma, where traditional peripheral venous access is difficult or impossible and emergency central venous access is essential but difficult due to the nature of the injuries sustained by the patient and the degree of shock and vasoconstriction (Lowther, 2011). Depending on the type of IO device used, they are inserted into the sternum, the proximal or distal tibia or the proximal humerus, where a network of 'canals' provides access to the central circulation (Day, 2011). They should be left in situ for no longer than 24 hours and must be removed as soon as traditional venous access has been established.

Indications for use

- Emergency vascular access in life-threatening situations.

Fact Box 16.1   IV therapy in the community and Vascular Access Teams

The provision of dedicated and highly skilled Vascular Access Teams working in hospitals and the community has become increasingly common in the United Kingdom. With increasing pressure on beds, drives to reduce unnecessary admissions and reduce length of stay, and patient desire to avoid hospital admission and receive treatment in the community, healthcare provision is increasingly becoming more and community focused in the primary and secondary care arenas. IV therapy can be safely managed in the community setting, promoting admission avoidance in the first instance or early discharge from hospital. Besides being more convenient for patients, it also reduces the risk of acquiring a healthcare-associated infection (HCAI), particularly from resistant organisms.

The pathogenesis of VAD-related BSIs (bacteraemia)

Colonisation is an essential prerequisite in the pathogenesis of cannula or catheter-related BSI, and results from contamination of the device during insertion and subsequent care. The point at which colonisation changes to infection is unclear but is thought to relate to the number of inoculating organisms, the type of organism, its virulence (see Chapter 5) and the length of time that the device is in situ. Cannula or catheter-related BSIs can be either endogenous or exogenous in origin (see Chapter 8).

Fact Box 16.2 Endogenous and exogenous device–related infections

Staphylococcus aureus and *Staphylococcus epidermidis* (see Chapter 20) are the common culprits implicated in endogenous infections (Pratt *et al.*, 2007), and they are known as pathogens of plastic (Dougherty, 1996), readily colonising IV devices and producing biofilm (see Chapter 5). Exogenous cannula or catheter infections occur as a result of cross-infection from organisms (particularly transient organisms) carried on the hands of healthcare staff or acquired from contact with the environment or contaminated equipment.

There are three ways in which cannula or catheter-related BSIs can occur:

- Skin microorganisms at the insertion site can contaminate the device on insertion, affecting the distal tip.
- Microorganisms can migrate along the cutaneous catheter track.
- Microorganisms can be transferred on the hands of healthcare workers and subsequently contaminate and colonise the cannula or catheter hub.

Bacteraemia

Fact Box 16.3 Prevalence of BSIs

In the HCAI Point Prevalence Survey undertaken in 2011 (Health Protection Agency, 2012), BSIs accounted for 7.3% of HCAIs in adults and 15.1% in children; 64% of patients had a peripheral or central VAD in the 48 hours prior to the onset of symptoms.

While potentially life-threatening BSIs can occur as a result of infection anywhere in the body, the majority are associated with VADs, particularly peripheral IVs and CVCs, and patients receiving IV therapy have a fourfold risk of developing bacteraemia (Elliott, 1993).

The presence of viable bacteria circulating in the bloodstream is called bacteraemia, and it can be transient, intermittent or constant. The bactericidal properties of the blood, including phagocytes, the complement pathway and antibodies, help to resolve many episodes of transient bacteraemia, which can arise following dental work, childbirth and procedures such as bronchoscopy and sigmoidoscopy (Elliott, 2011). The organisms responsible for these transient bacteraemias are normally the flora that reside at that particular site, and they are usually of low virulence (Bannister et al., 1996). Transient bacteraemias in particular often go undetected, and bacteraemia is not necessarily associated with fever and clinical signs of infection (Ray et al., 2010; Willey et al., 2011). However, if host defence mechanisms are successfully evaded, the patient will go on to develop signs of systemic infection.

Fact Box 16.4   Bacteraemia

Bacteraemia associated with VADs can result in metastatic spread to other body sites, giving rise to endocarditis, osteomyelitis and spinal and psoas abscesses, with potentially devasting implications for patients (Burgess et al., 2005; Cosgrove and Fowler, 2008; Paik et al., 2011). Fragments of bacterial biofilm (see Chapter 5) colonising the device may become dislodged, either shearing away naturally or as a result of pressure from the administration of an IV bolus injection, and enter the circulation, seeding at other sites.

Fact Box 16.5   Bacteraemia in renal patients

Vascular access is essential for dialysis, and while the preferred choice is the creation of an arteriovenous fistula or an arteriovenous graft, these can take as long as two years to become fully established and reach maturation, and in a small number of patients they may not be suitable. Vascular access therefore has to be obtained via a CVC. However, due to the long-term requirement for vascular access, renal patients are at significant risk of developing a potentially life-threatening bacteraemia. The risk of developing a meticillin-resistant *Staphylococcus aureus* (MRSA) bacteraemia in particular is 100-fold greater than the risk in the general population, and it is an additional eightfold higher in a renal patient with a CVC as opposed to a fistula (UK Renal Registry, 2008).

Phlebitis

Phlebitis, inflammation of the tunica intima (the innermost lining) of a superficial peripheral vein, is a common complication of peripheral IV cannulation, and is estimated to affect between 27% and 80% of patients with a peripheral cannula (Pandero et al., 2002). Box 16.2 summarises the risk factors for the development of phlebitis.

Box 16.2   Risk factors for the development of phlebitis

Patient risk factors

- Age
- Neutropenia
- Malnutrition
- Impaired circulation
- Peripheral neuropathy

Mechanical phlebitis

- Cannula size, material, length, insertion site, method of immobilisation and duration of insertion.

Chemical phlebitis

- Vessel-irritating drugs (due to the pH or osmolality of the infusate).

Infective phlebitis

- Inadequate skin decontamination prior to insertion
- Poor hand decontamination
- Lack of aseptic non-touch technique on insertion and/or on subsequent handling or access of the device
- Length of time the cannula remains in situ.

Source: Pandero *et al.*, 2002; Macklin, 2003; Lanbeck *et al.*, 2004; Higginson, 2011; Kaur *et al.*, 2011.

In infective phlebitis, microorganisms that either originated from the patient's own flora or were acquired exogenously access the vein (and potentially the bloodstream) via the cannula insertion site, and can give rise to the clinical signs given in Box 16.3.

Box 16.3   Clinical signs of phlebitis

- Pain at the cannula insertion site
- Pain on injection (i.e. administration of IV bolus) or infusion
- Erythema and swelling, visible along the track of the affected vein; the vein may become hardened (indurated).
- The skin around the insertion site or along the vein may feel warm to touch.
- Oozing or exudate from the insertion site.

Source: Macklin, 2003; Lanbeck *et al.*, 2004; Pandero *et al.*, 2004; Higginson, 2011; Kaur *et al.*, 2011.

Complications of phlebitis include bacteraemia, septicaemia and thrombophlebitis, where a blood clot develops in the affected vein.

Phlebitis is an avoidable complication of peripheral cannulation and can be prevented through close observation of the cannula insertion. The Visual Infusion Phlebitis (VIP) score or scale, which gives the cannula insertion site a score of 0–5, was developed in 1998 (Jackson, 1998) as an early indicator of the potential onset of phlebitis and a prompt as to when the cannula should be removed. Healthcare workers should be fully conversant with the use of the VIP score as part of routine cannula care (RCN, 2010).

The first VIP score should not be recorded on insertion – the insertion site will obviously appear healthy at that point. A score of **1** indicates possible early onset of phlebitis; **2** indicates the early stages of phlebitis (pain at the insertion site and/or erythema and swelling), and at this stage the cannula should be removed, the tip sent for microscopy and culture and the insertion site swabbed; and **3, 4** and **5** indicate mid-stage phlebitis, advanced phlebitis with early thrombophlebitis and advanced thrombophlebitis, respectively. With advanced thrombophlebitis, the patient will experience pain, swelling, induration of the venous cord (which will be palpable), pus at the insertion site and pyrexia.

Fact Box 16.6   Poor cannula management

If cannulae are managed appropriately, progression to mid-stage phlebitis and beyond should **not** occur. A score of 3 or above indicates poor cannula management and should be reported as an adverse incident and investigated via root cause analysis (RCA).

The insertion site should be inspected, and the VIP score recorded at least twice every 24 hours (e.g. once on the early shift and once on the night shift). See www.vipscore.net for further information and resources.

Reflection point

Undertake a simple audit of compliance of VIP score recording within your ward (patients currently with a cannula in situ and patients who have previously had a cannula inserted). How compliant have staff been recording the VIP score according to your local policy? What are the barriers to compliance, and how can they be overcome?

Best practice in the prevention of peripheral cannula infection

Initial considerations

- Is the need for a peripheral cannula clinically indicated? As cannulation is an invasive procedure that is fraught with potential complications for the patient, the decision to cannulate must be justified and this must be clearly documented in the patient's notes.

- If peripheral cannulation is considered likely to be difficult, or cannot be achieved, the Vascular Access Team should be contacted.
- If, before the patient is initially cannulated, it is considered likely that vascular access will be required beyond six days, consideration should be given at this initial stage to other more suitable VADs, such as a PICC. Again, the Vascular Access Team should be contacted for advice.
- The insertion time, date and site; cannula size; batch number; name of the person inserting the cannula and review and removal dates must be documented.

Skin decontamination

As discussed in this chapter, given that insertion of the cannula is the critical point during which contamination of the device is likely to occur, thorough decontamination of the patient's skin is crucial. Two percent chlorhexidine gluconate (CHG) in 70% isopropyl alcohol (IPA) is the agent of choice, and its use is endorsed by the EPIC Guidelines (Pratt *et al.*, 2007), the DH (2007a), the RCN (2010) and the Centers for Disease Control and Prevention (O'Grady *et al.*, 2011). Chloraprep® (2% chlorhexidine gluconate in 70% IPA) has largely been adopted nationally as the standard product for skin decontamination prior to the insertion of peripheral IV cannulae, central venous catheters and blood culture collection, having received a level 1 recommendation from the Department of Health and Health Protection Agency Rapid Review Panel in 2007.

The benefits of Chloraprep are summarised in Box 16.4.

241

Box 16.4   The benefits of Chloraprep® (2% chlorhexidine gluconate in 70% IPA)

- Although IPA achieves a 99.99% reduction in bacteria, it has no residual activity. CHG, however, carries on working for up to 48 hours after application.
- It is rapid acting and is effective in the presence of blood and serum.
- It has a broad spectrum of activity.
- The sponge applicator, used in a 'back-and-forth' motion, applies gentle friction to the skin, enabling Chloraprep to penetrate the first five cell layers of the skin.

Further information on the benefits of CHG, IPA and Chloraprep can be found at http://carefusion.co.uk.

Hand decontamination

As discussed in Chapter 12, hand hygiene is the single most important intervention that healthcare staff can undertake in order to prevent the spread of infection. Healthcare workers must decontaminate their hands in accordance with the 5 Moments for Hand Hygiene before cannulating the patient, and before contact with any part of the device, including changing the administration set or infusion.

Aseptic non-touch technique (ANTT)

Cannulation and manipulation of the device (i.e., changing the administration set, changing the infusion and administering bolus injections) must be undertaken using ANTT. There is a Fact Sheet (16.1) on the companion website.

Early detection of phlebitis

The cannula insertion must be inspected at least twice daily for signs of infusion phlebitis using the VIP scale (or score), and the cannula removed if the score is ≥ 2.

Box 16.5 summarises evidence-based best-practice points for the management of peripheral venous cannulae.

Box 16.5   Best-practice points regarding peripheral venous cannula management

- The cannula should be removed or re-sited at 96 hours. **Note**: If this is not possible due to poor venous access, this should be recorded in the medical or nursing notes and the Vascular Access Team informed. The patient should not be left without venous access if it is required. For 'difficult' cannulations, the intervention of the Vascular Access Team should be sought at the earliest opportunity.
- IV administration sets should be changed when the cannula is replaced; at 72 hour intervals; at the end of the infusion or within 24 hours of initiating the infusion when administering lipid emulsions.
- Blood administration sets should be changed on completion of the transfusion or every 12 hours (whichever is the soonest).
- Intermittent administration sets should be changed every 24 hours if remaining connected to the cannula or discarded after each use if disconnected. **Note:** Where fluids or drugs have been disconnected partway through infusion, the administration set **must** be discarded and a new administration set connected. Under no circumstances must the administration set be reconnected.
- Keep the number of lines and ports to the absolute minimum.
- Use a needle-free system to access the injection site.
- The use of bandages around the device should be avoided where possible. If a bandage is used, it must be removed at least twice a day to allow visual inspection of the insertion site.
- Splints should be used to secure the cannula only if it has been inserted in or around an area of flexion. They should be removed and the site, along with the patient's circulatory status, assessed at regular intervals. This assessment should be documented.
- When the site is accessed (i.e. prior to bolus injection), the portal should be disinfected using a 2% chlorhexidine in 70% alcohol single-use wipe to prevent the entry of microorganisms via the portal.
- The cannula should be flushed at least daily, and pre and post drug administration, with 5–10 ml normal saline (0.9%) to maintain patency.

- The cannula site dressing should be changed if it becomes damp, soiled or loosened. The dressing should be changed using ANTT, and the skin cleaned with alcoholic chlorhexidine.
- As well as checking the VIP score, the site should also be checked to ensure that the cannula has not become dislodged, and for signs of infiltration and extravasation.
- Peripheral cannulae should not be used for routine blood sampling. A fresh stab for venepuncture should be made.
- If the cannula has been inserted in an emergency situation where aseptic technique has been compromised, it should be re-sited within 24 hours.

Source: Pratt *et al.*, 2007; RCN, 2010.

Reflection point

Read a copy of your local policy for the insertion and management of peripheral IV cannulae, and observe a peripheral cannula being inserted. Are the insertion and the ongoing care of the cannula in accordance with the policy?

Chapter summary: key points

- VADs are complex, and their insertion and ongoing management and maintenance are skilled procedures that should be undertaken only by healthcare staff who have been trained and assessed as competent (see Chapter 2).

- Peripheral venous cannulation is the most commonly performed invasive procedure in hospitals.

- There are wide-ranging complications associated with VADs.

- The majority of bloodstream infections, which are potentially life-threatening, are associated with VADs, and are largely associated with poor device management.

- Phlebitis is a common, but avoidable, complication of peripheral cannulation and can occur as a result of endogenous or exogenous contamination of the cannula.

- Hand hygiene, ANTT and skin decontamination are integral components of effective VAD insertion and management.

- All VADs should be managed according to evidence-based best-practice guidelines.

Further resources are available for this book, including interactive multiple choice questions. Visit the companion website at:

www.wiley.com/go/fundamentalsofinfectionprevention

References

Bannister B.A., Begg N.T., Gillespie S.H. (1996). The nature and pathogenesis of infection. In: *Infectious Diseases*. Blackwell Science Ltd, London: 1–21.

Bion J., Richardson A., Hibbert P., Beer J., Abrusci T. *et al.* (2012). Matching Michigan: a 2-year stepped interventional programe to minimise central venous catheter blood stream infections in intensive care units in England. *British Medical Journal* Quality and Safety; accessed at http://dx.doi.org/10.1135/bmjqs-2012-001325

Burgess C.M., Wolverson A.S., Dale M.T. (2005). Cervical epidural abscess: a rare complication of intravenous cannulation. *Anaesthesia.* 60 (6): 606–608.

Cosgrove S.E., Fowler V.G. (2008). Management of meticillin-resistant *Staphylococcus aureus* bacteraemia. *Clinical Infectious Diseases.* 46 (Suppl. 5): S386–S393.

Cowley K. (2004). Making the right choice of vascular access device. *Professional Nurse.* 19 (10): 43–46.

Day M. (2011). Intraosseous devices for intravascular access in adult trauma patients. *Critical Care Nurse.* 31 (2): 76–88.

Department of Health (DH) (2007a). *High Impact Intervention No 2: Peripheral Intravenous Cannula Care Bundle*. Department of Health, London.

Department of Health (DH) (2007b). *High Impact Intervention No 3: Renal Dialysis Catheter Care Bundle*. Department of Health, London.

Department of Health (DH) (2007c). *High Impact Intervention No 1: Central Venous Catheter Care Bundle*. Department of Health, London.

Dougherty L. (1996). Intravenous management. In: Mallett J., Bailey C. (Eds.). *The Royal Marsden Hospital Manual of Clinical Nursing Procedures*. 4th ed. Blackwell Science Ltd, London: 311–337.

Elliott T.S.J. (1993). Line-associated bacteraemias. *CDR Review.* 3 (7): R91–R96.

Elliott T. (2011). Bacteraemia and bloodstream infection. In: Elliott T., Cassey A., Lambert P., Sandoe J. (Eds.), *Medical Microbiology and Infection: Lecture Notes*. 5th ed. Wiley-Blackwell, London: 229–232.

Hadaway L. (2012). Short peripheral intravenous catheters and infections. *Journal of Infusion Nursing.* 35 (4): 230–240.

Health Protection Agency (2012). *English National Point Prevalence Survey on Healthcare Associated Infections and Antimicrobial Use, 2011: Preliminary Data*. Health Protection Agency, London.

Higginson R. (2011). Phlebitis: treatment, care and prevention. *Nursing Times.* 107 (36): 18–21.

Jackson A. (1998). A battle in vein: infusion phlebitis. *Nursing Times.* 94 (4): 68–71.

Kaur P., Thakur R., Kaur S., Bhalla A. (2011). Assessment of risk factors of phlebitis amongst intravenous cannulated patients. *Nursing and Midwifery Nursing Journal.* 7 (3): 106–114.

Kelly L.J. (2009). The family of vascular access device. *Journal of Infection Prevention*. 10 (Suppl. 1): S7–S12.

Lanbeck P., Odenholt I., Paulsen D. (2004). Perception of risk factors for infusion phlebitis among Swedish nurses: a questionnaire study. *Journal of Infusion Nursing*. 27 (1): 24–30.

Lowther A. (2011). Intraosseous access and adults in the emergency department. *Nursing Standard*. 25 (48): 35–38.

Macklin D. (2003). Phlebitis, a painful complication of peripheral intravenous catheterization that may be prevented. *American Journal of Nursing*. 103 (2): 55–60.

National Clinical Guideline Centre (2012). *Partial Update of NICE Clinical Guideline 2. Infection: Prevention and Control of Healthcare Associated Infections in Primary and Community Care*. National Institute for Health and Clinical Excellence (NICE), London.

O'Grady N.P., Alexander M., Burns L.A., Dellinger E.P., Garland J. *et al.* (2011). *Guidelines for the Prevention of Intravascular Catheter-Related Infections, 2011*. Centers for Disease Control and the Healthcare Infection Control Practices Advisory Committee (CDC/HICPAC), Atlanta, GA.

Paik J.C., Killian M.E., Feldhaus J.J., Estrada C. (2011). A dreaded complication of MRSA infection. *International Journal of Case Reports and Images*. 2 (3): 17–20.

Pandero A., Ioham G., Taj J., Mackay N., Shorten G. (2002). A dedicated intravenous cannula for post-operative use: effect on incidence and severity of phlebitis. *Anaesthesia*. 57: 921–925.

Pikwer A., Åkeson J., Lindgren S. (2011). Complications associated with peripheral or central routes for central venous cannulation. *Anaesthesia*. 67: 65–71.

Pratt R.J., Pellowe C.M., Wilson J.A., Loveday H.P., Harper P. *et al.* (2007). EPIC2: national evidence-based guidelines for preventing healthcare-associated infections in NHS hospitals in England. *Journal of Hospital Infection*. 65 (Suppl. 1): S1–S64.

Ray C.G., Ryan K.J., Drew W.L. (2010). Intravascular infections, bacteraemia and endotoxemia. In: Ryan K.J., Ray G.C. (Eds.), *Sherris Medical Microbiology*. 5th ed. McGraw-Hill Medical, New York: 959–970.

Royal College of Nursing (RCN) (2010). *Standards for Infusion Therapy*. The RCN IV Therapy Forum. 3rd ed. January. Royal College of Nursing, London.

Sado D.M., Deakin C.D. (2005). Local anaesthetic for venous cannulation and arterial blood gas samples: are doctors using it? *Journal Royal Society Medicine*. 98 (4): 158–160.

Saini R., Agnihotri M., Gupta A., Walia I. (2011). Epidemiology of infiltration and phlebitis. *Nursing and Midwifery Research Journal*. 7 (1): 22–33.

UK Renal Registry (2008). *The Eleventh Annual Report, December 2008*. www.renalreg.com (accessed 20 December 2012)

Webster J., Lloyd S., Hopkins T., Osborne S., Yaxley M. (2007). Developing a research base for intravenous peripheral cannula re-sites (DRIP Trial): a randomised controlled trial of hospital in-patients. *International Journal of Nursing Studies*. 44: 664–671.

Willey J.M., Sherwood L.M., Woolverton C.J. (2011). Infection and pathogenicity. In: *Prescott's Microbiology*. 8th ed. McGraw-Hill International Edition, New York: 739–759.

17

The prevention and management of catheter-associated urinary tract infections

Contents

Fundamentals of Infection Prevention and Control: Theory and Practice, Second Edition. Debbie Weston.
© 2013 John Wiley & Sons, Ltd. Published 2013 by John Wiley & Sons, Ltd. Companion Website: www.wiley.com/go/fundamentalsofinfectionprevention

Introduction

Urinary tract infections (UTIs) account for 1–3% of all General Practitioner consultations, and have been identified as the second most common clinical indication for antibiotic prescribing in primary and secondary care (Morgan and McKenzie, 1993), accounting for 17.2% of all healthcare-associated infections (Health Protection Agency [HPA], 2012). Ninety-seven percent of healthcare-associated urinary tract infections are associated with instrumentation such as catheterisation (Hooton, 2010), which is an accepted and commonplace healthcare intervention. Two-thirds of bacteraemias of known source are associated with device-related infections (Public Health Laboratory Service, 1999), so it is obvious that catheters represent a serious threat to patients. So great is the risk they pose that the EPIC2 guidelines clearly state that 'catheterising patients places them in significant danger of acquiring a urinary tract infection. The longer a catheter is in place, the greater the danger' (Pratt *et al.*, 2007). In other words, urinary catheters can kill.

This chapter looks at the economic burden and the incidence of catheter-associated urinary tract infections, along with the pathogenesis and diagnosis of infection, and evidence-based best-practice recommendations for the management of urinary catheters and infection prevention.

Learning outcomes

After reading this chapter, the reader will be able to:

- Understand how and why catheter-associated urinary tract infections occur.

- Understand the significance of bacteriuria.

- Be able to list the clinical features of a urinary tract infection in non-catheterised and catheterised patients.

- Be able to list the key elements of best practice in relation to catheter-associated urinary tract infection.

The economic burden of catheter-associated urinary tract infections, and the prevalence of urinary catheters in healthcare

The United Kingdom

Just over a decade ago, it was estimated that urinary tract infections (UTIs) cost the NHS an estimated £124 million per annum, equating to 800 000 lost bed days and incurring an additional cost of £1327 per patient, blocking a hospital bed for an extra six days, making them a huge drain on NHS resources as well as patient care (Plowman *et al.*, 2000). The NHS Institute for Innovation and Improvement have corrected these costs for inflation and estimated the annual cost per patient to have increased to £1964 (www.institute.nhs.uk). Crow *et al.* (1998) estimated the prevalence of catheterised patients in UK hospitals at 12.6%. At the time of the *Third National Prevalence Survey* (Hospital Infection Society and Infection Control Nurses Association, 2007), 31.6% of patients had a urinary catheter either present on the day of the survey or within the previous seven days. *The English National Point Prevalence Survey on Healthcare-associated Infections and Antimicrobial Use* (HPA, 2012) identified that 43% of patients with a UTI had a catheter in situ within the previous seven days

The prevalence of urinary catheters has been estimated to be between 0.5% and 40% in the community setting (McNulty *et al.*, 2003; NICE, 2003). A study by McNulty *et al.* in 2008, of the prevalence of urinary catheters in 14 large care homes, found that patients were rarely catheterised by care home staff; the decision to catheterise residents was generally taken if residents were admitted to hospital, and was considered by care home staff to have been undertaken because there were insufficient staff on the wards to attend to the needs of the patients. A study undertaken in 2009 by Lomas *et al.* found that a staggering 57% of care home residents acquired a catheter in hospital that was not removed on discharge.

The United States

In the United States, 15–25% of patients in hospital are estimated to receive short-term urinary catheters (Gould *et al.*, 2009). UTIs account for 35% of all HCAIs, are estimated to cost $565 million per year and contribute to 8205 deaths annually (www.cdc.gov). Changes to the Centers for Medicare and Medicaid Services Reimbursement System mean that hospitals do not receive payment for catheter-associated urinary tract infections (CAUTIs) that were not present on admission to hospital, as CAUTI is viewed as a preventable problem (Would and Kramer, 2007; Bernard *et al.*, 2012). Box 17.1 lists some of the common indications for catheterisation.

Box 17.1   Indications for catheterisation

- Acute urinary retention
- Chronic urinary retention (as a last resort)
- Urinary obstruction
- Monitoring urine output in critically ill patients
- Incontinence with sacral sore(s) or to aid wound healing (sacral, perianal or perineal wounds)
- Intractable incontinence as a last resort (where all other methods of management have been tried and have failed)
- Terminally ill or palliative care
- Urine measurement during and post surgery
- Where the patient requires prolonged immobilisation (e.g. unstable thoracic or lumbar spine fractures, or pelvic fractures)
- For bladder irrigation if haematuria or clot retention is present
- Urodynamic study
- The instillation of medication (e.g. chemotherapy).

Source: Cravens and Zweig, 2000; Hart, 2008; Nazarko, 2008; Gould *et al.*, 2009; Doughty and Kisanga, 2010; RCN, 2012.

Reflection point

How many patients within your place of work currently have an indwelling urinary catheter? What is the clinical indication for catheterisation?

The pathogenesis of CAUTIs

Box 17.2 describes the various host defence mechanisms that provide protection against UTI.

Box 17.2 Protection against UTI – host defence mechanisms

Urinary flow
White blood cells on bladder surface
IgA antibody on bladder wall (see Chapter 8)
Exfoliation (shedding) of bladder epithelial cells
Mucin layer on bladder wall – prevents bacterial adherence
Urinary pH and osmolality.

Source: Graham, 2010; Hooton, 2010.

249

Although the urethra is colonised with bacteria, urine proximal to the distal urethra is normally sterile. In individuals who are not catheterised, and assuming that there is no known defect of the genito-urinary system, the urethra remains closed, protecting the bladder which is also sterile, except when urine is being voided. The regular emptying of the bladder and the hydrodynamic force of voiding urine flush away microorganisms.

Fact Box 17.1 Men versus women

In men, the length of the urethra (18–20 cm) offers some protection from the potentially uropathogenic colonic and genital flora that colonise the perineum, making them less susceptible to UTIs. Women, on the other hand, have a short urethra (4 cm) which is in very close proximity to the perineum, and are more prone to endogenous infections, as bacteria can be transiently displaced into the bladder during sexual intercourse, resulting in cystitis (Hooton, 2010; Ray et al., 2010).

The presence of the catheter, which is essentially a foreign body, forces the urethra open and makes it unable to close to protect the bladder. It also interferes with the flushing effect of the urine and the regular and complete emptying of the bladder. Crucially, the catheter forms a bridge between the naturally sterile bladder and the external environment, where it effectively acts as a gateway, or ladder, for the ascending passage of bacteria. The catheter retention balloon prevents complete emptying of the bladder as the catheter drainage holes are sited above the level of the balloon, and there is therefore a small residual volume of urine in the bladder (Hashmi *et al.*, 2003; Wilson, 2006; Barford and Coates, 2009), where bacteria could potentially multiply. The retention balloon can also damage the lining of the bladder if it is under- or over-inflated, irritating the lining of the bladder and interfering with the correct positioning of the bladder tip by resting against the bladder mucosa in an area known as the delicate trigone, where it can cause the equivalent of a small pressure sore (Godfrey and Evans, 2000; Robinson, 2001).

Fact Box 17.2   Bacteriuria

Of those catheterised patients who have had a catheter in situ for longer than seven to 10 days, 50% will develop bacteria in their urine (bacteriuria, or bacterial colonisation of the urine). Although bacteriuria is often symptomatic, it can lead to microbial invasion of the tissues, with 20–30% of patients going on to develop a symptomatic UTI. Between 1% to 4% will develop a bacteraemia (bacteria in the bloodstream but without systemic signs of infection), and of these 13–30% will subsequently die (Saint and Lipsky, 1999; Pratt *et al.*, 2001).

Although most of the organisms causing CAUTI are derived from the patient's own flora, they can also be acquired exogenously via the hands of healthcare staff, which may be contaminated with antibiotic-resistant organisms.

Microorganisms can gain entry to the urinary tract via three main routes:

- Contamination of the distal tip of the catheter on insertion will introduce bacteria into the bladder and colonise the distal urethra.
- Once the catheter has been inserted, bacteria colonising the distal urethra can migrate up and along the outside of the catheter.
- If the catheter drainage bag, the sampling port or the junction between the bag and the catheter becomes contaminated, bacteria can migrate up through the lumen of the catheter.

Catheters and their associated drainage systems provide a wonderful environment for bacteria as they support the growth of bacterial biofilms (see Chapter 5). Once in situ, the catheter becomes encrusted with proteins and electrolytes from the urine, and these serve as a conditioning film which encourages microbial attachment (Trautner and Darouiche, 2004).

Fact Box 17.3   Catheters and biofilm formation

The bacteria secrete a polysaccharide matrix consisting of sugars and proteins which encase them, affording protection from the effects of antibiotics and host immune defence mechanisms such as phagocytosis (Neidhardt, 2004). The presence of bacteria such as *Proteus*, *Pseudomonas* and *Klebsiella* encourages biofilm formation, parts of which can shear off, detach and seed to other parts of the catheter or to the bladder (Jacobsen *et al.*, 2008) or other body sites. When the catheter is removed, biofilm may be visible around the catheter tip as a slimy coating. Encrustation is not always as easily spotted as it may be inside the catheter lumen (Simpson, 2001).

Bacterial causes of UTIs

More than 95% of UTIs occurring in patients with short-term urinary catheters are caused by a single bacterial species, whereas infections in patients with long-term catheters are generally polymicrobial and increasingly likely to be multidrug resistant (Strohl *et al.*, 2001; Perez *et al.*, 2007). Some bacterial causes of UTIs include:

- *Escherichia coli* (see Chapter 10)
- *Klebsiella* (see Chapter 10)
- *Pseudomonas* spp. (see Chapter 10)
- *Staphylococcus saprophyticus* (see Chapter 20)
- *Proteus mirabilis* (see Fact Sheet 1.6 on the companion website)
- *Serratia* (see Fact Sheet 9.3 on the companion website).

Clinical features of UTIs

Uncatheterised patients

Detecting a UTI in an uncatheterised patient is relatively straightforward. In cases of cystitis, which has an abrupt onset, the symptoms are due to inflammation and irritation of the bladder mucosa as well as the mucosal surface of the urethra. This gives rise to frequency of urination (micturition) which is often accompanied by a feeling of urgency, dysuria (pain on urinating), suprapubic or loin pain or tenderness and a temperature. In severe cases, the urine may be blood stained (haematuria) as well as cloudy and malodorous.

Pyelonephritis is a more severe infection affecting the kidney and the upper renal tract, which can lead to kidney damage and the onset of septic shock (see Chapter 9). Symptoms include flank pain, a temperature which exceeds 38 °C and rigors. As the infection progresses, the patient may develop diarrhoea and vomiting.

Catheterised patients

UTI is less apparent in patients who are catheterised as the key symptoms of frequency and pain on urinating are absent. While suprapubic tenderness and cloudy, malodorous urine may be present, these features are not reported in all cases, and in elderly patients fever may be the first symptom, along with confusion or delirium (Tambyah and Maki, 2000). National clinical guidance from the Scottish Intercollegiate Guidelines Network (2012) recommends the following actions in the event of a catheterised patient presenting with a fever:

- Look for associated localising loin or suprapubic tenderness, or other systemic signs of infection.
- Exclude other potential sources of infection.
- Obtain a urine sample for culture, microscopy and sensitivity.
- Consider commencing antibiotic therapy, taking into account the severity of the presenting symptoms and any co-morbidities.

Given that the prevalence of bacteriuria in catheterised patients is virtually 100% if the catheter has been in situ for three to four weeks, the results are not clinically significant in the absence of clinical symptoms (Morgan and McKenzie, 1993), and specimens should be sent for laboratory culture **only** if the patient has clinical sepsis, **not** because the appearance or smell of the urine suggests that bacteriuria is present (Scottish Intercollegiate Guidelines Network, 2013; HPA, 2009). 'Dip sticking' must not be used to diagnose urinary tract infection in catherterised patients. Treatment of asymptomatic bacteriuria can lead to the emergence of drug-resistant bacteria, a significant problem particularly as it is known that CAUTIs comprise perhaps the largest institutional reservoir of antibiotic-resistant organisms (Maki and Tambyah, 2001).

Diagnosis

Unsurprisingly, urine specimens comprise the largest single category of specimens examined in most medical microbiology laboratories (Morgan and McKenzie, 1993). Laboratory confirmation of a UTI is dependent upon the examination of a sample of normally sterile urine and the detection of bacteria and the accompanying inflammatory response which is evident by the number of white blood cells present in the sample (Ryan, 2004). Chapter 6 describes how a catheter specimen of urine (CSU) should be obtained. Although counts of $>10^5$ CFU bacteria/mL of urine are considered to indicate UTI (HPA, 2009; Ray et al., 2010), bacterial counts of $\geq 10^2$ CFU/mL of urine are considered to be of clinical significance in catheterised patients as periurethral contamination of the specimen is unlikely (Sobel and Kaye, 2004).The results need to be carefully interpreted alongside the clinical symptoms.

Clinical considerations: Best practice in the prevention of CAUTIs

For more information on this topic, see Pratt et al. (2001, 2007), Department of Health (DH) (2012), National Clinical Guideline Centre (2012) and Royal College of Nursing (RCN, 2012).

Fact Box 17.4   Department of Health safety thermometer: Catheters and UTIs

The NHS Safety Thermometer is a quality improvement tool for the measuring, monitoring and analysis of four recognised 'harm' events that occur at the point of care, and that are part of the Commissioning, Quality and Innovation (CQUIN) payment programme. The data that are collected will, over time, enable national baselines to be established regarding these four events and lead to improvements in care. Catheters and UTIs are one of the events measured, and participating organisations are required to collect data on all patients on one day of the month relating to treatment for a UTI and the presence of indwelling urinary catheters.

See http://www.ic.nhs.uk/services/nhs-safety-thermometer and DH (2012).

Avoid catheterisation

The best method of prevention is to avoid catheterisation where at all possible and consider alternative methods (Pratt et al., 2001, 2007; DH, 2007; National Clinical Guideline Centre, 2012; RCN, 2012). Trovillion et al. (2011), developed a list of indicators, known as the HOUDINI protocol, to be used when assessing the need for catheterisation, and they advised that catheterisation should be undertaken **only** in the presence of one or more of the following conditions: obvious haematuria (visible blood in the urine), urinary obstruction, urology surgery, open sacral or perineal decubitus ulcer in conjunction with incontinence, monitoring of fluid input and output (fluid balance), patients receiving nursing care or end-of-life care only, and immobility. A pilot study implementing the HOUDINI protocol in three medical wards at an acute general hospital in England found that it gave nursing staff greater confidence in deciding when to remove urinary catheters (Adams *et al.*, 2012).

Reflection point

Does your organisation employ a Continence Advisor?
How widely are alternative methods of catheterisation and bladder drainage used (e.g. supra-pubic catheters, convenes and flip-flo valves)?

Guidance published by the RCN in 2008 clearly states that risk avoidance (don't catheterise), risk reduction (consider intermittent, as opposed to indwelling, catheterisation) and justification for catheter insertion are key to protecting patients from CAUTIs. With regard to justifying the need for catheterisation, the RCN are emphatic that it is unprofessional of nursing staff to catheterise a patient even if it is requested as a medical intervention, without undertaking a clinical risk assessment of their own, and that 'Nursing has no defence in stating "the Doctor told me to do it"'.

Competency

Catheterisation is a skilled procedure, and appropriate education and training followed by supervised practice and successful demonstration of competency in accordance with policy are required to ensure evidence-based best practice. Healthcare Assistants must also be trained in catheter maintenance. See Chapter 2 for further discussion of competency.

Prevent trauma

The EPIC 2 guidelines (Pratt *et al.*, 2007) recommend the use of lubricant gels to facilitate the insertion of urinary catheters. Although these have been used for many years in male catheterisations to facilitate the passage of the catheter along the long male urethra, their use during female catheterisations has not been consistent, with the general consensus being that as the female urethra is shorter the discomfort experienced on catheterisation is less (Woodhead, 2005).

Fact Box 17.5   National Patient Safety Alert

Between January 2006 and September 2009, there were 114 incidents in hospital and community care settings where female-length catheters were inserted in men. Complications included severe pain, penile swelling, retention of urine and bleeding (of varying severity). Two patients developed acute renal failure, and two went on to develop impaired renal function.

Source: Data from NPSA, 2009.

The urethra in both men and women is flat and ribbon-like, has a good blood and nerve supply and contains collagen which reduces its elasticity, making it susceptible to trauma during catheterisation. The use of a single-use lubricant gel that has anaesthetic, antiseptic and bacteri-cidal properties, inserted into the urethra approximately five minutes before the procedure takes place, dilates the urethra, reduces pain and discomfort, increases patient compliance and reduces the risk of infection occurring as a result of a traumatic catheterisation (RCN, 2012).

Prevent contamination

Aseptic non-touch technique (ANTT) must be used for catheter insertion and all catheter-related interventions (see Fact Sheet 16.1 on the companion website). Hands must be decontaminated before any contact with the catheter and drainage system. Urine specimens must be taken only from the sampling port.

The use of silver catheters

The broad-spectrum antibacterial properties of silver have long been recognised (Sagripanti, 1992). The Department of Health Rapid Review Panel gave the Bardex IC silver alloy–coated hydrogel-coated catheter (manufactured by CR Bard) a level 1 recommendation in 2004. The catheter, which contains a layer of gold and palladium over a layer of silver, reduces microbial adherence to the catheter which minimises biofilm formation, and inhibits the migration of bacteria along the catheter surface and into the bladder (Ahearn et al., 2000). The short-term use of silver catheters has been implemented in many organisations as part of routine CAUTI prevention, but they should not be viewed as a quick fix. They are not a cure for existing infections, but they can be utilised as a preventive measure in conjunction with sound clinical practice.

Box 17.3 lists other best-practice considerations with regard to urinary catheter management.

Box 17.3   Other best-practice considerations

- Secure the catheter to the thigh or the abdomen using an adhesive pad or a restraining strap in order to prevent the catheter from dragging and causing trauma.
- Maintain a closed system; use a link-drainage bag overnight.
- Ensure that the drainage bag is positioned below the level of the bladder in order to prevent urinary reflux.
- Ensure that the bag and the drainage tap are not in contact with the floor.
- Change the urinary drainage bag every seven days.
- Use a clean container to empty the catheter.
- Document all catheter-related interventions.
- **Remove the catheter as soon as possible.**

Reflection point

Obtain a copy of your organisation's Catheterisation Policy or Guidelines. How well is the Policy or Guideline adhered to? How is compliance with the Policy or Guideline audited?

Chapter summary: key points

- Ninety-seven percent of UTIs are associated with instrumentation such as catheterisation.

- Catheters potentially pose a serious risk to patients.

- Between 13% to 30% of patients who develop a bacteraemia secondary to a CAUTI are likely to die.

- Dip sticking must not be used to diagnose infection in catheterised patients – treatment of asymptomatic bacteriuria leads to the emergence of drug resistance.

- Catheter-associated UTIs (CAUTIs) comprise the largest institutional reservoir of antibiotic-resistant organisms, which has implications for treatment and patient care.

- The best method of preventing CAUTIs is to avoid catheterisation where at all possible and consider alternative methods of bladder drainage.

- Where catheterisation can be justified, it must be undertaken by appropriately trained staff who have been assessed as competent.

255

Further resources are available for this book, including interactive multiple choice questions. Visit the companion website at:

www.wiley.com/go/fundamentalsofinfectionprevention

References

Adams D., Bucior H., Day G., Rimmer J. (2012). HOUDINI: make that catheter disappear – nurse led protocol. *Journal of Infection Prevention*. 13 (2): 44–46.

Ahearn D.G., Grace D.T., Jennings M.J., Borazjani R.N., Boles K. *et al.* (2000). Effects of hydrogel/silver coatings on in vitro adhesion to catheters of bacteria associated with urinary tract infections. *Current Microbiology*. 41 (2): 120–125.

Barford J.M.T., Coates A.R.M. (2009). The pathogenesis of catheter-associated urinary tract infection. *Journal of Infection Prevention*. 10 (2): 50–56.

Bernard S.M., Hunter K.F., Moore K.N. (2012). A review of strategies to decrease the duration of indwelling urethral catheters and potentially reduce the incidence of catheter associated urinary tract infections. *Urologic Nursing*. 32 (1): 29–37.

Cravens D.D., Zweig S. (2000). Urinary catheter management. *American Family Physician*. 61 (2): 369–376.

Crow R., Mulhall A., Chapman R. (1998). Indwelling catheterisation and related nursing practice. *Journal of Advanced Nursing*. 13 (4): 489–495.

Department of Health (DH) (2007). *High Impact Intervention. Urinary Catheter Care Bundle*. Department of Health, London. www.clean-safe-care.nhs.uk (accessed 20 December 2012)

Department of Health (DH) (2012). *Delivering the NHS Safety Thermometer CQUIN 2012/13. A Preliminary Guide to Measuring 'Harm Free' Care*. Department of Health, London.

Doughty D., Kisanga J. (2010). Regulatory guidelines for bladder management in long-term care. *Journal of Wound, Ostomy, and Continence Nursing*. 37 (4): 399–411.

Godfrey H., Evans A. (2000). Management of long-term urethral catheters: minimising complications. *British Journal of Nursing*. 9 (2): 74–81.

Gould C.V., Umscheid C.A., Agarwal R.K., Kuntz G., Pegues D.A. and the Healthcare Infection Control Practices Advisory Committee (HICPAC) (2009). *Guideline for Prevention of Catheter-Associated Urinary Tract Infections*. Centers for Disease Control and Prevention, Atlanta, GA.

Graham C. (2010). Investigation of urine samples. In: Ford M. (Ed.), *Medical Microbiology*. Oxford University Press, Oxford: 117–141.

Hart S. (2008). Urinary catheterisation. *Nursing Standard*. 22 (27): 44–48.

Hashmi S., Kelly E., Rogers S.O., Gates J. (2003). Urinary tract infections in surgical patients. *American Journal of Surgery*. 186: 53–56.

Health Protection Agency (HPA) (2009). *National Standard Method. BSOP14: Investigation of Urine*. Health Protection Agency, London.

Health Protection Agency (HPA) (2012). *English National Point Prevalence Survey on Healthcare-associated Infections and Antimicrobial Usage: Preliminary Data*. Health Protection Agency, London.

Hooton M. (2010). Nosocomial urinary tract infections. In: Mandell G.L., Bennett J.E., Dolin R.D. (Eds.), *Mandell's Principles and Practices of Infectious Diseases*. 6th ed. Churchill Livingstone Elsevier, London. http://expertconsult.com (accessed 20 December 2012)

Hospital Infection Society and Infection Control Nurses Association (2007). *The Third Prevalence Survey of Healthcare-associated Infections in Acute Hospitals in England, 2006. Report for the Department of Health (England)*. Hospital Infection Society, London.

Jacobsen S.M., Stickler D.J., Mobley H.L.T., Shirtliff M.E. (2008). Complicated catheter-associated urinary tract infections due to *Escherichia coli* and *Proteus mirabilis*. *Clinical Microbiology Reviews*. 21 (1): 26–59.

Lomas, G.M., Howell-Jones R., McNulty C.A.M. (2009). Identifying key factors that affect care home catheterisation rates: changing practice through audit. *Journal of Infection Prevention*. 10 (2): 66–69.

Maki D., Tambyah P.A. (2001). Engineering out the risk for infection with urinary catheters. *Emerging Infectious Diseases*. 7 (2): 342–347.

McNulty C., Bowen J., Howell-Jones R., Walker M., Freeman E. (2008). Exploring reasons for variation in urinary catheterisation in care homes: a qualitative study. *Age and Ageing*. 37 (6): 706–710.

McNulty C., Freeman E., Smith G., Gunn K., Foy C. *et al.* (2003). Prevalence of urinary catheterization in UK nursing homes. *Journal of Hospital Infection*. 55 (2): 119–123.

Morgan M.G., McKenzie H. (1993). Controversies in the laboratory diagnosis of community acquired urinary tract infection. *European Journal of Clinical Microbiology & Infectious Diseases*. 12 (7): 491–504.

National Clinical Guideline Centre (2012). *Partial Update of Clinical Guideline 2: Infection: Prevention and Control of Healthcare Associated Infections in Primary and Community Care*. National Institute for Health and Clinical Excellence (NICE), London.

National Patient Safety Agency (2009). *Female Urinary Catheters Causing Trauma to Adult Males*. Rapid Response Report NPSA/2009/RRR02. April. National Patient Safety Agency, London.

Nazarko L. (2008). Reducing the risk of catheter associated urinary tract infection. *British Journal of Nursing*. 17 (16): 56–58.

Neidhardt F.C. (2004). Bacterial processes. In: Sherris J.C., Ryan K.J., Ray G.C. (Eds.). *Sherris Medical Microbiology: An Introduction to Infectious Diseases*. 4th ed. McGraw-Hill, London: 27–51.

Perez F., Endimian A., Hujer K.M., Bonomo R.A. (2007). The continuing challenge of ESBLs. *Current Opinion in Pharmacology*. 7 (5): 459–469.

Plowman R., Graves N., Griffin M., Roberts J., Swan A.V. *et al.* (2000). *The Socio-economic Burden of Hospital Acquired Infection*. Public Health Laboratory Service, London.

Pratt R.J., Pellowe C.M., Loveday H.B., Robinson M., Smith G.W. and the EPIC Guidelines Development Team (2001). The EPIC Project: developing national evidence-based guidelines for preventing healthcare associated infections. *Journal of Hospital Infection*. 47 (Suppl.): S1–S82.

256

Pratt R.J., Pellowe C.M., Wilson J.A., Loveday H.P., Harper P.J. *et al.* (2007). EPIC2: national evidence-based guidelines for preventing healthcare-associated infections in NHS hospitals in England. *Journal of Hospital Infection*. 65 (Suppl. 1): S1–S64.

Public Health Laboratory Service (1999). *Surveillance of Hospital-Acquired Bacteraemias in English Hospitals 1997–1999*. Public Health Laboratory Service, London.

Ray C.G., Ryan K.J., Drew W.L. (2010). Urinary tract infections. In: Ryan K.J., Drew C.G. (Eds.). *Sherris Medical Microbiology*. 5th ed. McGraw Hill Medical, New York: 939–944.

Robinson J. (2001). Urethral catheter selection. *Nursing Standard*. 7 (15): 39–42.

Royal College of Nursing (RCN) (2008). *Catheter Care: RCN Guidance for Nurses*. Royal College of Nursing, London.

Royal College of Nursing (RCN) (2012). *Catheter Care: RCN Guidance for Nurses*. Royal College of Nursing, London.

Ryan K.J. (2004). Urinary tract infections. In: Sherris J.C., Ryan K.J., Ray G.C. (Eds.). *Medical Microbiology: An Introduction to Infectious Diseases*. 4th ed. McGraw-Hill, London: 867–879.

Sagripanti J.L. (1992). Metal based formulations with high microbial activity. *Applied Environmental Microbiology*. 58 (9): 3157–3162.

Saint S., Lipsky B. (1999). Preventing catheter-related bacteriuria: should we? Can we? How? *Archives of Internal Medicine*. 159: 800–808.

Scottish Intercollegiate Guidelines Network (2012). *Management of Suspected Bacterial Urinary Tract Infection in Adults: A National Clinical Guideline*. SIGN Publication 88. Scottish Intercollegiate Guidelines Network, Edinburgh.

Simpson L. (2001). In dwelling urethral catheters. *Nursing Standard*. 15 (46): 47–53.

Sobel J.D., Kaye D. (2004). Urinary tract infections. In: Mandell G.L., Bennett J.E., Dolin R.D. (Eds.), *Mandell's Principles and Practices of Infectious Diseases*. 6th ed. Churchill Livingstone, Edinburgh. http://ppidonline.com (accessed 26 February 2013)

Strohl W.A., Rouse H., Fisher D. (2001). Enteric Gram-negative rods. In: Harvey R.A., Champe P.A. (Eds.), *Lippincott's Illustrated Reviews: Medical Microbiology*. Lippincott, Williams and Wilkins, London: 175–191.

Tambyah P.A., Maki D.G. (2000). The relationship between pyuria and infection in patients with indwelling urinary catheters: a prospective study of 761 patients. *Archives of Internal Medicine*. 160 (5): 673–677.

Trautner B.W., Darouiche R.O. (2004). Catheter-associated infections: pathogenesis affects prevention. *Archives of Internal Medicine*. 164: 842–850.

Trovillion E.W., Skyles J.M., Hopkins-Broyles D., Recktenwald A., Faulkner K. *et al.* (2011). *Development of a nurse-driven protocol to remove urinary catheters*. Abstract 592. SHEA 2011 Annual Scientific Meeting, April 1–4, Dallas, TX.

Wilson J. (2006). Preventing infections associated with urethral catheters. In: *Infection Control in Clinical Practice*. 3rd ed. Bailliere Tindall Elsevier, London: 215–228.

Woodhead S. (2005). Use of lubricant in female urethral catheterisation. *British Journal of Nursing*. 14 (9): 1022–1023.

Would H.L., Kramer A.M. (2007). Non-payment for harms resulting from medical care: catheter associated urinary tract infections. *JAMA*. 298: 2782–2784.

18

The prevention and management of surgical site infections

Contents

Fundamentals of Infection Prevention and Control: Theory and Practice, Second Edition. Debbie Weston.
© 2013 John Wiley & Sons, Ltd. Published 2013 by John Wiley & Sons, Ltd. Companion Website: www.wiley.com/go/fundamentalsofinfectionprevention

Introduction

Wound or surgical site infections (SSIs) are a common but potentially avoidable complication following any surgical procedure during which the skin is breached and opportunistic resident or transient microorganisms gain entry to the wound. They are associated with significant distress to the patient and are often interpreted as a marker of poor standards of care, particularly in relation to standards and practices within the operating theatre. While most wounds heal without complication, complications can range from a relatively 'trivial' wound discharge to systemic illness and a potentially life-threatening infection (Scanlon, 2005), and up to one-third of deaths that occur post-operatively may be attributable to SSIs (Astagneau *et al.*, 2001). They frequently affect only the superficial tissues, but more serious infections can affect the deeper tissues or other parts of the body manipulated during the procedure. The majority of SSIs become apparent within 30 days of an operative procedure, with most occurring between the fifth and 10th post-operative days. Where a prosthetic implant is used, SSIs affecting the deeper tissues may occur up to 12 months after the operation.

This chapter begins by looking at the prevalence and definitions of SSI. This is followed by the common bacterial causes of SSI and the pathogenesis of infection. The chapter concludes with a summary of the best-practice recommendations regarding the prevention and management of SSIs from the Department of Health (DH, 2007) and the NICE Clinical Guideline, *Surgical Site Infection: Prevention and Treatment of Surgical Site Infection*, which was published by the National Collaborating Centre for Women's and Children's Health in 2008. SSI surveillance is covered in Chapter 3.

Learning outcomes

After reading this chapter, the reader will be able to:

- Understand the three different levels used to define SSIs.

- Describe the three stages of wound healing and the importance of the inflammatory response.

- List at least four bacterial causes of SSIs.

- Describe three risk factors for the development of SSIs.

- List the clinical features of SSIs.

- Describe the four categories of wounds.

- Understand the best-practice recommendations for the prevention of SSIs.

The prevalence of surgical site infections

Table 18.1 displays the prevalence of surgical site infections (SSIs) in England, Northern Ireland, Scotland and Wales in 2011–2012 as identified in National HCAI Point Prevalence Surveys.

Table 18.1   Surgical site infection prevalence as identified by National HCAI Point Prevalence Surveys in England, Northern Ireland, Scotland and Wales

Fourth English National Point Prevalence Survey (Health Protection Agency, 2011a)	SSI prevalence: 15.7%
Second Northern Ireland National Point Prevalence Survey (Public Health Agency, 2012)	SSI prevalence: 19%
Welsh Point Prevalence Survey (Public Health Wales NHS Trust, 2011)	SSI prevalence: 19.6%
Second Scottish National Point Prevalence Survey (Health Protection Scotland, 2012)	SSI prevalence: 18.6%

The prevention of SSIs: Compliance with the Health and Social Care Act 2008

With regard to the prevention of SSIs, Trusts must (DH, 2010):

- Have in place and operate effective management systems for the prevention and control of healthcare-associated infections (HCAIs) which are informed by risk assessments and analysis of infection incidents.
- Ensure that patients presenting with an infection, or who acquire an infection during their care, are identified promptly and receive appropriate management and treatment to reduce the risk of transmission.
- Have and adhere to appropriate policies and protocols for the prevention and control of HCAIs.

Defining SSIs

The Centers for Disease Control and Prevention (CDC) (Garner, 1984) and the Health Protection Agency (2011b) describe three levels of SSIs:

1. **Superficial incisional**: affecting the skin or subcutaneous tissue. These infections occur within 30 days of surgery and may by indicated by localised signs such as redness, pain, heat or swelling at the site of incision, or by the drainage of pus.
2. **Deep incisional**: affecting the fascial and muscle layers. These infections occur within 30 days of surgery unless a prosthetic implant is in place, in which case infection may be apparent within a year of surgery. Infection may be indicated by the presence of pus or an abscess, fever with tenderness of the wound, or a separation of the edges of the incision, exposing the deeper tissues.

3. **Organ or space infection**: This involves any part of the anatomy other than the incision that is opened or manipulated during the surgical procedure, for example a joint or the peritoneum. Infections occur within 30 days without an implant, or within a year with an implant. Organ or space infections may be indicated by the drainage of pus or the formation of an abscess, detected by histopathological or radiological examination, or during re-operation.

The process of wound healing

Wound healing is a complex process of which there are three main phases which overlap in time (Li *et al.*, 2007):

- **Inflammation** (see Chapter 8):
  - Early (the first 24 hours): This begins with haemostasis (the process whereby bleeding stops) through vasoconstriction (the narrowing, or constriction, of the muscular wall of arteries and blood vessels), thrombin formation (part of the coagulation cascade that slows bleeding) and the clumping together of platelets in the blood to form a clot. Platelets release cytokines that directly influence white blood cell activity and direct them to the wound site.
  - Late (24–72 hours): This involves the release of vasodilators and other agents which increase the permeability of the local capillary bed, allowing serum and white blood cells to be released into the area surrounding the wound, and enabling the removal of bacteria and tissue debris. This creates a local inflammatory response, giving rise to pain, swelling, heat and redness at the wound site, but these should not be interpreted as signs of infection.
- **Regeneration:** This occurs over the next few days to weeks, with the repair of damaged cells and tissues and the formation of epithelium to cover the surface of the wound, along with the growth of granulation tissue which fills the wound space (Li *et al.*, 2007).
- **Maturation:** This is the final phase of wound healing and is also referred to as the 'remodelling' phase (Li *et al.*, 2007); it can take up to two years to complete. Granulation tissue strengthens and matures into scar tissue which gradually thins and shrinks. Over time, the tensile strength ('stretchability') of the scar tissue improves, but only to 80% of that of normal skin.

The pathogenesis of SSIs

The development of an SSI depends on contamination of the wound site at the end of a surgical procedure, and specifically relates to the pathogenicity and number of microorganisms present, balanced against the host's immune response.

Endogenous infection

The microorganisms that cause SSIs are usually derived from the patient and, being present on the skin or in an opened viscus (internal organ), migrate from one body site to another. When a viscus such as the large bowel is opened, tissues are likely to become contaminated by a whole range of microorganisms, which may act together to cause an SSI.

Reflection point

Patients can transfer their own resident body flora to different body sites on their hands, and potentially contaminate their wound. What advice is given to patients within your place of work regarding 'touching' their wound?

Exogenous infections

These occur when microorganisms from instruments or the operating theatre environment contaminate the site of operation, when microorganisms from the environment contaminate a traumatic wound or when microorganisms gain access to the wound after surgery and before the skin has healed.

Fact Box 18.1   SSIs and exogenous infection

Dancer *et al.* (2012) reported a sudden increase of SSIs in orthopaedic patients undergoing elective joint replacement. Following an extensive investigation that examined all aspects of clinical practice, there was evidence that surgical sets had become wet or dampened following autoclaving and that poor instrument-handling practices within the sterilisation department contributed to contamination of the sets.

Microorganisms from a distant source of infection, principally through haematogenous spread via the bloodstream, can cause an SSI by attaching to prosthesis or another implant inserted into the operative site, although infections by this route are rare. Skin squames can be carried in dust on air currents and can settle on open wounds if wounds are dressed while activities such as bed making or ward cleaning are in progress. The use of electric fans in ward areas can also disseminate dust and skin squames, and they should be used with caution.

Fact Box 18.2   The implications of SSI

The development of an SSI after elective (planned) 'clean' joint replacement or cataract surgery is known to have potentially devastating effects on patients (Dancer *et al.*, 2012). Patients contracting an infection following the replacement of a major joint, such as the hip or knee, may require prolonged courses of antibiotics. If the prosthesis itself is infected, it may require a two-stage revision, involving removal of the cement, removal of the infected prosthesis and debridement of infected tissue, followed at a later date by the insertion of a new joint. This increases length of stay and exposes the patient further to the risks of developing other HCAIs. Infection following cataract surgery can cause endopthalmitis, which may result in either complete loss of vision in the affected eye or reduced visual fields. There is a Fact Sheet (18.1) on the companion website.

Bacterial causes of SSIs

The main bacterial causes of SSIs are shown in Box 18.1.

Box 18.1   The main bacterial causes of surgical site infections

Staphylococcus aureus (including meticillin-resistant *S. aureus* [MRSA])
Pseudomonas aeruginosa
Klebsiella spp.
Proteus spp.
Clostridium perfringens
Bacteroides spp.
Group A streptococcus
Enterobacteriaceae

(see Fact Sheets 1.6, 3.3 and 3.8 on the companion website for further information regarding some of these organisms)

Risk factors for the development of SSIs

Patient susceptibility

Regarding patient susceptibility, age, underlying illness, disease or infection, as well as malnutrition, smoking, obesity and medication (e.g. steroids which suppress the immune response, or antibiotics which can alter the body flora) are acknowledged risk factors for the development of any infection (National Collaborating Centre for Women's and Children's Health, 2008; Bibi *et al.*, 2011; Wloch *et al.*, 2012). Associated co-morbidities at the time of surgery increase the risk of post-operative wound infection.

Fact Box 18.3   The ASA score

The American Society of Anesthesiologists (ASA, 1963) devised a pre-operative risk score (the ASA score) to identify those patients most at risk. Patients are given a score of 1–5, with 1 representing the lowest risk (a normal, healthy patient) and 5 the highest risk (patient not expected to survive 24 hours with or without surgery).

Emergency versus elective surgery

Patients undergoing elective (planned) surgery are generally in a better state of health and better prepared pre-operatively than those who require emergency surgery. One study found that the infection rate following emergency surgery was 25.2% compared to 7.6% for elective cases (Satyanarayana *et al.*, 2011).

Wound classification

Wounds are classified into different categories according to their origin (Garner, 1984):

- **Clean wounds** are surgical wounds which are created under controlled conditions using an aseptic technique. At the time of surgery, there is no inflammation present and sites such as the gastro-intestinal (GI) tract which contain their own flora are not breached.
- **Clean-contaminated wounds** are surgical wounds which extend into the GI, respiratory, genital or urinary tract but without contamination of the wound occurring.
- **Contaminated wounds** include those that arise as a result of trauma, a major break in sterile technique or contamination as a result of spillage from the GI tract, or where inflamed tissue is encountered but without the presence of pus.
- **Dirty or infected wounds** are contaminated with foreign material (e.g. dirt or debris) or the contents of perforated viscera. Infected wounds may contain necrotic devitalised tissue.

Duration of surgery

The duration of surgery is defined as the time between skin incision and skin closure (Leong *et al.*, 2006). When tissues are exposed to the air during surgery, there is a risk that bacteria carried on airborne particles can settle in the wound, on surgical instruments or on the hands of operating staff. The majority of microorganisms are from the staff present in the theatre and the dispersal of microorganisms increases with movement, and this represents the biggest risk in joint replacement surgery.

It has been estimated that each person sheds approximately 10 000 microorganisms per minute when they are at rest, increasing to 50 000 per minute during periods of activity (Howarth, 1985), so the number of staff present at the time of surgery should be limited to essential personnel only. In order to further reduce airborne transmission and contamination of the wound, operating theatres should have at least 20 air changes an hour, equating to one air change every three minutes, which will reduce airborne contamination to 37% of its former level (Dharan and Pittett, 2002). In orthopaedic surgery, the use of laminar flow systems in conjunction with high-efficiency particulate air (HEPA) filters in orthopaedic theatres has been shown to significantly reduce infection rates (Garner, 1984). However, Gastmeier *et al.* (2012) suggest that the efficacy of laminar flow is debatable, and that it has actually been implicated as a risk factor for SSIs.

Surgical technique

Poor surgical technique can lead to contamination of the site (e.g. perforation of the bowel will contaminate the operative site with anaerobic gut flora), prolong the duration of surgery and damage tissues and blood and oxygen supply to the area (Garner, 1984).

Presence of foreign material

Prosthetic implants, sutures and drains have all been found to increase the risk of post-operative infection. Without a suture, 6.5 million bacteria would be required to initiate an infection, but in the presence of just one suture, only 100 bacteria are required (Wilson, 2006). Prosthetic implants including those used in orthopaedic and cardiac surgery 'attract' organisms such as coagulase-negative staphylococci which produce biofilm and adhere to implanted material.

Length of hospital stay, and time interval between admission and surgery

The majority of patients for routine elective surgery are now admitted on the day of operation, having had pre-operative investigations such as full blood count, electrocardiogram (ECG) and X-rays carried out in the pre-assessment clinic. This has the benefit of reducing bed occupancy. Plus the less time the patient is in hospital before surgery, the less opportunity there is for the patient's normal body flora to be replaced by hospital pathogens (Cruse and Ford, 1980).

Pre-operative hair removal

Pre-operative shaving with a razor has been identified as a major contributing factor to wound infection (Cruse and Ford, 1973; Tkach *et al.*, 1979). Nicks and cuts on the skin's surface reduce its integrity, and liberate resident dermal bacteria into the operative field, making the skin environment more favourable to bacterial proliferation (McIntyre and McCloy, 1994).

Antibiotic prophylaxis

Approximately 30–50% of all antibiotics prescribed in hospitals are for the prevention of SSIs (Satyanarayana *et al.*, 2011). The first three hours is considered to be the critical period during which bacterial contamination of the wound leading to infection can occur (Howarth, 1985), and antibiotics may be administered peri-operatively and during surgery to minimise the risk (Scottish Intercollegiate Guidelines, 2008). The administration of antibiotic prophylaxis depends on:

- The patient's risk of developing a post-operative surgical wound infection
- The severity of the consequences of an infection (in patients with an orthopaedic implant, the implant and possibly the joint may have to be removed)
- The effectiveness of the antibiotic and the potential consequences of administration, such as the risk of developing *Clostridium difficile* and pseudomembranous colitis.

The antibiotics used for surgical prophylaxis are chosen to target the pathogens that commonly cause infections in specific types or sites of wounds, and they are administered at induction, as near to the time of incision as possible, and during surgery. The timing of administration is important – the aim is to achieve the correct concentrations of the drug in the blood and in the tissues at the time of surgery and to maintain them while the procedure is taking place.

Box 18.2 describes the clinical features of SSIs.

Box 18.2   Clinical features of SSIs

- Inflammation and tenderness at the incision site. If the infection is deep seated, the pain is generally more severe (described as throbbing). The surrounding tissues are often oedematous, and any discharge from the site can be purulent and malodorous, particularly if anaerobic bacteria are present.
- Pyrexia, which indicates that an inflammatory response is taking place in response to the infection

Continued

265

- Discolouration at the wound margin and friable granulation tissue which bleeds easily
- Complete wound dehiscence following abdominal surgery with visible loops of bowel appearing through the incision is a surgical emergency, and the patient needs to be swiftly returned to the operating theatre.

Best-practice recommendations for the prevention of SSIs

Box 18.3 summarises some of the key recommendations of the DH's *Saving Lives High Impact Intervention Care Bundle to Prevent Surgical Site Infection* (DH, 2007), and the NICE Clinical Guideline for the prevention and management of SSIs (National Collaborating Centre for Women's and Children's Health, 2008, which is due to be updated in 2013). The full NICE Guideline, which details the evidence base for each recommendation, can be accessed at http://www.nice.org.uk/nicemedia/pdf/CG74NICEGuideline.pdf.

Note on skin preparation: The current NICE Guideline recommends either an aqueous or an alcohol based preparation, such as povidone-iodine or chlorhexidine gluconate. Chloraprep® 2% chlorhexidine in 70% IPA received a level one recommendation from the Rapid Review Panel in 2005 (and again in 2011 following the introduction of 'tinted' Chloraprep®), although it is not used nationally for surgical skin prep. Whichever product is used, Trusts should ensure that it is licensed as a medicinal product, meaning that it is suitable for its intended purpose. A product used for skin prep that is actually a biocide will be suitable for 'hygienic' use only, not for 'prevention' (i.e. not for the prevention of SSI), and if used for skin disinfection could be considered to be used 'improperly'. Another point to note is that where alcohol-based solutions are applied using soaked gauze, it can soak drapes and pool underneath the patient, which could potentially lead to skin irritation and chemical burns and, in the worse case scenario, risk of fire and serious injury to the patient if diathermy is used.

Box 18.3   Best-practice recommendations for the prevention of SSIs

- Patients and carers should be offered information and advice on how to care for their wound after discharge.
- Patients and carers should be offered information about how to recognise a SSI and who to contact if they are concerned.
- Patients should be screened for MRSA and, if positive, decolonised prior to surgery.
- Advise patients to shower or have a bath (or help patients to shower, bathe or bed-bath) using soap, either the day before or on the day of surgery.
- When hair removal is indicated, it must be undertaken as close to the time of surgery as possible, using electric clippers with a single-use disposable head.
- Staff should keep their movements in and out of the operating theatre to a minimum.

- Do not use nasal decontamination with topical antimicrobial agents aimed at eliminating *S. aureus* routinely to reduce the risk of SSIs.
- Mechanical bowel preparation should not routinely be used to reduce the risk of SSIs.
- The operating team should wash their hands prior to the first operation on the list using aqueous aseptic surgical solution, with a single-use brush or pick for the nails, and ensure that their hands and nails are visibly clean.
- Before subsequent operations, hands should be washed using either an alcoholic hand rub or an antiseptic surgical solution.
- If hands are soiled, they should be washed again with an antiseptic surgical solution.
- Artificial nails, nail polish and jewellery may conceal underlying soiling and impair hand decontamination, and must not be worn. The operating team should remove hand jewellery before operations.
- Antibiotic prophylaxis should be given to patients before:
    - Clean surgery involving the placement of a prosthesis or implant
    - Clean-contaminated surgery
    - Contaminated surgery.
- Antibiotics should not be used routinely for clean non-prosthetic uncomplicated surgery.
- Antibiotics should be prescribed in accordance with local Trust guidelines.
- A single dose of antibiotic prophylaxis should be given on induction.
- Antibiotics should be given to patients having surgery on a dirty or infected wound.
- If an incise drape is required, use an iodophor-impregnated drape unless the patient has an iodine allergy.
- The operating team should wear sterile gowns in the operating theatre during the surgery.
- The use of reusable or disposable drapes and gowns does not influence the risk of SSIs.
- Consideration should be given to wearing two pairs of sterile gloves when there is a high risk of glove perforation and the consequences of contamination of the operative field can be serious.
- Prepare the skin at the surgical site immediately before incision using an antiseptic (aqueous or alcohol-based) preparation: povidone–iodine or chlorhexidine are most suitable.
- If diathermy is to be used, antiseptic skin preparations must be dried by evaporation, and pooling of alcohol-based preparations avoided.
- Do not use diathermy for surgical incisions to reduce the risk of SSIs.
- Maintain patient temperature in line with 'inadvertent peri-operative hypothermia'.
- Maintain optimal oxygenation during surgery. In particular, give patients sufficient oxygen during major surgery and in the recovery period to ensure that a haemoglobin saturation of more than 95% is maintained.
- Maintain adequate perfusion during surgery.
- Do not give insulin routinely to patients who do not have diabetes to optimise blood glucose post-operatively as a means of reducing the risk of SSIs.
- Do not use wound irrigation to reduce the risk of SSIs.
- Do not use intracavity lavage to reduce the risk of SSIs.

Continued

- Cover surgical incisions with an appropriate dressing (e.g. a semi-permeable film membrane with or without an absorbent island) at the end of the operation for a period of 48 hours.
- An **aseptic non-touch technique** should be used for changing or removing surgical wound dressings.
- Sterile saline can be used for wound cleansing up to 48 hours following surgery.
- Patients should be advised that they can shower 48 hours after surgery.
- Tap water can be used for wound cleansing after 48 hours if the surgical wound has separated or has been surgically opened to drain pus.
- Refer to the Tissue Viability Team for advice on appropriate dressings for the management of wounds healing by secondary intention.
- Do not use Eusol and gauze, or moist cotton gauze or mercuric antiseptic solutions, to manage surgical wounds that are healing by secondary intention.
- When an SSI is suspected (e.g. cellulitis), the patient should be prescribed an antibiotic that covers the likely causative organism.
- Eusol and gauze, or dextranomer or enzymatic treatments, should not be used for debridement of SSIs.
- A structured approach to wound care (including pre-operative assessments to identify individuals with potential wound-healing problems) is required in order to improve overall management of surgical wounds.

Reflection point

Clinical practice

As stated in the introduction to this chapter, most SSIs become apparent 5–10 days post-operatively, by which time the majority of patients are likely to have been discharged. What information is given to patients and carers regarding problems with the wound occurring post discharge?

Chapter summary: key points

- Surgical site infections are potentially avoidable.

- SSIs account for 15.7% of all HCAIs in England.

- They can have devastating long-term effects and may account for up to one-third of post-operative deaths.

- Associated co-morbidities at the time of surgery increase the risk of post-operative SSIs.

- The majority of SSIs occur between the fifth and 10th post-operative day.

- Approximately 30–50% of all antibiotics prescribed in hospitals are for the prevention of SSIs.

- Healthcare staff should implement best-practice recommendations for the prevention of SSIs.

Further resources are available for this book, including interactive multiple choice questions. Visit the companion website at:

www.wiley.com/go/fundamentalsofinfectionprevention

References

American Society of Anesthiologists (ASA) (1963). New classification of physical status. *Anaesthesiology*. 21: 111.

Astagneau P., Rioux C., Golliot F., Brucker G. and the INCISO Network Society Study Group (2001). Morbidity and mortality associated with surgical site infections: results from the 1997–1999 INCISO survey. *Journal of Hospital Infection*. 48: 267–274.

Bibi S., Channa G.A., Siddiqui T.R., Ahmed W. (2011). Frequency and risk factors of surgical site infections in general surgery ward of a tertiary care hospital of Karachi, Pakistan. *International Journal of Infection Control*. 7 (3):http://www.ijic.info/article/6098 (20 December 2012)

Cruse P.J.E., Foord R. (1973). A five-year prospective study of 23,649 surgical wounds. *Archives of Surgery*. 107 (2): 206.

Cruse P.J.E., Foord R. (1980). The epidemiology of wound infection: a 10 year prospective study of 62,939 surgical wounds. *Surgical Clinics of North America*. 60 (1): 27–40.

Dancer S.J., Stewart M., Coulombe C., Gregori A., Virdi M. (2012). Surgical site infections linked to contaminated surgical instruments. *Journal of Hospital Infection*. 81 (4): 231–238.

Department of Health (DH) (2007). *High Impact Intervention. Care Bundle to Prevent Surgical Site Infection*. Department of Health, London.

Department of Health (DH) (2010). *The Health and Social Care Act 2008. Code of Practice on the Prevention and Control of Infections and Related Guidance*. Department of Health, London.

Dharan S., Pittett D. (2002). Environmental controls in operating theatres. *Journal of Hospital Infection*. 51 (2): 79–84.

Garner J. (1984). *Guideline for Prevention of Surgical Wound Infections*. http://www.cdc.gov/ncidod/hip/Guide/surwound.htm (accessed 20 December 2012)

Gastmeier P.M., Breier A.C., Brandt C. (2012). Influence of laminar airflow on prosthetic joint infections: a systematic review. *Journal of Hospital Infection*. 81: 73–78.

Health Protection Agency (2011a). *English National Point Prevalence Survey of Healthcare Associated Infections and Antimicrobial Use, 2011: Preliminary Data*. Health Protection Agency, London.

Health Protection Agency (2011b). *Protocol for the Surveillance of Surgical Site Infection*. Version 5. Health Protection Agency and Surgical Site Infection Surveillance Service, London.

Health Protection Scotland (2012). *Scottish National Point Prevalence Survey of Healthcare Associated Infections and Antimicrobial Prescribing, 2011*. Health Protection Scotland, Glasgow.

Howarth F.H. (1985). Prevention of airborne infection during surgery. *The Lancet*. 1 (8425): 386–388.

Leong G., Wilson J., Charlett A. (2006). Duration of operation as a risk factor for surgical site infection: comparison of English and US data. *Journal of Hospital Infection*. 63: 255–262.

Li J., Chen J., Kirsner R. (2007). Pathophysiology of acute wound healing. *Clinics in Dermatology*. 25: 9–18.

McIntyre F.J., McCloy R. (1994). Shaving patients before surgery a dangerous myth? *Annals Royal College of Surgeons of England*. 76: 3–4.

National Collaborating Centre for Women's and Children's Health (2008). *Surgical Site Infection: Prevention and Treatment of Surgical Site Infection. Clinical Guideline*. National Institute for Health and Clinical Excellence (NICE), London.

Public Health Agency (2012). *Northern Ireland Point Prevalence Survey of Hospital Acquired Infections and Antimicrobial Use 2012*. November. Public Health Agency, Belfast.

Public Health Wales NHS Trust (2011). *Point Prevalence Survey of Healthcare Associated Infections, Medical Device Usage and Antimicrobial Usage. 2011 – Wales*. Public Health Wales, Cardiff.

Satyanarayana V., Prashanth H.V., Basavaraj B., Kavyashree A.N. (2011). Study of surgical site infections in abdominal surgeries. *Journal of Clinical and Diagnostic Research*. 5 (5): 935–939.

Scanlon E. (2005). Wound infection and colonisation. *Nursing Standard*. 19 (24): 57–67.

Scottish Intercollegiate Guidelines Network (2008). *Antibiotic Prophylaxis in Surgery: A National Clinical Guideline*. SIGN Publication 45, July. Scottish Intercollegiate Guidelines Network, Edinburgh.

Tkach J.R., Shannon A.M., Beastrom R. (1979). Pseudofolliculitis due to pre-operative shaving. *AORN Journal*. 30 (5): 881–884.

Wilson J. (2006). Preventing wound infection. In: *Infection Control in Clinical Practice*. 3rd ed. Bailliere Tindall Elsevier, London: 179–198.

Wloch C., Wilson J., Lamagni T., Harrington P., Charlett A., Sheridan E. (2012). Risk factors for surgical site infection following caesarean section in England: results from a multicentre cohort study. *British Journal of Obstetrics and Gynaecology*. 119 (11): 1324–1333.

19

The prevention and management of hospital and community-acquired pneumonia

Contents

Fundamentals of Infection Prevention and Control: Theory and Practice, Second Edition. Debbie Weston.
© 2013 John Wiley & Sons, Ltd. Published 2013 by John Wiley & Sons, Ltd. Companion Website: www.wiley.com/go/fundamentalsofinfectionprevention

Introduction

Pneumonia is the most severe and life-threatening of all respiratory tract infections, affecting patients both in the community and in acute healthcare settings. In intensive care units, where it is strongly associated with endotracheal intubation and mechanical ventilation, it has a case fatality rate of 20–70% (Chastre and Fagon, 2002; Masterton *et al.*, 2008; Craven and Chroneou, 2009), and in the 2011 English National Point Prevalence Survey on Healthcare-associated Infections, 45.3% of healthcare-associated infections (HCAIs) in intensive therapy units were defined as pneumonia or lower respiratory tract infections, accounting for 22.8% of all HCAIs in total and holding the number one 'spot' in the HCAI league table (Health Protection Agency, 2011). In 2007, the Department of Health published a care bundle, consisting of six regular and two ongoing elements of care aimed at reducing ventilator-associated pneumonia (Department of Health, 2007), and this was adopted by Intensive Care Units as part of the Saving Lives High Impact Interventions in order to prevent HCAIs (see Chapter 1).

This chapter looks at community and hospital-acquired pneumonia, covering definitions, patient risk factors, diagnosis, management and prevention, and refers to national guidance and best-practice recommendations.

Learning outcomes

After reading this chapter, the reader will be able to:

- Understand the definitions of community-acquired, hospital-acquired and ventilator-associated pneumonia.

- List some of the host defence mechanisms that protect individuals against respiratory tract infections in general.

- Identify the host risk factors for the development of community and hospital-acquired pneumonia.

- List some of the common causative organisms.

- List the common investigations that are undertaken, and understand the significance of the CURB-65 score.

- Describe the preventative measures for community and hospital-acquired pneumonia.

Definition of pneumonia

Pneumonia is a generally severe respiratory tract infection. It affects the lung tissue (parenchyma) and is associated with consolidation of the affected area, which may affect one or both lungs, and the presence of an inflammatory exudate within the alveoli. It can affect adults and children but is more commonly associated with the elderly.

Respiratory tract host defence mechanisms

In spite of the fact that the respiratory tract is constantly exposed to gases, fumes, particles and microorganisms, it is extremely well protected. Box 19.1 lists some of the host defence mechanisms (see Chapter 8) that protect the respiratory tract from invasion by microorganisms.

Box 19.1   Host defence mechanisms of the respiratory tract

Nasal hairs
Ciliated epithelium
Mucociliary blankets
Saliva
Cough reflex
Swallow reflex
IgA antibody
Complement
Dendritic cells
Alveolar macrophages
Phagocytes.

Microorganisms causing pneumonia

Community and hospital-acquired pneumonia can be caused by bacteria, viruses and fungi. In cases where the primary cause is viral, as a result of influenza or **varicella zoster** infection, for example (see Chapter 5), or HIV (see Chapter 24), secondary bacterial or fungal infections can develop. Box 19.2 summarises the common bacterial, viral and fungal causes of pneumonia.

Box 19.2   Common bacterial, viral and fungal causes of pneumonia

Bacteria

Streptococcus pneumoniae
Staphylococcus aureus (including meticillin-resistant *S. aureus* [MRSA]; see Chapter 20)
Haemophilus influenzae
Escherichia coli (see Chapter 10)
Klebsiella pneumoniae (see Chapter 10)
Serratia (see Fact Sheet 9.3 on the companion website)
Pseudomonas aeruginosa (see Chapter 10)
Legionella (see Fact Sheet 1.3 on the companion website).

Viruses

Influenza A and B
Respiratory syncitial virus
Rhinoviruses (see Chapter 5)
Coxsackieviruses (see Chapter 5).

Fungi

Pneumocystis jiroveci (formerly known as *P. carinii*) – a complication of AIDS (see Chapter 24).

Boxes 19.3 and 19.4 list the clinical features of pneumonia and the routine investigations that are undertaken.

Box 19.3   Clinical features of pneumonia

The onset may be over hours to days.

- Symptoms of a lower respiratory tract illness (cough and at least one other respiratory tract symptom, e.g. dyspnoea, pleural pain and/or tachyapnoea)
- New (not pre-existing) focal chest signs on examination
- At least one systemic feature (sweating, shivers, aches and pains and/or temperature >38 °C)
- No other explanation for illness.

Source: Data from Donowitz, 2009; Lim *et al.*, 2009.

275

Box 19.4   Routine investigations

Chest X-ray
Oxygen saturation
Blood gas
C-reactive protein (CRP) (see Chapter 8)
White cell count (see Chapter 8)
Full blood count
Sputum for culture and sensitivity (see Chapters 6 and 7)
Urine for *Legionella* antigen testing (see Fact Sheet 1.3 on the companion website)
Blood culture (see Chapters 6 and 7).

Community-acquired pneumonia

Community-acquired pneumonia (CAP) can be defined as pneumonia that is not associated with care in community or acute healthcare settings (i.e. the person with pneumonia is not a resident or patient within a nursing or residential home or other community care facility, or a hospital in-patient setting). Box 19.5 lists the risk factors for CAP, and Box 19.6 lists the organisms that are commonly implicated.

Box 19.5   Risk factors for CAP

Age
Chronic pulmonary or cardiac disease
Diabetes
Renal failure
Immunocompromised

Box 19.6   Common microorganisms causing CAP

S. aureus, including MRSA (see Chapter 20)
S. pneumoniae
H. influenzae
Legionella
Influenzas A and B

S. pneumoniae is the most common pathogen identified overall. *Legionella* and *S. aureus* are the most common pathogens isolated in patients with CAP severe enough to warrant admission to an Intensive Care Unit (Lim *et al.*, 2009).

Fact Box 19.1   CAP and the CURB-65 score

The British Thoracic Society guidelines (Lim *et al.*, 2009) recommend use of the CURB-65 score to assess the severity of pneumonia, which in turn should inform treatment. It can also be used as a predictor of mortality, as the higher the score the higher the likelihood that the patient will die. The CURB-65 assessment should be undertaken by the Medical Team on all patients admitted with CAP in particular, but it can also be undertaken for hospital-acquired pneumonia. 1 point is allocated for the presence of each of the following criteria. A score of 2 or more is an indicator of severe infection and a poor outcome:

Confusion
Urea >7 mmol
Respiratory rate ≥30/minute
Blood pressure: low systolic (≤90 mmHg) or diastolic (≤ 60 mmHg)
Age ≥ 65.

Reflection point

Is there documented evidence that the CURB-65 score is routinely used by medical staff at your workplace?

Treatment of CAP

'Blind therapy' with amoxicillin and metronidazole is often commenced initially as the number of organisms responsible for causing pneumonia can make the antibiotic treatment of CAP a therapeutic challenge (Donowitz, 2009). In uncomplicated CAP (previously 'healthy' chest and admission to the intensive therapy unit [ITU] not required), doxycline or amoxicillin may be prescribed orally. In severe cases, amoxicillin (cefuroxime if penicillin allergy) and clarithromycin may be prescribed in combination.

Hospital-acquired or ventilator-associated pneumonia

Hospital-acquired pneumonia (HAP) is defined as pneumonia occurring more than 48 hours after admission to hospital (Masterton *et al.*, 2008), or, in the case of ventilator-associated pneumonia (VAP), occurring within 48–72 hours of intubation (Craven and Chroneou, 2009). Box 19.7 lists the risk factors for the development of HAP and VAP, and Box 19.8 lists the organisms that are commonly implicated.

The risk of VAP is estimated to be 3% per day during days 1–5 of ventilation, decreasing to 2% during days 5–10, and then 1% each day thereafter (Cook *et al.*, 1998).

277

Box 19.7 Risk factors for HAP and VAP

- Mechanical ventilation for >48 hours
- Duration of ITU stay or hospital admission
- Severity of underlying illness
- Co-morbidities
- Age
- Malnutrition
- Immunosuppression
- History of alcohol or substance misuse
- Pre-existing chronic lung disease
- Administration of antibiotics (alteration of normal body flora; colonisation with drug-resistant bacteria)
- Naso-gastric tube insertion
- Aspiration
- Surgery involving the head, neck, thorax or upper abdomen

Continued

- Restricted mobility due to age, trauma, surgery or prolonged bed rest
- Exposure to contaminated respiratory devices
- Transmission of pathogens on the hands of healthcare staff or from contaminated equipment.

Source: Data from Lynch, 2001; Chastre and Fagon, 2002; Craven and Chroneou, 2009.

Box 19.8   Common bacterial and fungal causes of HAP and VAP

S. aureus, including MRSA (see Chapter 20)
S. pneumoniae
H. influenzae
P. aeruginosa (see Chapter 10)
Moraxella catarrhalis
Acinetobacter species (see Chapter 10)
Serratia species (see Fact Sheet 9.3 on the companion website.)
K. pneumonia (see Chapter 10)
E. coli (see Chapter 10)
Legionella is a less common cause of HAP.
Candida species and *Aspergillus fumigatus* – in patients who are immunocompromised as a result of transplant, or severely neutropenic (see Chapter 9 and Fact Sheet 9.1 on the companion website).

Source: Data from American Thoracic Society and the Infectious Diseases Society of America, 2005; Craven and Chroneou, 2009.

Fact Box 19.2   Sensitivity of microorganisms

Antibiotic-sensitive pathogens are commonly implicated in early-onset HAP (e.g. pneumonia occurring within five days of admission) (Carven and Chroneou, 2009), whereas pneumonia acquired after this period is more likely to be multidrug resistant, as the longer the patient is in hospital the wider the exposure to resistant pathogens (Lynch, 2001).

The pathogenesis of infection

In order for HAP to develop, host defences must be breached so that pathogens can successfully enter and colonise the lower respiratory tract. In order to accomplish this, they have to overcome mechanical (innate immune response mechanisms, such as cilliated epithelium and mucus), cellular (e.g. leukocytes and macrophages) and humoral (antibody and complement) host immune defences (American Thoracic Society and the Infectious Diseases Society of America, 2004).

- The most common cause of HAP is the aspiration of nasopharyngeal and oropharyngeal secretions. This can occur in patients with impaired cough or swallowing reflexes and through vomiting.
- In mechanically ventilated patients, the endotracheal (ET) tube provides a direct route of entry into the normally well-protected respiratory tract. Organisms colonising the oropharynx may be carried into the trachea during intubation, and the process of intubation itself can cause local trauma and inflammation, which increases colonisation of the trachea with resident organisms as well as pathogens (Craven and Chroneou, 2009). In addition, the lumen of the ET tube supports the growth of bacteria which grow within a biofilm (see Chapter 5), and biofilm formation within the ET tube may be a contributing factor in the development of VAP (Craven and Chroneou, 2009). Procedures such as suctioning may result in dislodging biofilm-encased bacteria which may be transported to the alveoli (Adair et al., 1999).
- Secretions pool above the inflated cuff of the endotracheal tube and often contain Gram-negative bacilli and S. aureus which colonise the upper respiratory tract in patients who have been in hospital for longer than five days.
- Once the secretions have been aspirated into the lower respiratory tract, they cause inflammation and infection in the terminal bronchioles and alveoli in the lung, filling the alveolar spaces with fluid instead of air, preventing gases exchange and resulting in consolidation (Dunn, 2005).
- The outcome is dependent upon the number and types of organisms that gain entry to the lower respiratory tract and the efficiency of host immune defence mechanisms.

279

Diagnosis – Clinical Pulmonary Infection Score (CPIS) (Masterton et al., 2008)

- Core temperature >38.3 °C
- Raised or lowered white cell count (>10 000/mm^3 or <4000/mm^3)
- Purulent tracheal secretions and/or new or persistent infiltrations on chest X-ray which are otherwise unexplained
- Worsening gaseous exchange and increased oxygen requirements.

Fact Box 19.3   The collection of specimens – HAP and VAP

The collection of a specimen of sputum or endotracheal aspirate is considered to be of limited microbiological value as it can become contaminated during collection by flora colonising the upper respiratory tract, and the organism(s) detected may not actually be the causative agent(s). Potential pathogens will be most heavily concentrated deep within the lung, and to this end, bronchoscopy-assisted lavage (BAL) or bronchoscopy-directed protected specimen brushings (PSBs) are considered to be the most rapid and least invasive sampling methods for the detection of VAP (Masterton et al., 2008).

Aspiration pneumonia

Aspiration pneumonia can be both community and hospital-acquired and is caused by inhalation of 'foreign' material such as food, drink, medication and vomit, along with neurological conditions and disorders (see Box 19.9).

Box 19.9   Risk factors for aspiration pneumonia

- Altered neurological state – that is, loss of consciousness following trauma, drinking large amounts of alcohol, coma, sedation or anaesthesia
- Neurological disorders and disease – for example, stroke or myasthenia gravis
- Impaired swallow reflex
- Gastro-oesophageal reflux and gastro-oesophageal stricture.

Prevention of HAP and VAP – best-practice recommendations

The best-practice recommendations given in Boxes 19.10 and 19.11 include guidance published by the Department of Health (2007), the British Society for Antimicrobial Chemotherapy (Masterton *et al.*, 2008) and the American Thoracic Society and the Infectious Diseases Society of America (2004), along with papers by Kress *et al.* (2000), Dodek *et al.* (2004) and Machin (2005).

Box 19.10   Best-practice recommendations – general preventative measures for HAP and VAP

- Adequate post-operative pain relief to facilitate deep breathing, coughing and mobilisation
- Chest physiotherapy
- Early mobilisation post-operatively
- Hand decontamination in accordance with the 5 Moments for Hand Hygiene (see Chapter 12) to prevent the exogenous transmission of microorganisms acquired from contact with other patients or the environment
- Isolation or cohort nursing of patients known to be colonised or infected with microorganisms in order to reduce the risk of cross-infection to other patients (see Chapter 11)
- Correct use of personal protective equipment (PPE) (see Chapter 13)
- Ensure that all respiratory therapy equipment is decontaminated appropriately in between patients according to manufacturer's instructions (i.e. single use, single-patient use, cleaned, disinfected or sterilised).

- Change anaesthetic tubing and filters if an anaesthetic machine is used on a patient with a known infection.
- Use single-use spirometry mouth pieces.
- Consider use of the semi-recumbent position (30–45 °C) if the patient does not have to be supine.
- In patients who require enteral feeding, keep the patient in the semi-recumbent position whilst the feed is in progress to prevent aspiration.
- Assist patients who have difficulty swallowing with eating, drinking and the swallowing of oral medication to prevent aspiration.
- Ensure that naso-gastric tubes and enteral feeding tubes are sited correctly to prevent aspiration.
- Help preserve gastric acid function and prevent reflux.
- Vaccination against *S. pneumoniae* in 'at-risk' patient groups, and staff vaccination against influenza (to prevent patient cross-infection).

Fact Box 19.4   Nebulisers

In 2004, the Medicines and Healthcare Products Regulatory Agency issued a Medical Device Alert (MDA) regarding the possible transmission of *Legionella* from nebulisers. Where nebulisers are single-patient use (as opposed to single use), the nebuliser must be thoroughly cleaned and dried before re-use, to ensure that no water is left 'standing' in the nebuliser 'acorn', which could then be aerosolised and disseminated. In intensive care units, the nebuliser acorn should be single-use only and disposed of after each use.

281

Box 19.11   Preventative measures – ventilated patients

- Semi-recumbent positioning (if safe for the patient) with elevation of the head of the bed to 30–45 °C (decreases the risk of aspiration from gastro-intestinal contents and/or oropharyngeal or nasopharyngeal secretions)
- Maintain the semi-recumbent position when the patient is transferred from the ITU to a ward.
- Use non-invasive (NI) rather than mechanical ventilation (MV), and oral intubation rather than naso-tracheal intubation where possible.
- Avoid re-intubation.
- Sedation holding – daily interruption of sedation reduces the duration of ventilation.
- Airway humidification – use of heat and moisture exchangers (HMEs) to prevent drying out of the respiratory mucosa, rather than heat humidifiers (HHs). Use sterile water. Change the HME when it becomes visibly soiled.

Continued

- Management of ventilator circuit – change when visibly soiled.
- Use a sterile technique for performing endotracheal suction to prevent contamination of the suction catheter before it is introduced into the trachea; use each suction catheter only once.
- Change suction equipment weekly unless contaminated.
- Nebulisers, where used as part of the ventilator circuit, should be single-use only.
- Adjust the rate and volume of enteral feeding in order to avoid gastric distension and reduce the risk of aspiration.

Chapter summary: key points

- Pneumonia is the most severe and life-threatening of all respiratory tract infections, affecting patients both in the community generally (with no history of community or acute sector healthcare) and in community and acute healthcare settings.

- In intensive care units, it is strongly associated with endotracheal intubation and mechanical ventilation.

- Pneumonia can be caused by a wide range of bacteria and viruses, as well as fungi, and there are wide-ranging risk factors depending on whether it is community or hospital acquired.

- There are numerous interventions that healthcare workers can implement in order to reduce the risk of 'general' hospital-acquired pneumonia, and pneumonia associated with ventilation.

Further resources are available for this book, including interactive multiple choice questions. Visit the companion website at:

www.wiley.com/go/fundamentalsofinfectionprevention

References

Adair C.G., Gorman S.P., Feron B.M., Byers L.M., Jones D.S. *et al.* (1999). Implications of endotracheal biofilm for ventilator-associated pneumonia. *Intensive Care Medicine*. 25: 1072–1076.

American Thoracic Society and the Infectious Diseases Society of America (2004). Guidelines for the management of adults with hospital-acquired, ventilator-associated and healthcare-associated pneumonia. *American Journal of Respiratory and Critical Care Medicine*. 171: 388–416.

Chastre J., Fagon J.Y. (2002). Ventilator-associated pneumonia. *American Journal of Respiratory and Critical Care Medicine*. 165 (7): 867–903.

Cook D.J., Walter S.D., Cook R.J., Griffith L.E., Guyatt G.H. *et al.* (1998). Incidence of and risk factors for ventilator-associated pneumonia in critically ill patients. *Annals of Internal Medicine*: 129–440.

Craven D.E., Chroneou A. (2009). Nosocomial pneumonia. In: Mandell G.L., Bennett J.E., Dolin R.D. (Eds.), *Mandell, Douglas and Bennett's Principles and Practice of Infectious Diseases*. http://expertconsult.com (accessed 20 December 2012)

Department of Health (2007). *High Impact Intervention No. 5. Care Bundle for Ventilated Patients (or Tracheostomy Care Where Appropriate)*. Department of Health, London.

Dodek P., Keenhan S., Cook D., Heyland D., Jaka M. *et al.* (2004). Evidence-based clinical practice guideline for the prevention of ventilator-associated pneumonia. *Annals of Internal Medicine*. 141 (4): 305–313.

Donowitz G.R. (2009): Acute pneumonia. In: Mandell G.L., Bennett J.E., Dolin R.D. (Eds.), *Mandell's Principles and Practices of Infectious Diseases*. 7th ed. Churchill Livingstone Elsevier, London. Expert Consult online: http://expertconsult.com (accessed 26 February 2013)

Dunn L. (2005). Pneumonia: classification, diagnosis and nursing management. *Nursing Standard*. 19 (42): 50–54.

Health Protection Agency (2011). *English National Point Prevalence Survey on Healthcare-associated Infections and Antimicrobial Use*. Health Protection Agency, London.

Kress J.P., Pohlman A.S., O'Connor M.F., Hall J.B. (2000). Daily interruption of sedative infusions in critically ill patients undergoing mechanical ventilation. *New England Journal of Medicine*. 342 (20): 1471–1477.

Lim W.S., Baudonin S.V., George R.C., Hill A.T., Jamieson C. *et al.* (2009). Guidelines for the management of community-acquired pneumonia in adults: update 2009. *Thorax*. 64 (Suppl. 3): iii1–iii55.

Lynch J.P. (2001). Hospital-acquired pneumonia: risk factors, microbiology and treatment. *Chest*. February. 119 (2; Suppl.): 373S–384S.

Machin J. (2005). Tracheostomy care and laryngeal voice rehabilitation. In: Mallett J., Bailey C. (Eds.), *The Royal Marsden Hospital Manual of Clinical Nursing Procedures*. 4th ed. Blackwell Science, London: 550–564.

Masterton R.G., Galloway A., French G., Street M., Armstrong J. *et al.* (2008). Guidelines for the management of hospital-acquired pneumonia in the UK: report of the Working Party of Hospital-Acquired Pneumonia of the British Society for Antimicrobial Chemotherapy. *Journal of Antimicrobial Chemotherapy*. 62: 5–34.

Medicines and Healthcare Products Regulatory Agency (2004). *Reusable Nebulisers*. MDA/2004/020. Medicines and Healthcare Products Regulatory Agency, London.

Part Four

Specific organisms

20

Stapylococcus aureus (including MRSA)

Contents

Fundamentals of Infection Prevention and Control: Theory and Practice, Second Edition. Debbie Weston.
© 2013 John Wiley & Sons, Ltd. Published 2013 by John Wiley & Sons, Ltd. Companion Website: www.wiley.com/go/fundamentalsofinfectionprevention

Introduction

No organism has had such an extraordinary media profile over the last 15 years as meticillin-resistant *Staphylococcus aureus* (MRSA). Extensive media coverage increased the profile of MRSA, caused considerable public anxiety and forced the issues of antibiotic-resistant organisms, dirty hospitals and poor compliance with infection control to the top of the political agenda. Healthcare workers generally are not unfamiliar with MRSA but may be unfamiliar with the virulence factors that *S. aureus* possesses, which means that MRSA colonisation can never be viewed as trivial. This chapter looks at *S. aureus* and its virulence factors, the evolution of MRSA, the significance of MRSA colonisation and infection, the emergence of community-acquired MRSA and the problems associated with Panton–Valentine leukocidin (PVL)–producing strains of *S. aureus* and MRSA. It also discusses screening, decolonisation and the infection control management of positive patients, and concludes with best-practice recommendations for the prevention of MRSA colonisation, infection and bacteraemia in acute and community and primary care settings.

Learning outcomes

After reading this chapter the reader will be able to:

- Understand the clinical significance of staphylococcal or MRSA infection.

- Be able to list the patient risk factors for MRSA infection or colonisation, as well as common body sites for MRSA carriage or colonisation, and understand the importance of patient screening.

- Understand how to administer the topical decolonisation protocol.

- Be able to describe the infection control precautions that need to be taken in order to reduce the risk of transmission to other patients.

287

Staphylococcus aureus

Staphylococci are Gram-positive, catalase-positive, facultative anaerobes, measuring 0.5–1.5 μm in diameter. Cultured on agar or in broth for 12–24 hours at 37 °C, they produce golden-yellow colonies ('golden staph') with a smooth shiny surface and grow in grape-like clusters (from 'staphyle', Greek for 'bunch of grapes'), in pairs, in chains or singly (Humphreys, 2007; Que and Moreillon, 2010). They are characterised by the ability to clot plasma (see Chapter 7), and in the laboratory, the catalase test is carried out to distinguish the organism from Streptococci (Health Protection Agency, 2011).

Of the 36 species of Staphylococci, 16 are found in humans (Que and Moreillon, 2010), although only three are considered to be pathogenic:

- *Staphylococcus aureus* (including meticillin-resistant *Staphylococcus* aureus (MRSA)) – discussed in detail in this chapter.

- *Staphylococcus epidermidis*, which forms part of the normal skin flora in large numbers and is frequently associated with infections involving invasive indwelling devices such as intravenous (IV) cannulae, urinary catheters and prosthetic implants.
- *Staphylococcus saprophyticus*, a common cause of cystitis in women.

S. aureus causes a wide range of infections, ranging from mild to potentially life-threatening (Box 20.1).

Box 20.1   Infections caused by *S. aureus*

Localised skin infections (boils, styes and abscesses)
Deep-seated infections (osteomyelitis, septic arthritis)
Acute endocarditis
Meningitis
Pneumonia (see Chapter 19)
Healthcare-associated infections (HCAIs) (wound infections and infections associated with invasive devices)
Toxin-mediated infections (toxic shock syndrome and food poisoning)

S. aureus is carried by 20–30% of the population, either as part of the resident skin flora (see Chapter 8) or intermittently, colonising the skin (including skin folds, the hairline, the perineum and the umbilicus) and the anterior nares (inside the nostrils). The anterior nares are the primary reservoir for *S. aureus* carriage as there are very few host defences (Klutymans *et al.*, 1997). It can also colonise chronic wounds such as varicose and decubitus ulcers, and can be shed or dispersed in large quantities, particularly from patients with chronic skin conditions such as eczema or psoriasis (patients with a high staphylococcal burden are often referred to as 'shedders'). Dust, consisting of skin squames and cloth fibres from clothing, can contaminate the environment (Humphreys, 2007).

S. aureus possesses many virulence factors (Humphreys, 2007; Que and Moreillon, 2010):

- Surface proteins facilitate colonisation of the host tissues. Surface protein A (*spa*) in the cell wall is a significant virulence factor as it inhibits the activation of the complement cascade (Levinson, 2010) (see Chapter 8).
- Invasins (leukocidin, kinases and hyaluronidase) assist the spread of the organism through the tissues.
- The bacterial cell wall, together with protein A, protects the bacteria against phagocytosis, along with other components which assist it in evading host immune defences (see Chapter 8).
- *S. aureus* can form biofilm (see Chapter 5), which can be a particular problem in the event of a prosthetic device–related infection following a hip or knee replacement.
- Teichoic and lipoteichoic acid (LPS) are major components of the Gram-positive bacterial cell wall (see Chapter 5). As well as facilitating adherence to mucosal cells, they also play a role in inducing septic shock (Levinson, 2010) (see Chapter 9).
- *S. aureus* produces potent toxins, commonly referred to as super-antigens (see Chapter 5), which are potent activators of the immune system and trigger an immune response by the host that is actually responsible for many of the signs and symptoms of *S. aureus* infections.

288

- Enterotoxins A, B, C, E and G are produced by approximately one-half of all *S. aureus* isolates and are the principle cause of vomiting and diarrhoea in cases of staphylococcal food poisoning. If contaminated food is ingested, the enterotoxins bind to receptors in the upper gastro-intestinal tract, stimulating the vomiting centre in the brain and inducing nausea, vomiting and diarrhoea within 1–6 hours of eating.
- Toxic shock syndrome toxin (TSST-1) causes toxic shock, manifesting as a high fever; a widespread rash resembling sunburn which leads to skin desquamation, vomiting and diarrhoea, hypotension and multi-organ failure. It has been particularly associated with tampon use (see www.toxicshock.com).
- Epidermolytic toxins (A and B) cause blistering skin diseases, the most dramatic of which is scalded skin syndrome, sometimes seen in small children where parts of the skin blister and slough away (Humphreys, 2007).

Meticillin-resistant *Staphylococcus aureus*

The evolution of MRSA

Chambers and Deleo (2009) propose that MRSA has emerged in four waves, and that the first wave arose from a clone of *S. aureus* known as phage-type 80/81.

Fact Box 20.1   Clones

Clones are strains of bacteria that are descended from a single common ancestor (mother cell). Within clones, there are descendants (lineages). There is variation amongst clones and strains as a result of mutation, recombination (hospital-acquired and community-acquired strains combining) and the acquisition or loss of genes (Rodriguez-Noriega *et al.*, 2009).

According to Chambers and Deleo (2009), the first wave began when *S. aureus* developed resistance to penicillin soon after penicillin was introduced into clinical practice, producing an enzyme called penicillinase which rendered the antibiotic ineffective (see Chapter 10). Antibiotics that were stable against penicillinase were developed during the 1950s and 1960s. The first of these was methicillin (which was renamed in 2005 as meticillin), a semi-synthetic derivative of penicillin which was introduced in 1959. Phage type 80/81 gradually disappeared with the introduction of meticillin, although penicillinase production was seen amongst other strains of *S. aureus*.

Fact Box 20.2   Meticillin

Although meticillin is no longer used to treat infections, it is used in the laboratory to test *S. aureus* for susceptibility to flucloxacillin. Resistant strains of *S. aureus* are still referred to as meticillin resistant, which means the same as flucloxacillin resistant. Flucloxacillin should not be prescribed for patients who are MRSA positive, or who have a history of MRSA. Ordinary strains of *S. aureus* that are not meticillin resistant are referred to as meticillin-sensitive *Staphylococcus aureus* (MSSA).

The introduction of meticillin heralded the onset of the second wave of MRSA (Chambers and Deleo, 2009), with the emergence of meticillin resistance and the isolation and identification in 1963 of a strain of MRSA known as COL, which was isolated from a patient in Colindale, London (now home of the Health Protection Agency Staphylococcal Reference Laboratory), and belonged to the first clone of MRSA, the 'archaic' clone. Outbreaks of MRSA were subsequently seen across England (Duckworth, 1993; Newsom, 2004) and Europe (Chambers and Deleo, 2009). The archaic clone gave rise to other MRSA clones and the emergence of other resistant descendants, constituting the third wave and a global MRSA pandemic in hospitals. During the late 1980s and early 1990s, epidemic strains (clones) EMRSA15 and EMRSA16 emerged. EMRSA16 originated in Kettering, Northamptonshire, during 1991–1992 and caused an outbreak that affected more than 400 patients and cost in excess of £400 000, seeding the spread of MRSA across the country (National Audit Office, 2000; Department of Health [DH], 2002).

The fourth wave was 'invasion' of the community and the emergence of community-acquired clones (Chambers and Deleo, 2009).

Fact Box 20.3   The MRSA resistance gene

The MRSA resistance gene (*mecA*) is carried on a mobile (transferrable) gene known as Staphylococcal Chromosome Cassette mec (SCCmec), which was probably acquired by *S. aureus* from another species of bacteria (species unknown). There are five types of SCCmec – types I–III are associated with hospital strains, whilst types IV and V are commonly associated with community strains (Robinson and Enright, 2005).

290

'Typing' MRSA

In order to distinguish between clones and identify their genealogy (family tree), molecular typing using either pulse field gel electrophoresis (PFGE) or multilocus sequence typing (MLST) have been the essential tools. PFGE involves the use of an electric current to separate large fragments of DNA in order to determine its sequence or code (see Chapter 7) and compare it to the DNA sequence of other MRSA isolates. MLST involves sequencing DNA fragments of seven key 'housekeeping' genes (genes that are essential for cellular function). As mentioned in Chapter 7, *spa* typing (analysis of the staphylococcal protein A gene) is another tool used to identify MRSA strains and clones.

Fact Box 20.4   MRSA in animals

Staphylococci can colonise the skin and mucous membranes of animals as well as humans, and MRSA has emerged in domestic pets, horses and livestock, with some veterinary MRSA infections likely to have been human in origin and associated with healthcare facilities (Cuny *et al.*, 2010).

In 2003, livestock-associated MRSA clonal complex (CC) 398 was first identified in a human, although it was previously associated only with pigs and cattle (Garcia-Alvarez *et al.*, 2011).

National guidance on the control of MRSA was first issued in 1986 by a combined working party of the Hospital Infection Society and the British Society for Antimicrobial Chemotherapy, and reviewed again in 1990 (Working Party Report), 1998 (Duckworth *et al.*) and 2006 (Coia *et al.*; Gemmell *et al.*)

The clinical importance of MRSA infection, and risk factors associated with MRSA colonisation and infection

Colonised and infected patients are the primary reservoir of MRSA infection for others, and while most patients with MRSA are colonised rather than infected, MRSA colonisation can predispose patients to developing invasive disease, particularly if the patient is in a high-risk patient group (see Box 20.2).

Box 20.2 'High-risk' patients for developing MRSA infection

- Patients who are undergoing surgical interventions and procedures, particularly orthopaedic surgery
- Patients with invasive devices such as vascular access devices (see Chapter 16), urinary catheters (Chapter 17) and wound drains , which can facilitate entry of MRSA into the bloodstream
- Patients in renal units receiving haemodialysis
- Patients in high-dependency, critical and intensive care units
- Oncology and chemotherapy patients
- Known colonised patients undergoing invasive procedures.

Patients and their relatives are often upset when they are told that they have MRSA, often equating MRSA carriage and colonisation with infection. It is important that healthcare workers are able to make the distinction clear between carriage and colonisation and infection.

MRSA carriage and colonisation: MRSA is found on the skin or mucous membranes; there are no clinical signs of infection or tissue invasion. People can be carriers of MRSA intermittently or for prolonged periods of time but without any adverse effects to themselves.

MRSA infection: There are clinical signs and symptoms of infection (see Chapter 8), or MRSA has been isolated from a sterile body site.

Not all infections are severe, and not all patients require treatment with antibiotics. Where antibiotics are indicated, MRSA infection can be difficult to treat because of its antibiotic resistance, and the cost of treating hospital-acquired MRSA infections is high. This is due to the cumulative cost of increased in-patient stay, extra diagnostic procedures and the use of expensive antibiotics such as vancomycin and teicoplanin. For this reason, steps are taken within the hospital setting to control the spread of MRSA and to protect those patients who are most vulnerable to infection (e.g. ITU patients), those with joint replacements or other prosthetic implants, and neutropenic patients.

Although the majority of patients with MRSA are merely colonised, and are not ill and do not require antibiotic therapy, a significant proportion of patients do develop infection, including invasive infection, which may result in death. Control of MRSA is also necessary because of the recent emergence of vancomycin-intermediate and resistant *S. aureus* (VISA and VRSA, respectively).

Community-acquired MRSA (CA-MRSA)

Although the acquisition of MRSA has always been linked to hospitals, and it is commonly and unhelpfully referred to in the media as the 'hospital superbug', there has been an increase in recent years in the number of people acquiring serious life-threatening MRSA and MSSA infections who have no prior history of exposure to the healthcare setting (Gonzalez *et al.*, 2006). Box 20.3 lists the indications for CA-MRSA.

Box 20.3   Indications for CA-MRSA

MRSA detected within 48 hours of admission to hospital
No previous history of MRSA colonisation or infection
No significant medical history within the previous year
No admissions to hospital within the previous year
No admissions to nursing or residential homes, community hospitals or other care facilities
    (e.g. hospice) within the previous year
No history of dialysis or surgery
No indwelling invasive devices (e.g. a urinary catheter)
In cases of infection – often spontaneous (e.g. not linked to an invasive indwelling device) and
    generally the site of infection is the skin (e.g. cellulitis or abscesses).
Different antibiotic susceptibilities on laboratory testing.

Source: www.cdc.gov; data from HPA, 2008.

Resistant and sensitive strains of *S. aureus* can produce a toxin called Panton–Valentine leukocidin (PVL) which destroys white blood cells. Although PVL-producing strains have been in existence for a hundred years and have emerged worldwide, they have risen to prominence over the last decade (Health Protection Agency, 2008; Royal College of Nursing, 2011). Community strains of MRSA have been found to be more likely to produce PVL than the strains which are commonly found in hospitals.

Fact Box 20.5   USA300

In the United States, the USA300 community clone emerged over a decade ago in Pennsylvania and Missouri, where it was responsible for causing skin and soft tissue infections in college football players and prisoners (Tenover and Goering, 2009). It swiftly became problematic and within five years established itself as the predominant community clone, responsible for severe invasive infections including necrotising fasciitis (see Fact Sheet 3.3 on the companion website), and osteomyelitis, endocarditis, bacteraemia and necrotising pneumonia (Tenover and Goering, 2009). It has become a particularly 'fit' clone, expanding from the community into hospitals (Health Protection Agency, 2008).

PVL-producing strains can cause severe invasive infections, the most lethal of which is necrotising pneumonia, which presents as a rapidly progressive, haemorrhagic, necrotising, community-acquired pneumonia in previously young, fit and healthy individuals, and is rapidly fatal (Holmes *et al.*, 2005; Morgan, 2005). Patients with invasive PVL infections require aggressive management in an intensive care unit and combination antibiotic therapy.

Box 20.4 summarises the risk factors for *S. aureus* and MRSA PVL infection.

293

Box 20.4   Risk factors for *S. aureus* and MRSA PVL infection

The Centers for Disease Control (CDC, Atlanta, United States) refer to the '5 C's' (Gorwitz *et al.*, 2006):

- **C**ontaminated items
- **C**lose contact
- **C**rowding
- **C**leanliness
- **C**uts and other compromised skin integrity.

High-risk settings include:

- Households
- Close-contact sports such as rugby, judo and wrestling
- Military training camps
- Gyms
- Prisons.

Control of MRSA

Screening

294

The purpose of screening for MRSA is to detect those individuals with asymptomatic MRSA carriage or colonisation, as they represent the most important reservoir of MRSA in healthcare facilities (Grundmann *et al.*, 2006). Supplementary guidance on screening was issued by the DH in 2006 to further reduce the risk of MRSA colonisation and the incidence of MRSA bacteraemias, and again in 2008. Box 20.5 identifies the patients who should be screened.

Box 20.5   Patients who should be screened for MRSA on admission

- All emergency admissions within 24 hours of admission to hospital (this will 'capture' admissions from 'high-risk' areas such as nursing and residential homes, as well as patients who have frequent emergency admissions)
- All elective surgical admissions, either at the Pre-assessment or Admission appointment **or** on admission to the ward if there has been no pre-assessment
- All oncology and haematology patients attending for chemotherapy (frequency of screening will be determined locally)
- All renal patients attending for haemodialysis (frequency of screening will be determined locally)

Data from DH, 2006.

Box 20.6 lists the patients who do not require admission screening (DH, 2008).

Box 20.6   Patients who do not require admission screening

Ophthalmology day cases
Dental day cases
Endoscopy day cases (e.g. gastroscopy, colonoscopy and bronchoscopy)
Minor dermatological procedures
Children (paediatric patients) unless in a high-risk group (e.g. known to have associated co-morbidities or transferred from another hospital)
Maternity admissions unless elective or emergency caesarean section
Patients attending for day case medical procedures
Patients attending for routine medical and surgical out-patient appointments.

Source: Data from Department of Health, 2008.

Box 20.7 summarises the body sites that should be screened.

Box 20.7   Body sites to be screened

Anterior nares
Axillae (nose and axilla if screening is undertaken using enrichment broth – see Chapter 6)
Groin and perineum (may not form part of routine screens)
All skin lesions and skin breaks, including pressure sores
All wounds
Sites of indwelling invasive devices such as lines and drains
Sputum if expectorating
Tracheostomy sites
Percutaneous endoscopic gastrostomy (PEG) sites
Urine if catheterised
Umbilicus in neonates

295

Staff screening

The screening of healthcare staff for MRSA carriage is no longer undertaken routinely, and is required only if there is evidence of cross-infection occurring to patients or if the strain of MRSA is unusual (e.g. evidence of spread of a community-acquired strain within a healthcare setting). It is recognised that staff can acquire MRSA transiently during the course of their duties (e.g. transient nasal carriage), but this is generally lost very quickly, and nasal carriage among staff carries little risk in terms of transmission to patients. However, staff with skin lesions may be colonised with MRSA, and if staff screening is requested, any skin breaks and skin lesions should be included in the screen. The implementation of staff screening needs to be carefully planned, with staff screened at the beginning of a shift and not halfway through or at the end, in order to minimise the possibility of detecting transient carriage, and it may be undertaken in conjunction with both the Occupational Health Department and the Infection Prevention and Control Team (IP&CT). Although MRSA-positive healthcare staff generally can continue to work, there are exceptions (e.g. theatre staff), and local policy may require certain staff groups to refrain from working until they have completed a five-day course of the decolonisation protocol, and/or possibly oral antibiotics until they have had one negative screen. The IP&CT and the Occupational Health Team will advise.

Treatment of MRSA colonisation and infection

Topical agents such as an antibiotic nasal cream (e.g. Bactroban or Naseptin) in conjunction with a disinfectant body wash (e.g. Hydrex, Octenisan® or Prontoderm®) are used to eradicate or reduce nasal and/or skin carriage. While there is no evidence to suggest that it is always possible to completely eradicate MRSA, and patients can recolonise either with the same strain or through acquisition of a new one, the use of these topical agents can decrease MRSA carriage in the short term, reducing the risk of transmission to other patients within the healthcare environment, as well as reducing the risk to the patient of developing an infection. How effective the decolonisation regimen is depends in part on the presence of 'foreign bodies' such as clips or sutures and invasive indwelling devices, and wounds or skin lesions. For elective patients who are MRSA-positive, the course of decolonisation treatment should be completed as close to the date of surgery as possible.

It is important that the 'decol' is applied or administered according to the manufacturer's instructions in order that its efficacy is not reduced (see Box 20.8).

Box 20.8   How to apply the topical MRSA 'decolonisation protocol' consisting of nasal cream and topical skin disinfectant

Nasal decolonisation

A 'pea-sized' amount of 2% mupirocin (Bactroban nasal cream) **or** Naseptin® nasal cream (containing neomycin and chlorhexidine) should be applied to the inner surface of each nostril (anterior nares) by healthcare staff, either on the tip of a cotton-bud or a gloved finger, three or four times daily respectively for **five days only**. Where possible, the patient should be encouraged to pinch the nostrils together and then sniff – the patient should be able to taste the cream at the back of the throat after application. If the patient is applying the cream, it is important that he or she is shown how to do it.

In some Trusts, Naseptin may be prescribed only for mupirocin-resistant strains of MRSA, while in others, mupirocin may not be used at all because of concerns around mupirocin resistance.

Topical decolonisation

Chlorhexidine gluconate (Hydrex or Hibiscrub) or Octenisan® baths and showers, or bed baths and washes daily, for five days. The product must be applied to wet skin like a liquid soap or bath or shower gel. **It must not be diluted in a bowl of water or poured into the bath** (it will be diluted and its effectiveness will be reduced). It must remain in contact with the skin for at least one minute, then rinsed thoroughly. **Special attention much be paid to known carriage sites on the skin, including any superficial skin breaks**. For patients with eczema, dermatitis or other skin conditions, attempts should be made to treat the underlying skin condition, and advice on a suitable eradication protocol should be sought from a Dermatologist. Oilatum bath additive, or Oilatum plus, may be used for these patients but should be prescribed only on the advice of a Dermatologist.

The hair must be washed at least twice during the five-day course and rinsed well. Ordinary conditioner and other hair products can then be used.

Following the baths or washes, patients should have clean clothing and bed sheets.

Allow two treatment-free days before re-screening. The decolonisation protocol should not be recommenced.

Discharge prior to completion of the decolonisation protocol

Patients should always finish the full five-day course and, if discharged home before the course is completed, they should be advised to complete it at home if possible (e.g. if they are able to self-administer or have a carer who can assist). Patients being discharged to nursing or residential homes should complete the course after discharge – the Manager must be informed.

If a patient is found to be MRSA-positive after discharge, decolonisation in the community is generally **not** indicated. The IP&CT will have arrangements in place regarding the notification of General Practitioners, and Community Infection Control Teams if the patient has been discharged to a nursing or residential home.

Patients with an MRSA infection

Patients with an infection will be treated with the appropriate antibiotic, depending upon the antibiotic susceptibilities of the MRSA strain involved.

Vancomycin: Deep-seated or severe infections are treated with vancomycin, which has long been the antibiotic of choice. The dose is adjusted in the elderly and/or those patients with renal impairment. Too much vancomycin can be potentially toxic, and too little can be sub-therapeutic, so serum blood levels are recorded pre-dose and 1–2 hours post dose every three days, and the dose decreased or increased as required. There are increasing concerns about bacterial resistance to vancomycin among enterococci and staphylococci, with resistance to vancomycin recorded in both sensitive and resistant strains of *S. aureus*, which obviously has implications for the treatment of not only MRSA but also other infections.

Teicoplanin: Penetrates tissues including skin, fat and bone. Teicoplanin blood assays are performed only where there is severe deep-seated infection and/or renal impairment.

Linezolid: A newer antibiotic which is increasingly being prescribed for the treatment of severe infections.

MRSA clearance

Once the patient has had three complete sets of negative screens taken on three consecutive occasions seven days apart, he or she can generally be considered to be 'MRSA clear'. However, some patients never achieve 'clearance' and may be permanently or intermittently colonised. Even if 'clearance' is achieved during an in-patient hospital stay, the patient should be screened regularly until discharge.

Patients undergoing surgery and invasive procedures

- Prior to any planned surgery, efforts should be made to minimise the risk of infection through topical and systemic decolonisation, and prophylactic antibiotics effective against MRSA, where appropriate. Antibiotic prophylaxis is **not** required routinely for **all** MRSA-positive patients. However, MRSA-positive patients undergoing implant surgery (e.g. orthopaedic implants or vascular grafts) must routinely be given a single dose of IV teicoplanin (400 mg). In the event of any queries regarding antibiotic prophylaxis, the Consultant Microbiologist must be contacted.
- The patient's medical team or Pre-admission Clinic staff should inform the theatre coordinator that the patient has MRSA infection or colonisation. The medical team should also consult the Microbiologist to discuss chemoprophylaxis and inform the theatres of the known or suspected case.
- Vancomycin or teicoplanin should be given prophylactically to cover implant surgery (e.g. joint replacement) in colonised or infected patients, following discussions with a Consultant Microbiologist.
- There is no absolute requirement to place the patient last on the list, as patients with MRSA can be safely managed using standard precautions. However, this may be local policy. In all cases, the Theatre Co-coordinator or Nurse in Charge, as well as the Surgeon, should be informed. Extraneous equipment should be removed from the theatre, and theatre personnel should be kept to a minimum.

Discharge of patients

- Patients with MRSA should be discharged promptly from hospital when their clinical condition allows. It is essential that patients, their relatives and their carers are provided with an MRSA Information Leaflet, and informed that there is no risk of infection to healthy relatives and contacts outside the hospital, and that normal social interaction should not be compromised.
- Patients should be advised that if they are re-admitted to hospital at any time, they should inform admitting staff that they have previously been identified as a carrier of MRSA in order to ensure that they are appropriately managed.
- There is no indication for routine screening before hospital discharge to the community. However, in certain high-risk areas, such as elective orthopaedic surgery, pre-discharge screening may be indicated and requested by the IP&CT.
- Carriage of MRSA is **not** a contraindication to the transfer of a patient to a nursing or convalescent home, and should **not** delay the patient's discharge.
- The risk of cross-infection from an MRSA-colonised or infected patient to other patients in an ambulance environment is minimal. Good infection control practices and routine cleaning should be sufficient to prevent cross-infection.
- MRSA carriers may be transported in the same ambulance as others without special precautions other than changing the bedding of the carrier. However, if transporting a potentially

heavy disperser (e.g. with large skin lesions), the patient should be transported alone and the handling staff should wear a disposable apron and gloves, decontaminate their hands with alcohol hand rub following the removal of the apron and gloves and before direct contact with another patient, and wipe down surfaces in contact with the patient with detergent wipes.

- High-risk patients (those susceptible to infection, e.g. neutropenic) should not be transported in the same ambulance as a known MRSA-positive patient.
- Patients with MRSA can be discharged home via a hospital car. No special precautions are required, and there is no evidence that ambulance staff or hospital drivers or their families are put at risk by transporting patients with MRSA. No additional cleaning of the ambulance, or hospital car, is required after transporting an MRSA-positive patient.

Clinical practice points: the infection control management of MRSA-positive patients

General points

- Patient care must not be compromised by control measures.
- Isolation room doors should be kept closed whenever possible to minimise spread to adjacent areas (see Chapter 11).
- Patients in rooms without en-suite facilities **can** use the ward bath or shower (which must be cleaned after use).
- Healthcare staff do not need to wear protective clothing unless they are having direct physical contact with the patient or their immediate environment (see Chapter 13). Visitors are not required to wear protective clothing but must be asked to decontaminate their hands on entering and leaving the room.
- Healthcare staff must decontaminate their hands according to the 5 Moments for Hand Hygiene (see Chapter 12).
- Equipment (e.g. sphygmomanometers, stethoscopes, lifting slings and physiotherapy exercise machines) used on patients with MRSA infection and colonisation should be single-patient use or designated for MRSA patients. Multiple-patient use items must be decontaminated appropriately before use on another patient in accordance with local policy or manufacturer's instructions (see Chapter 15).
- Movement of patients within the hospital should be kept to a minimum wherever possible to minimise the risk of spread, but should not compromise other aspects of patient care such as rehabilitation. There should be joint working between the IP&CT and Bed Managers in planning patient admissions, transfers, discharges and movements between wards, departments and other healthcare facilities.
- If patients have open wounds or lesions, these should be covered where possible and applicable with an impermeable dressing.
- In the event of a patient being transferred to another ward, or to another department for investigations, it is the responsibility of the Nurse in Charge of the ward to ensure that the receiving ward is aware of the patient's MRSA status.
- Visits by MRSA-positive patients to other departments should be kept to a minimum. If this is necessary, for either investigation or treatment, prior arrangements should be made with the staff of the receiving department, so that infection control measures for that department can be implemented.

- Deceased bodies require no additional precautions other than Standard Precautions. The normal Last Offices procedure is appropriate. There is negligible risk to mortuary staff or undertakers provided that standard infection control precautions are employed. Body bags are not required.

Best-practice recommendations for the prevention of MRSA colonisation, infection and bacteraemia (Acute Trusts)

- Screen all emergency admissions within 24 hours of admission.
- Screen all elective surgical admissions either at their Pre-assessment appointment or on admission to the ward (within 24 hours of admission).
- Screen all hospital in-patients every seven days until discharge.
- Ensure that screens include all appropriate body sites (audit compliance).
- Consider implementing discharge screening on wards in the event of clusters of MRSA.
- Ensure that patients with MRSA are either isolated or cohort-nursed appropriately according to local policy and that equipment is dedicated for that patient's use.
- Audit compliance with screening on a monthly basis.
- Collate the numbers of hospital-acquired MRSA colonisations (patients with negative admission screens) per ward and division every month, and report to the Divisions and Trust Board monthly.
- Where there are two or more hospital-acquired colonisations on a ward in a month, hold a meeting with the Ward Manager and Matron to review compliance with policy and clinical practice, and review environmental cleanliness.
- Ensure that all staff who administer the topical MRSA decolonisation protocol (nasal cream and skin disinfectant) undergo an annual competency assessment.
- Ensure that all staff who obtain MRSA screens and swabs are competent in the process (to avoid contamination of specimens).
- Ensure that antibiotics, where indicated, are prescribed in accordance with local antimicrobial prescribing guidelines or policy, and that any prophylaxis before surgery is effective against MRSA.
- Do not insert vascular access devices or urinary catheters unless their insertion can be justified on clinical grounds, in which case they must be managed only by staff who are competent in their insertion and/or management and ongoing care, in strict accordance with policy, and must be removed at the earliest opportunity. All device-related interventions must be recorded and documented.
- Audit compliance with hand hygiene – the 5 Moments and personal protective equipment (PPE) use.
- Ensure that a patient's MRSA status is communicated at handover.
- On discharge, ensure that the patient's MRSA status is recorded on the discharge letter or Electronic Discharge Notification (EDN) if the patient is MRSA-positive.
- In the event of a cluster of ward-acquired cases, serious infection or MRSA bacteraemia, hold a root cause analysis (RCA) or post infection review (PIR), ensuring that compliance with clinical practice is investigated thoroughly.

Reflection point

How are staff made aware of MRSA-positive patients who are nursed on the open ward? This is particularly important for on-call Medical Teams who will not always know patients from other areas and who may prescribe antibiotics or take blood cultures.

Best-practice recommendations for the prevention of MRSA colonisation, infection and bacteraemia (community and primary care)

- MRSA-positive patients in nursing and residential homes do not need to be confined to their room and segregated from other residents.
- Audit compliance with hand decontamination in accordance with the 5 Moments and PPE use.
- Ensure that staff (including the GP and Community Nursing staff) are aware of the residents' MRSA-positive status. This is particularly important if the patient develops signs of infection (e.g. a respiratory, urinary tract or wound infection) and is prescribed antibiotics.
- In the event of infections not responding to antibiotics, ensure that this is escalated appropriately and that the appropriate clinical specimens are obtained.
- Ensure that the environment and equipment are cleaned to a generally high standard and that audits of cleaning and decontamination are undertaken.
- Do not catheterise residents without having considered alternative methods. Only staff who are competent in the management and ongoing care of catheters should have contact with the catheter and drainage system.
- If the resident is admitted to hospital, ensure that the resident's positive MRSA status is communicated to hospital staff.
- In the event of an MRSA bacteraemia or serious infection, hold a root cause analysis (RCA) or post infection review (PIR), ensuring that compliance with clinical practice is investigated thoroughly.

Chapter summary: key points

- *Staphylococcus aureus* and MRSA possess numerous virulence factors and are capable of causing a diverse range of infections, some of which are potentially life-threatening.

- *S. aureus* is carried by 20–30% of the population, either as part of the resident skin flora (see Chapter 8) or intermittently, colonising the skin (including skin folds, the hairline, the perineum and the umbilicus) and the anterior nares (inside the nostrils).

- Staphylococci can colonise the skin and mucous membranes of animals as well as humans, and MRSA has emerged in domestic pets, horses and livestock, and is probably human in origin.

Continued

- Resistant and sensitive strains of *S. aureus* can produce a toxin called Panton–Valentine leukocidin (PVL) which destroys white blood cells.

- Community-acquired MRSA has occurred in individuals with no prior history of healthcare contact.

- Colonised and infected patients are the primary reservoir of MRSA infection for others, and while most patients with MRSA are colonised rather than infected, MRSA colonisation can predispose patients to developing invasive disease.

- The purpose of screening for MRSA is to detect those individuals with asymptomatic MRSA carriage and colonisation, as they represent the most important reservoir of MRSA in healthcare facilities.

Further resources are available for this book, including interactive multiple choice questions. Visit the companion website at:

www.wiley.com/go/fundamentalsofinfectionprevention

References

Barrett S.P., Mummery R.V., Chattopadhyay B. (1998). Trying to control MRSA causes more problems than it solves. *Journal of Hospital Infection*. 39 (2): 85–93.

Chambers H.F., Deleo F.R. (2009). Waves of resistance: *Staphylococcus aureus* in the antibiotic era. *Nature Reviews Microbiology*. September 7 (9): 629–641.

Coia J.E., Duckworth G.J., Edwards D.I., Farrington M., Fry C. *et al.* for the Joint Working Party of the British Society of Antimicrobial Chemotherapy, the Hospital Infection Society and the Infection Control Nurses Association (2006). Guidelines for the control and prevention of meticillin-resistant Staphylococcus aureus (MRSA) in healthcare facilities *Journal of Hospital Infection*. 63S: S1–S44.

Cuny C., Friedrich A., Kozytska S., Layer F., Nubel U. (2010). Emergence of meticillin-resistant *Staphylococcus aureus* (MRSA) in different animal species. *International Journal of Medical Microbiology*. 300: 109–117.

Department of Health (DH) (2002). *Getting Ahead of the Curve. A Strategy for Combating Infectious Diseases (including Other Aspects of Health Protection)*. Report by the Chief Medical Officer. Department of Health, London.

Department of Health (DH) (2006). *Screening for Meticillin-resistant Staphylococcus aureus (MRSA) Colonisation: A Strategy for NHS Trusts: A Summary of Best Practice*. Department of Health, London.

Department of Health (DH) (2008). *MRSA Screening – Operational Guidance 2*. Department of Health, London.

Duckworth G.J. (1993). Diagnosis and management of meticillin-resistant *Staphylococcus aureus* infection. *British Medical Journal*. 307 (6911): 1049–1053.

Duckworth G., Cookson G., Humphreys H., Heathcock R. (1998). Revised meticillin-resistant *Staphylococcus aureus* infection control guidelines for hospitals. Report of a Working Party for the British Society of Antimicrobial Chemotherapy, the Hospital Infection Society and the Infection Control Nurses Association. *Journal of Hospital Infection*. 39 (4): 253–290.

Garcia-Alvarez L., Holden M.T.G., Lindsay H., Webb C.R., Brown D.F. (2011). Meticillin-resistant *Staphylococcus aureus* with a novel mecA homologue in humans and bovine populations in the UK and Denmark: a descriptive study. *The Lancet*. (11): 70126–70128. doi:10.1016/S1473:3099

Gonzalez B.E., Rueda A.M., Shelburne S.A., Musher D.M., Hamill R.J., Hulten K.G. (2006). Community-acquired strains of meticillin-resistant *Staphylococcus aureus* as the cause of healthcare-associated infection. *Infection Control Hospital Epidemiology*. 27 (10): 1051–1056.

Gorwitz R.J., Jernigan D.B., Powers J.H., Jernigan J.A. and participants in the Centers for Disease Control and Prevention Convened Experts' Meeting on Management of MRSA in the Community (2006). *Strategies for Clinical Management of MRSA in the Community: Summary of an Experts Meeting Convened by the Centers for Disease Prevention and Control*. Centers for Disease Control and Prevention, Atlanta, GA.

Grundmann H., Aires-de-Sousa M., Boyce J., Tiemersma E. (2006). Emergence and resurgence of meticillin-resistant *Staphylococcus aureus* as a public health threat. *Lancet*. 368: 874–885.

Health Protection Agency (2008). *Guidance on the Diagnosis and Management of PVL-associated* Staphylococcus aureus *Infections (PVL-SA) in England*. Report prepared by the PVL sub-group of the Steering Group on Healthcare Associated Infections. Health Protection Agency, London.

Health Protection Agency (2011). *UK Standards for Microbiology Investigations. Catalase Test*. TP8 Issue 2.2. Health Protection Agency, London.

Holmes A., Ganner M., McGuane S., Pitt T.L., Cookson B.D., *et al.* (2005). *Staphylococcus aureus* isolates carrying Panton–Valentine leukocidin genes in England and Wales: frequency, characterisation and association with clinical disease. *Journal of Clinical Microbiology*. 43 (5): 2384–2390.

Hospital Infection Society and the British Society for Antimicrobial Chemotherapy (1986). Guidelines for the control of meticillin-resistant *Staphylococcus aureus*. *Journal of Hospital Infection*. 7 (2): 193–201.

Humphreys H. (2007). Staphylococcus. In: Greenwood D., Slack R., Peutherer J., Barer M. (Eds.), *Medical Microbiology. A Guide to Microbial Infections: Pathogenesis, Immunity, Laboratory Diagnosis and Control*. 17th ed. Churchill Livingston Elsevier, London: 172–177.

Klutymans J., van Belkum A., Verbrugh H. (1997). Nasal carriage of *Staphylococcus aureus*: epidemiology, underlying mechanisms and associated risks. *Clinical Microbiology Reviews*. 10 (3): 505–520.

Levinson W. (2010). Gram-positive cocci. In: *Review of Medical Microbiology and Immunology*. 11th ed. McGraw-Hill Lange, New York: 94–107.

Morgan M. (2005). Editorial: *Staphylococcus aureus*, Panton-Valentine leukocidin and necrotising pneumonia. *British Medical Journal*. 331 (7520): 793–794.

National Audit Office (2000). *The Management and Control of Hospital-Acquired Infection in Acute NHS Trusts in England*. Report by the Comptroller and Auditor General. HC 230 Session 1999–2000, 17 February. National Audit Office, London.

Newsom S.W.B. (2004). MRSA and its predecessor–a historical overview. Part three: the rise of MRSA and EMRSA. *British Journal of Infection Control*. 5 (2): 25–28.

Que Y-A., Moreillon P. (2010). *Staphylococcus aureus* (including staphylococcal toxic shock). In: Mandell G.L., Bennett J.E., Dolin R.D. (Eds.), *Mandell's Principles and Practices of Infectious Diseases*. 6th ed. Churchill Livingstone Elsevier, London. http://expertconsult.com (accessed 20 December 2012)

Robinson D.A., Enright M.C. (2003). Evolutionary models of the emergence of meticillin-resistant *Staphylococcus aureus*. *Antimicrobial Agents and Chemotherapy*. 47 (12): 3926–3934.

Rodriguez-Noriega E., Seas C., Guzman-Blanco M., Meija C., Alvarez C. *et al.* (2009). Evolution of meticillin-resistant *Staphylococcus aureus* clones in Latin America. *International Journal of Infectious Diseases*. doi:10.1016/ijid.2009.08.018

Royal College of Nursing (2011). *Panton-Valentine Leukocidin-Positive* Staphylococcus aureus *(PVL-SA)*. RCN Guidance for Healthcare Professionals. Royal College of Nursing, London.

Teare E.L., Barrett S.P. (1997). Stop the ritual of tracing colonised patients. *British Medical Journal*. 314: 665–666.

Tenover F.C., Goering R.V. (2009). Meticillin-resistant *Staphylococcus aureus* strain USA300: origin and epidemiology. *Journal of Antimicrobial Chemotherapy*. 64: 441–446.

Working Party Report (1990). Guidelines for the control of epidemic meticillin-resistant *Staphylococcus aureus*. *Journal of Hospital Infection*. 16 (4): 351–377.

21

Tuberculosis

Contents

Fundamentals of Infection Prevention and Control: Theory and Practice, Second Edition. Debbie Weston.
© 2013 John Wiley & Sons, Ltd. Published 2013 by John Wiley & Sons, Ltd. Companion Website: www.wiley.com/go/fundamentalsofinfectionprevention

Introduction

In 1993, the World Health Organization (WHO) declared tuberculosis (TB), known to be a preventable and curable infectious disease, a global emergency (http://www.who.int/topics/tuberculosis/en). Over 95% of new cases of TB and deaths occur in developing countries. In the United Kingdom, 9000 new cases of TB are reported annually, mostly in inner cities and particularly London (http://www.hpa.org.uk/Topics/InfectiousDiseases/InfectionsAZ/Tuberculosis), which has a highly mobile population, the highest proportion of HIV-related cases and the highest rates of drug-resistant strains. Prompt recognition of symptoms, confirmation of cases and the appropriate infection control precautions to minimise spread are key to preventing and controlling tuberculosis.

This chapter focuses on the prevention and control of tuberculosis in the United Kingdom, with reference to the revised 'national guidelines' (National Institute for Health and Clinical Excellence [NICE], 2011), referred to in this chapter as the 'NICE guidelines'. The chapter examines the organism *Mycobacterium tuberculosis*, with particular emphasis on the pathogenesis, diagnosis and treatment of infectious respiratory tuberculosis. Infection with environmental opportunistic mycobacteria and non-respiratory tuberculosis is discussed briefly, and specific problems associated with multidrug-resistant disease and the link between TB and HIV are also explained.

Note: It is not possible to cover all aspects of TB management in all healthcare settings in one chapter, and therefore this chapter only covers the management of respiratory tuberculosis in relation to hospitals. Readers seeking in-depth information regarding the diagnosis, management and contact tracing of children and adults, including the homeless, new entrants to the United Kingdom and healthcare employees, in all other settings should refer to the full NICE Guideline (2011), together with new NICE guidance for *Identifying and Managing TB among Hard-to-Reach Groups* (NICE, 2012), and Royal College of Nursing guidance on *Tuberculosis Case Management and Cohort Review* (Royal College of Nursing, 2012).

305

Learning outcomes

At the end of this chapter, the reader will be able to:

- Understand, and be able to describe, the pathogenesis of infection with respiratory tuberculosis.

- Understand the difference between, and the clinical significance of,

  - infection with respiratory tuberculosis

  - non-respiratory tuberculosis

  - environmental opportunistic mycobacteria.

- Be able to describe the risk factors for, and the implications of, infection with multidrug-resistant tuberculosis.

- Understand the actions of the drugs used to treat tuberculosis.

- Understand the infection control precautions that need to be implemented in the hospital setting when caring for a patient with respiratory tuberculosis.

Background

Tuberculosis, or TB, an age-old disease which has been identified in the skeletal remains of prehistoric humans and the spines of Egyptian mummies (Zink *et al.*, 2003), has historically had many names – consumption, white plague, phthisis and scrofula, to name but a few – and it is now the second commonest infectious cause of death in the world after HIV/AIDS. While it can affect virtually any area of the body, respiratory tuberculosis is the most clinically important disease.

Fact Box 21.1   TB facts

- No country has ever eliminated TB.
- Thirteen percent of cases of TB occur in people living with HIV.
- In 2010, 8.8 million people contracted TB and there were 1.4 million deaths.
- In 2009, approximately 10 million children were orphaned due to parental deaths from TB.
- In 2010, 70 000 children died from TB.
- The TB mortality rate has decreased by 40% between 1990 and 2010.
- Since 1995, 7 million lives have been saved through the directly observed therapy strategy (DOTS) and the WHO Stop TB Strategy.

Source: Data from WHO, 2011.

Fact Box 21.2   Mycobacteria

There are over 80 species of mycobacteria (Grange, 2003), and those which are human pathogens belong to a group of organisms known as the *Mycobacterium tuberculosis* complex (MTC), consisting of *M. tuberculosis*, *Mycobacterium bovis*, *Mycobacterium africanum* and *Mycobacterium microti*.

M. tuberculosis is the principle cause of infectious tuberculosis in humans, with pulmonary disease the most clinically significant illness.

Mycobacteria are slender, obligate, aerobic Gram-positive rods (bacilli) with no capsule.

They are motile and non-spore forming, and compared to most other bacterial pathogens which divide every hour, mycobacteria are slow growers, dividing once every 16–24 hours and forming visible colonies on solid agar at 3–6 weeks (Ryan and Drew, 2010).

The bacterial cell wall consists of 60% lipids, and this high lipid content means that the organism cannot be identified by the traditional method of Gram-staining; the Ziehl–Nelson (ZN) stain technique used to identify the waxy bacterial cell wall is described in Chapter 7.

Opportunistic mycobacteria

Some species of mycobacteria are environmental opportunists (see Box 21.1) isolated from water, soil, dust, milk, animals and birds. Although they are of low virulence and low-grade pathogenicity, they can cause a wide range of opportunistic infections in immunocompromised individuals, particularly those with HIV infection or pre-existing chronic pulmonary disease. Human-to-human transmission is very rare, and even if environmental mycobacteria are isolated from the sputum, the normal notification and contact-tracing procedures that would be initiated in the event of infection with *M. tuberculosis* do not apply.

The detection of environmental mycobacteria (see Box 21.1) is not always clinically significant, and only those who are immunocompromised through HIV infection or with underlying pulmonary disorders require treatment for opportunistic mycobacterial infections.

Box 21.1 Environmental opportunistic mycobacteria

Mycobacterium kansasii (the most common opportunistic mycobacterial pathogen isolated in England and Wales), *Mycobacterium xenopi* and *Mycobacterium avium complex* cause lung disease which clinically is very similar to the respiratory disease caused by *M. tuberculosis* (British Thoracic Society, 1999). *M. xenopi* was first isolated from a xenopus, or African claw-footed frog (Grange, 2007), and is commonly isolated in individuals infected with HIV (Jiva *et al.*, 1997).

Mycobacterium chelonae: These have been isolated from bronchoscopes, where the water supply feeding into the endoscopy washer-disinfector had contaminated the rinse water, and have also been isolated from clinical specimens such as bronchial washings (British Society of Gastroenterology, 2003).

Mycobacterium fortuitum: These are found in contaminated tap water, rivers, lakes, soil and dust; have been increasingly isolated in patients with AIDS (Smith *et al.*, 2001).

Mycobacterium malmonense: These were first isolated in Malmö, Sweden (Henriques *et al.*, 1994); they are frequently isolated from individuals with pulmonary disease (Grange, 2007).

Mycobacterium scrofulaceum: These are associated with cervical lymphadenitis (Grange, 2007).

Mycobacterium marinum: also known as 'fish tank granuloma' and 'fish fancier's finger' (Grange, 2007); commonly affects keepers of tropical fish and users of swimming pools, and causes superficial skin infections.

Mycobacterium ulcerans: the only species of mycobacteria to produce a toxin; associated with tissue necrosis (Grange, 2007).

Mycobacterium abscessus: associated with wound infections. An outbreak of *M. abscessus* was identified in 20 Americans who had plastic surgery (abdominoplasties) in the Dominican Republic in the 1990s (Furuya *et al.*, 2007).

Non-respiratory tuberculosis

Tuberculosis can affect almost any area of the body, commonly affecting the central nervous system (TB meningitis), the abdomen, the renal and genital tract, bones and joints (including the spine), lymph nodes and the skin.

It gives rise to general non-specific symptoms such as fatigue, weight loss, fever and night sweats, together with clinical features specific to the site of infection.

Individuals with non-respiratory tuberculosis are generally considered to be non-infectious and do not require isolation, but respiratory involvement must be investigated and excluded.

In the case of tuberculosis affecting the lymph nodes or skin where there may be open discharging lesions or cavities which require irrigating, aerosol-generating procedures (see Chapter 13) should be avoided in open ward areas.

Treatment of non-respiratory tuberculosis includes the standard six-month four-drug regimen with anti-tuberculosis drugs, as discussed later in this chapter.

The pathogenesis of tuberculosis infection

The initial site of TB infection is usually the lung, and it takes place through the inhalation of TB bacilli, which are expelled in small droplets of moisture from infected individuals through coughing, talking and sneezing. These airborne droplets contain just a few viable bacilli, but as they are released into the air, water evaporates from the surface of the droplets and they become much smaller, forming droplet nuclei with a more concentrated bacterial count.

Fact Box 21.3   Droplet nuclei

Droplet nuclei can float in room air for several hours, and it has been estimated that a single cough can generate as many as 3000 infected droplet nuclei (Fitzgerald *et al.*, 2009), with inhalation of less than 10 bacilli sufficient to initiate pulmonary infection in a susceptible individual (Plorde, 2004).

The inhaled droplet nuclei implant into alveoli in the middle and lower lung fields, areas of the lung that receive the highest air flow, where they are attacked and engulfed by non-specific alveolar macrophages. While phagocytosis will destroy some of the TB bacilli (see Chapter 8), others will survive and replicate within the macrophages but without harming the host. Most of the infected macrophages will die, releasing a new generation of bacilli and cell debris and initiating a cycle of infection, bacterial replication and host cell death.

Bacilli may be transported within the macrophages through the lymphatic system to the lymph nodes draining the affected site, where they may be disseminated via blood and lymph tissue to other sites such as the liver, spleen, bone, brain and kidneys, giving rise to clinical disease affecting any of these organs, known as non-respiratory tuberculosis. Secondary foci may develop in the lymph nodes in the hilum of the lung.

The pathogenesis of respiratory tuberculosis infection

In respiratory TB, a local inflammatory lesion called the Ghon focus develops in the middle or lower lung field. This develops into a granuloma, a feature of chronic infection consisting of infected macrophages, lymphocytes and fibroblasts, which walls off and isolates the site of infection within the lung. As the macrophages within the granuloma are metabolically active, they consume oxygen, and the centre of the granuloma becomes necrotic, producing a hostile environment in which the majority of the bacilli will die. Bacterial replication subsequently becomes inhibited, infection is arrested and over time the granuloma may become calcified. The 'infected' individual has no idea that they have TB, and in most people an efficient and effective immune response can contain the infection. In fact, 90–95% of initial infections do not progress to clinical disease, with the individual in the asymptomatic or dormant (latent) phase. However, not all of the bacilli contained in the alveolar macrophages within the granuloma are destroyed; 'persisters' may survive for months or years, and clinical disease can subsequently develop later in life. Box 21.2 lists the high-risk groups and individuals for having or contracting respiratory TB.

Box 21.2   High-risk groups for having, or contracting, respiratory TB

People with human immunodeficiency virus (HIV)
People who are immunocompromised
Drug abusers and alcoholics
Group II homeless:
- Rough sleepers
- Night shelters
- Bed and breakfast dwellers.

Immigrants from:
- The Indian subcontinent
- South-east Asia
- The Middle East
- South and Central America
- Africa
- Eastern Europe.

Close contacts of infectious cases
The very young and elderly
Certain groups of people with latent TB are at increased risk of going on to develop active TB, including people who:
- Are HIV-positive
- Are injecting drug users
- Have had solid organ transplantation
- Have had a jejunoileal bypass
- Have chronic renal failure or are receiving haemodialysis
- Have had a gastrectomy
- Are receiving anti–tumour necrosis factor
- Have silicosis.

Source: Data from NICE, 2011.

Fact Box 21.4   Pre-disposing factors (from primary infection to active disease)

The pre-disposing factors leading from primary infection to active disease are not always evident but are thought to be related to the number of infecting bacilli inhaled, and the efficiency of the host's immune response, which may become compromised by an underlying illness or disease, increasing age, alcoholism, malnutrition or stress (Plorde, 2004). In individuals who are immunocompromised as a result of HIV infection or following transplant surgery, the interval between infection and the development of active disease is considerably shorter (Grange, 2003).

Post-primary (reactivation) TB

Active clinical disease occurring after the initial primary infection is known as post-primary, or reactivation, TB. Here, the granuloma becomes more necrotic and takes on a tumour-like appearance, called a tuberculoma, which eventually erodes into the bronchi, leading to the formation of pulmonary cavities in the lung. Although the interior of the tuberculoma is not very conducive to the replication of the bacilli, the oxygen-rich environment of the pulmonary cavity supports the growth of the bacilli, which can be found in huge numbers in the cavity walls (Pratt et al., 2005a). From there, the bacilli gain access to the sputum and the patient becomes infectious.

The general, non-specific clinical features of TB, along with the clinical features of respiratory disease, are presented in Box 21.3.

Box 21.3   Clinical features of TB and respiratory TB

Non-specific features

Generally 'unwell'
Anorexia and weight loss
Fever and drenching night sweats
Enlarged lymph glands.

Respiratory symptoms

A chronic cough, which may have been unresponsive to a course of antibiotics, becoming more productive
Shortness of breath
Chest pain
Haemoptysis.

Diagnosing tuberculosis

Healthcare workers should assume a high index of suspicion of any patient presenting with the above symptoms, even if another presumptive diagnosis has been made. Tuberculosis is known as one of the 'great imitators' (Gladwin and Trattler, 2003) and mis-diagnosis can put other patients at risk and obviously delay the onset of treatment for the patient. As discussed in Chapter 6, the definitive method of confirming TB infection is through the detection of acid-fast bacilli in a clinical specimen, and the laboratory techniques used are described within Chapter 7.

A diagnosis of infectious respiratory tuberculosis is generally based upon a combination of a positive sputum smear, clinical features and chest X-ray findings. Box 21.4 identifies the different types of clinical specimens that may be obtained depending on the suspected site of infection.

Box 21.4   Clinical specimens for the diagnosis of TB

Sputum
Urine
Cerebral spinal fluid
Pleural fluid
Bronchial washings and aspirate
Tissue biopsy – taken at surgery, during investigative procedure and during post-mortem
Lymph node biopsy
Pus
Gastric aspirate
Blood.

311

The number of bacilli present in a clinical specimen can vary by the hour, so generally the more specimens collected, the higher the chance of detection.

Fact Box 21.5   Detection of bacilli in sputum

A diagnosis of infectious respiratory tuberculosis is made if 5000–10 000 acid-fast bacilli are detected in 1 ml of sputum (Pratt et al., 2005b; Fitzgerald et al., 2009).

Patients with bacilli detected in the sputum are said to have infectious or 'open' respiratory tuberculosis. If no bacilli are detected on the sputum smear, this does not exclude respiratory TB; patients may still be treated as positive based on the clinical features and also chest X-ray findings, but they are considered to be less infectious.

- **Sputum collection** (see Chapter 6)
- **Radiology**: Lesions, shadows, calcifications and cavities will be evident on chest X-ray. As lesions and shadows are also indicative of a diagnosis of lung cancer, a more detailed image of the lung fields can be provided by computed tomography (CT) or magnetic resonance imaging (MRI) scanning.

- **Polymerase chain reaction (PCR)**: PCR amplifies the bacterial DNA (see Chapter 7).
- **Skin testing and interferon-gamma testing**: The Mantoux test is predominantly used as a screening test to detect latent TB and recent TB infection (shown by conversion of the Mantoux from negative to positive), but it can also be used as an aid to diagnosis in the presence of clinical symptoms. A 0.1 ml solution of tuberculin purified protein derivative (PPD) is injected intradermally into the forearm, and the transverse diameter of the induration that arises at the injection site is read 48–72 hours later. Chapter 32 of the Department of Health's (DH) *Green Book* (http://www.immunisation.dh.gov.uk/green-book-chapters/chapter-32/; DH, 2006) describes the exact technique required for administering the Mantoux and interpreting the results (see Box 21.5). The test measures the degree of hypersensitivity to tuberculin, not immunity to TB, and the results need to be interpreted with care.

Box 21.5   Interpretation of the Mantoux test

An induration diameter of 15 mm or more suggests TB infection or disease, and the result should be viewed in the light of any clinical features that are suggestive of active disease.

A reaction of 6 mm or greater indicates an immune response which may be due to TB infection, infection with environmental mycobacteria, or a previous bacillus Calmette–Guérin (BCG) vaccination.

A skin reaction of 6 mm or less is reported as negative, indicating that the individual has no significant hypersentivity to tuberculin protein; in this situation, BCG vaccination may be given to unvaccinated individuals.

The result of the Mantoux may be affected, and the skin reaction suppressed, if the individual being tested has glandular fever, has any viral infection, is immunocompromised as a result of other disease or treatment, is on corticosteroid therapy, has had a live vaccine (viral) within the previous four weeks, or suffers from sarcoidosis.

- **Blood tests**: Three blood-based immunological tests are now commercially available in the United Kingdom – QuantiFERON-TB Gold, QuantiFERON TB In tube and T-SPOT. These detect tuberculosis antigens known as early secretion antigen target 6 (ESAT-6) and culture filtrate protein 10 (CFP-10), interferon gamma produced by T cells in specific response to *Mycobacterium tuberculosis*, which are not present in the BCG vaccine and are found in only a few strains of environmental mycobacteria.

Multidrug-resistant tuberculosis (MDR-TB)

Drug-resistant TB is becoming an increasing problem around the world, posing a major public health threat, for while it is no more virulent than 'ordinary' drug-sensitive disease, infection with a resistant strain prolongs the amount of time that the individual is infectious, compromises the effectiveness of treatment and increases the mortality rate. In addition, complex treatment regimens are required with more toxic, more expensive but less effective drugs, and each case has been estimated to cost in the region of £60 000–70 000 to treat (White and Moore-Gillan,

2000). Patients may initially be infected with a drug-resistant strain, or an initially drug-'sensitive' strain may become drug resistant as a result of inadequate treatment and poor patient compliance with therapy.

Two types of drug resistance have emerged in TB:

Multidrug-resistant tuberculosis (MDR-TB): This is defined by the World Health Organization (WHO) as resistance to at least rifampicin (the main killing, or bactericidal, drug) and isoniazid (the 'sterilising' drug). WHO estimate that there are at least 4 500 000 cases of MDR-TB worldwide in 109 countries, accounting for 4.3% of all TB cases. Over 40 000 of these are seen in African countries which have the highest prevalence of HIV. The former Soviet Union has a huge prison population, and of the 300 000 prisoners released each year who are infected with TB, 100 000 have a drug-resistant strain.

Extensively drug-resistant TB (XDR-TB): This is defined as MDR-TB plus resistance to (1) any fluoroquinolones and (2) at least one of three injectable second-line drugs – capreomycin, kanomycin and amikacin. Sixty-eight countries have now confirmed that they have, or have had, cases of XDR-TB, including the United Kingdom. While XDR-TB is still relatively rare, it poses a big risk to patients who are HIV positive, and there is always the possibility of community or hospital-acquired XDR-TB outbreaks.

For more information on MDR-TB and XDR-TB, see http://www.who.int/tb/challenges/mdr/tdrfaqs/en/index.html.

Box 21.6 lists the causes of drug-resistant TB; Box 21.7 lists the risk factors for the acquisition of drug-resistant TB.

Box 21.6   Causes of drug-resistant TB

Inadequate treatment of drug-sensitive strains: Poor prescribing practice, inadequate dose and inadequate duration of treatment

Poor patient compliance: Lack of patient understanding, poor communication between healthcare staff and patient and poor supervision

The treatment of drug-resistant disease continues for at least 18 months, often longer, and involves the use of multiple drugs, including antibiotics such as amikacin and capreomycin. Risk factors for the acquisition of drug-resistant tuberculosis are summarised in Box 21.7.

Box 21.7   Risk factors for the acquisition of drug-resistant TB

Previous drug treatment for TB

HIV-positive

Contact with a known case of MDR-TB

Failure of clinical response to treatment

Prolonged sputum smear (at four months) or culture positive (at six months) while on treatment.

Fact Box 21.6   Public health legislation

If a patient with infectious respiratory tuberculosis, particularly one with MDR-TB, refuses to comply with treatment, that individual may pose a risk to public health. For health protection purposes, the Consultant in Communicable Disease Control (CCDC) at the local Health Protection Unit (part of Public Health England) may consider it necessary to seek a magistrate's order for admission to hospital and detention under sections 37 and 38 of the Public Health (Control of Disease) Act 1984. Compulsory treatment of the patient, however, is not allowed.

TB and HIV

HIV-positive individuals are 50 times more likely to develop tuberculosis in a given year than those who are HIV-negative (www.who.int), and approximately 90% die within months of contacting tuberculosis, as the suppression of the immune system with HIV rapidly accelerates the progression of tuberculosis from latent infection to active disease.

Tuberculosis is harder to diagnose in someone who is HIV-positive as it can present in a non-specific, or atypical way, leading to misdiagnosis and a delay in treatment with rapidly fatal consequences.

Extra-respiratory disease and disseminated tuberculosis are more commonly seen in HIV-positive patients compared to other patient groups, and may co-exist alongside other opportunistic infections.

Hospital outbreaks of TB have occurred where as many as 40% of HIV-positive patients have developed active TB within 2 months of exposure to the index case (Daley *et al.*, 1992).

Fact Box 21.7   MDR-TB outbreaks in hospitals (London)

In the 1990s, two separate outbreaks of MDR-TB occurred in HIV units in two London teaching hospitals (Dooley *et al.*, 1992; Jarvis, 1993). One of the outbreaks resulted in the death of seven HIV-positive patients from MDR-TB (Breathnach *et al.*, 1998). HIV and TB patients should not be cared for together in the same ward environment.

The treatment of tuberculosis

Fact Box 21.8   TB sanatoria

Prior to the discovery of the antibiotic streptomycin during the 1940s, which became the mainstay of treatment of TB, patients were cared for in TB sanatoria which were often located in remote areas in the countryside. Fresh air, in all weathers, and bed rest were considered to be the 'cure' for tuberculosis, but where that failed, the diseased lung, or part of the lung, was often removed. The effectiveness of streptomycin against tuberculosis brought new hope, but the emergence of drug resistance has meant that it can be used only in combination with other antimicrobial agents.

The evidence-based 'gold standard' for the treatment of tuberculosis (see Box 21.8), both respiratory and non-respiratory disease, is a six-month four-drug regimen with isoniazid, rifampicin, pyrazinamide and either streptomycin or ethambutol (NICE, 2011).

Box 21.8   Treatment

Initial phase of treatment (2 months)

Aims to reduce the bacterial population as quickly as possible so that the patient becomes non-infectious as quickly as possible, and to prevent the emergence of drug resistance (Pratt *et al.*, 2005c).

Drugs, action and side effects

Isoniazid

Action: The principle 'killing' drug; destroys all replicating bacilli in the pulmonary cavity.
Side effects: Peripheral neuropathy in patients with HIV, diabetes, malnutrition, alcohol dependence and chronic renal failure.

Ethambutol or streptomycin

Streptomycin is given if isoniazid resistance is detected.
Action: Assists isoniazid.
Side effects (ethambutol): Visual disturbances (eye examination necessary before commencing treatment) – loss of acuity, colour blindness.

Rifampicin

Action: Targets less active bacilli within macrophages and inflammatory lesions; also sterilises pulmonary cavities.
Side effects: Transient disturbances in renal function; affects action of the oral contraceptive pill.

Pyrazinamide

Action: Targets less active bacilli within macrophages and inflammatory lesions; also sterilises pulmonary cavities.
Side effects: Can induce liver toxicity and may need to be discontinued; therefore prescribed for only two months.

Second phase of treatment (4 months): the continuation phase

Drugs

Isoniazid: Targets any bacilli that are rifampicin resistant.
Rifampicin: Kills dormant bacilli.

315

Contact tracing and screening (NICE, 2011)

The principle aim of contact tracing is to:

- Identify any associated cases of tuberculosis.
- Detect people with latent infection.
- Identify those who are not infected, and offer vaccination in order to prevent infection where appropriate.

It may also be a useful aid in detecting the source of infection in an outbreak situation where the index case is not obviously recognisable; this is of particular importance in cases of infectious respiratory tuberculosis.

Close contacts

Close contacts are defined as those from the same household, sharing a bedroom, kitchen, bathroom and/or sitting room with the index case. They may also include very close associates of the index case such as a partner or frequent visitors to the home. Occasionally, workplace contacts may also be classed as 'close contacts'.

Most occupational contacts come under the heading of 'casual contacts', and follow-up would usually be necessary only in any of the following circumstances:

- If the index case is sputum smear-positive and any of the contacts are felt to be unusually susceptible
- If the index case is considered to be highly infectious
- In the event of an outbreak.

In each case, the lifestyle of the index case needs to be carefully considered since other places of close contact may be revealed; for example, the index case may have recently been on a long-haul air flight, or may be living in a homeless shelter.

In-patient contact tracing

Within the hospital in-patient setting, there is always the possibility of a patient with active respiratory TB being mis-diagnosed, or just not detected, and being placed in the middle of an open ward. Although the risk of infectivity to other patients is considered to be small, each patient needs to be individually risk assessed, and decisions around the appropriate action to be taken should centre around:

- The degree of infectivity of the index case
- The length of time during which other patients were 'exposed' to the index case
- The proximity of the contact
- Whether any of the contacts were immunocompromised.

Patients in the same bay as the patient, as opposed to all patients on the ward, should be regarded as being at risk only if the index case was found to be sputum smear-positive with a productive cough and was in the bay for more than eight hours.

In the event of susceptible patients being on the same ward, but not necessarily in the same bay, as the index case, and the length of stay of the index case exceeding more than two days, individual patients should be risk assessed.

If an in-patient with smear-positive TB is found to have MDR-TB, or if exposed patients are HIV-positive, contact tracing should be undertaken in accordance with the recommendations within guidelines published by the Interdepartmental Working Group on Tuberculosis (1998).

Contact tracing and screening of healthcare workers

Although it is generally accepted that the incidence of tuberculosis in healthcare workers is no higher than in other members of the population at large, there is evidence to suggest that healthcare workers are at risk, particularly as staff have been recruited for employment within the NHS from countries where the burden of tuberculosis is high (Meredith *et al.*, 1996).

New employees who will either be having patient contact or be working with clinical specimens should undergo a health screen before they commence work, and the NICE guidance and new guidance from the Department of Health (2007) detail the processes that should be followed.

It is not recommended that the routine screening of healthcare workers following exposure to a patient with sputum smear-positive disease is undertaken unless the staff member concerned is considered to be at any significant risk. The NICE guidance recommends that after a 'TB incident' on a ward, staff are sent a 'one-off' reminder by the occupational health department, which details the signs and symptoms to look out for, and the importance of reporting any symptoms promptly.

Any healthcare worker who is concerned about having been exposed to tuberculosis would generally be advised to seek assurance from their own occupational health department. In the event of a healthcare worker being diagnosed with tuberculosis, from either occupational exposure or a community source, liaison between the treating physician, the occupational health department, the local Health Protection Unit (Public Health England) and the Infection Prevention and Control Team (IP&CT) is important.

If that member of staff has been working while they have been infectious, patients and colleagues who have had significant contact will need to be identified. It will not always be known how long the index case has been infectious for, so it is recommended that contacts be reviewed for the period of time that the index case has had a cough. In the event of this not being known, contacts should be traced back from the first three months preceding the first sputum smear or culture-positive results.

BCG vaccination

Fact Box 21.9   The BCG vaccination

The BCG vaccine, first used in 1921, contains live organisms modified from *M. bovis*. It was discovered by two scientists working at the Pasteur Institute in Paris, who isolated the organism from a cow with bovine tuberculosis, and over a period of several years the organism underwent numerous genetic changes which altered the original strain of *M. bovis*, producing what is now known as BCG. Its effectiveness has been the subject of much debate, and while it is not considered to be hugely effective in preventing respiratory TB, it does offer protection against more severe forms of disease such as TB meningitis, particularly in children.

Source: Salisbury *et al.*, 2006.

The BCG vaccine was introduced into the United Kingdom in 1953, and until the autumn of 2005 it was administered to schoolchildren between the ages of 10 and 14 as part of the schools' vaccination programme to prevent the acquisition of respiratory disease. However, the epidemiology of tuberculosis in the United Kingdom has changed significantly over the years, and in 2005 the Department of Health announced changes to the BCG vaccination programme. Within the United Kingdom, tuberculosis has changed from being a disease that affects the general population, to one that mostly affects high-risk group, and individuals requiring immunisation in the United Kingdom are listed in Box 21.9 as per the Department of Health *Green Book* (DH, 2006).

Box 21.9   BCG vaccination (UK): the immunisation of those at increased risk of developing severe disease and/or of exposure to TB infection

- All infants (aged 0 to 12 months) living in areas of the United Kingdom where the annual incidence of TB is 40/100 000 or greater, and all infants (0 to 12 months) with a parent or grandparent who was born in a country where the annual incidence of TB is 40/100 000 or greater.
- Previously unvaccinated children aged one to five years with a parent or grandparent who was born in a country where the annual incidence of TB is 40/100 000 or greater.
- Previously unvaccinated, tuberculin-negative children aged from six to under 16 years of age with a parent or grandparent who was born in a country where the annual incidence of TB is 40/100 000 or greater.
- Previously unvaccinated tuberculin-negative individuals under 16 years of age who are contacts of cases of respiratory TB.
- Previously unvaccinated, tuberculin-negative individuals under 16 years of age who were born in or who have lived for a prolonged period (at least three months) in a country with an annual TB incidence of 40/100 000 or greater.

Source: http://www.immunisation.dh.gov.uk/green-book-chapters/chapter-32/.

Clinical practice points: infection control precautions (drug-sensitive TB) (NICE, 2011)

General points

- All patients with TB should have risk assessments for drug resistance and HIV.

Reflection point

Review the medical notes and medical history of one of your patients with suspected or confirmed respiratory TB. Does the patient have any risk factors for MDR-TB? Has a risk assessment been made and documented? Is this in accordance with your hospital's TB Policy?

- Unless there is a clear clinical or socioeconomic need, such as homelessness, people with TB at any site of disease should not be admitted to hospital for diagnostic tests or for care.
- Any visitors to a child with TB in hospital should be screened as part of contact tracing, and kept separate from other patients until they have been excluded as the source of infection.
- No member of staff should enter the room unless they have had a BCG vaccination.
- The occupational health department should be informed of any confirmed cases of respiratory TB on a ward in order that the relevant checks on staff immunity can be made.
- Gloves and aprons are required only if contact with body fluids, including sputum, is anticipated.
- Only those visitors, including young children, who have already been in close contact with the patient before diagnosis should visit. Masks are not required.
- All waste contaminated with blood and body fluids, including sputum, should be treated as clinical waste.
- The room must be cleaned daily by Domestic Services Staff.

Patient isolation

See Chapter 11 for more information.

- A single room with a window ventilated to the outside is essential for the isolation of patients with suspected or confirmed respiratory TB. If the room is occupied by a patient who does not have TB, he or she must be moved out of the room and allocated a suitable bed elsewhere.
- The door must be kept closed and the appropriate isolation door sign must be displayed on the door.
- The room must have a toilet and wash hand basin (use of communal washing facilities is not permitted). It is therefore essential that particular rooms with en-suite facilities are designated within the hospital for nursing patients with respiratory tuberculosis, and arrangements must be made immediately to vacate the designated room if a patient with respiratory tuberculosis is admitted. Ideally, patients with respiratory TB should be nursed in negative-pressure isolation rooms.
- The patient must not leave the room other than for essential investigations and treatments. This must be discussed with the IP&CT and the Respiratory Physician and documented in the notes.
- Patients with respiratory TB must be separated from immunocompromised patients, by admission to either a single room on a separate ward or a negative-pressure room on the same ward.

Masks

See Chapter 13 for more information.

- Healthcare workers caring for people with TB are not required to wear masks **unless** MDR-TB is suspected **or** aerosol-generating procedures are being performed (NICE, 2011).

Reflection point

There may be disagreement locally amongst Respiratory and IP&C Teams with the recommendation from NICE (2011) regarding the wearing of masks, and in some Trusts, the recommendation may be that masks should routinely be worn for all episodes of contact with the patient. What does your local policy say regarding the wearing of masks? Have staff been fit-tested for a HEPA FFP3 mask? If so, who was responsible for undertaking this? Has a risk assessment been undertaken and a decision made to use FFP2 masks instead?

- Aerosol-generating procedures should be carried out in an appropriately engineered and ventilated area (not in an open ward environment) for all patients in whom TB is considered a possible diagnosis, in any setting. Healthcare workers undertaking these procedures must wear a HEPA FFP3 disposable respirator mask (e.g. Physiotherapists undertaking chest physiotherapy).
- Patients must always be educated to cough and sneeze into a tissue and are required to wear a surgical mask if it is necessary for them to leave the room before they have had two weeks of drug treatment. **Note**: In the event of the patient requiring oxygen via a Venuturi mask or nasal cannulae, the patient will be unable to wear a mask.
- TB patients admitted to a setting where care is provided for people who are immunocompromised, including those who are HIV-positive, should be considered infectious and, if sputum smear-positive, should stay in a negative-pressure room until:
  - The patient has had at least two weeks of appropriate multiple drug therapy and, if moving to accommodation (in-patient or home) with people who are immunocompromised, including those who are HIV-positive,
  - The patient has had at least three negative microscopic smears on separate occasions over a 14-day period; **and**
  - The patient is showing tolerance to the prescribed treatment and an ability and agreement to adhere to treatment; and either any cough has resolved completely, **or** there is definite clinical improvement on treatment, for example remaining apyrexial for a week.

Discontinuation of isolation

- Isolation may be discontinued after two complete weeks of anti-TB treatment containing rifampicin and isoniazid but must be discussed in the first instance with the Chest Physician.
- Three negative acid-fast bacilli smears are required prior to isolation discontinuing if:
  - The patient has been categorised as highly infectious by the IP&CT (more than 10% of contacts contract TB).
  - The patient is suspected or confirmed as having MDR-TB.
  - The patient is being transferred to an area with immunocompromised patients.

If the first two factors exist, negative-pressure isolation is recommended.

Patients may be discharged to their own home before the completion of two weeks of treatment if they no longer require hospitalisation for symptom control and home circumstances are satisfactory.

The GP and District Nurse (if appropriate) should be informed of the patient's diagnosis and treatment requirements.

The patient will be followed up post discharge by the Respiratory Physician and the TB Team (community).

Following discharge or transfer of the patient, the nursing staff must request an 'infection clean' of the room.

Infection control precautions for MDR-TB

- The appropriate isolation sign must be displayed on the door.
- Care must be carried out in the negative-pressure room until the patient is found to be non-infectious or non-resistant, and ideally until cultures are negative.
- Isolation must continue until the patient produces three negative sputum specimens on separate occasions over at least a 14-day period.
- Only relatives who have had contact with the patient prior to admission should visit. Masks are not required.

Masks

- Healthcare staff must wear a HEPA FFP3 disposable respirator mask during contact with a patient with suspected or known MDR-TB while the patient is considered to be infectious.
- Staff who have not been fit-tested and trained in performing an FFP3 pre-use fit check must not care for or have contact with patients with suspected or confirmed MDR-TB.

Discharge

- The decision to discharge a patient with suspected or known MDR-TB should be discussed with the IP&CT, the TB service, the CCDC and the GP, and secure arrangements for the supervision and administration of all anti-TB therapy should have been agreed with the patient and carers. A case conference to discuss discharge arrangements may be required.

Chapter summary: key points

- Tuberculosis represents a major threat to public health in developing countries, and there is a significant burden of TB in inner cities in the United Kingdom.

- It is a curable disease if diagnosed and treated promptly, and deaths from TB are preventable.

- Prompt recognition of symptoms, confirmation of cases and the appropriate infection control precautions to minimise spread are keys to preventing and controlling tuberculosis.

- Morbidity and mortality associated with TB are greatest in patients who are immunocompromised and/or who have MDR-TB.

- Not all patients with TB are infectious.

- Healthcare workers should have a high index of suspicion if a patient displays symptoms of TB even if an alternative diagnosis has been made.

Further resources are available for this book, including interactive multiple choice questions. Visit the companion website at:

www.wiley.com/go/fundamentalsofinfectionprevention

References

Breathnach A.S., de Ruiter A., Holdsworth G.M., Bateman N.T., O'Sullivan D.G. *et al.* (1998). An outbreak of multi-drug resistant tuberculosis in a London teaching hospital. *Journal of Hospital Infection.* 39 (2): 111–117.

British Society of Gastroenterology (2003). *BSG Guidelines for the Decontamination of Equipment for Gastrointestinal Endoscopy. The Report of a Working Party of the British Society of Gastroenterology Endoscopy Committee.* British Society of Gastroenterology, London.

British Thoracic Society (1999). Management of opportunistic mycobacterial infection: Joint Tuberculosis Committee Guidelines. *Thorax.* 55 (3): 210–218.

Daley C.L., Small P.M., Schecter G.F. (1992). An outbreak of tuberculosis with accelerated progression among persons infected with human immunodeficiency virus: an analysis using restriction-fragment-length polymorphisms. *New England Journal of Medicine.* 326 (4): 231–235.

Department of Health (DH) (2006). *Immunisation against Infectious Diseases. Department of Health, London.* http://www.dh.gov.uk/greenbook (accessed 22 January 2013)

Department of Health (DH) (2007): *Health Clearance for Tuberculosis, Hepatitis B and HIV: New Healthcare Workers.* Department of Health, London.

Dooley S.W., Villarino M.E., Lawrence M., Salvinas L., Amil S. *et al.* (1992). Nosocomial transmission of multi-drug resistant tuberculosis in a hospital unit for HIV infected patients. *Journal of the American Medical Association.* 267 (7): 2632–2635.

Fitzgerald D., Sterling T.R., Haas D.W. (2009). Mycobacterium tuberculosis. In: Mandell G.L., Bennett J.E., Dolin R.D. (Eds.), *Mandell's Principles and Practices of Infectious Diseases.* 7th ed. Churchill Livingstone Elsevier, London. http://expert.consult (accessed 17 October 2012)

Furuya E.X., Paez A., Srinivasan A., Cooksey R., Augenbraun M. *et al.* (2007). Outbreak of *Mycobacterium abscessus* wound infections among 'lipotourists' from the United States who underwent abdominoplasty in the Dominican Republic. *Clinical Infectious Diseases.* 15 April: 1181–1188.

Gladwin M., Trattler B. (2003). Mycobacterium. In: *Clinical Microbiology Made Ridiculously Simple.* 3rd ed. MedMaster Inc., Miami, FL: 102–110.

Grange J.M. (2003). Mycobacterium. In: Greenwood D., Slack R.C.B., Peutherer J.F. (Eds.), *Medical Microbiology: A Guide to Microbial Infections: Pathogenesis, Immunity, Laboratory Diagnosis and Control.* 16th ed. Churchill Livingstone, London: 200–214.

Grange J.M. (2007). Environmental mycobacteria: opportunist disease. In: Greenwood D., Slack R., Peutherer J., Barer M. (Eds.). *Medical Microbiology. A Guide to Microbial Infections: Pathogenesis, Immunity, Laboratory Diagnosis and Control.* 17th ed. Churchill Livingstone, London: 221–227.

Henriques B., Hoffner S.E., Petrini B., Juhlin I.M., Wåhlèn P. *et al.* (1994). Infection with *Mycobacterium malmoense* in Sweden. *Clinical Infectious Diseases.* 18 (4): 596–600.

Interdepartmental Working Group on Tuberculosis (1998). *The Prevention and Control of Tuberculosis in the United Kingdom: UK Guidance on the Prevention and Control of Transmission of HIV-related Tuberculosis and Drug-resistant, including Multiple-drug Resistant, Tuberculosis.* Department of Health, London.

Jarvis W.R. (1993). Nosocomial transmission of multi-drug resistant tuberculosis. *American Journal of Infection Control*. 22 (2): 146–151.

Jiva T.M., Jacoby H.M., Weymouth L.A., Kaminski D.A., Portmore A.C. (1997). *Mycobacterium xenopi*: innocent bystander or emerging pathogen? *Clinical Infectious Diseases*. 24: 226–232.

Meredith S., Watson J.M., Citron K.M., Cockcroft A., Darbyshire J.H. (1996). Are healthcare workers in England and Wales at increased risk of tuberculosis? *British Medical Journal*. 313 (7056): 522–525.

National Institute for Health and Clinical Excellence (NICE) (2011). *Tuberculosis: Clinical Diagnosis and Management of Tuberculosis, and Measures for Its Prevention and Control*. NICE Clinical Guideline 117. NICE, London.

National Institute for Health and Clinical Excellence (NICE) (2012). *Identifying and Managing tuberculosis among Hard-to-Reach Groups*. NICE Public Health Guidance 37. NICE, London. http://www.nice.org.uk/ph37 (accessed 12 October 2012)

Plorde J.J. (2004). Mycobacterium. In: Sherris J.C., Ryan K.J., Ray G.C. (Eds.), *Medical Microbiology: An Introduction to Infectious Diseases*. 4th ed. McGraw-Hill, London: 439–456.

Pratt R.J., Grange J.M., Williams V.G. (2005a). Immunity and immunopathology in tuberculosis. In: *Tuberculosis: A Foundation for Nursing and Healthcare Practice*. Hodder Arnold, London: 61–79.

Pratt R.J., Grange J.M., Williams V.G. (2005b). Diagnosis of tuberculosis and other mycobacterial diseases. In: *Tuberculosis: A Foundation for Nursing and Healthcare Practice*. Hodder Arnold, London: 95–108.

Pratt R.J., Grange J.M., Williams V.G. (2005c). The treatment of tuberculosis and other mycobacterial diseases. In: *Tuberculosis: A Foundation for Nursing and Healthcare Practice*. Hodder Arnold, London: 149–167.

Royal College of Nursing (2012). *Tuberculosis Case Management and Cohort Review: Guidance for Healthcare Professionals*. Royal College of Nursing, London.

Ryan K.J., Drew W.L. (2010). Mycobacteria. In: Ryan K.J., Ray C.G. (Eds.), *Sherris Medical Microbiology*. 5th ed. McGraw-Hill Medical, London: 489–506.

Salisbury D., Ramsay M., Noakes K. (2006). *Immunisation against Infectious diseases*, (chp 32) Department for Health, The Stationary Office.

Smith M.B., Schnadiva V.J., Boyars M.C., Woods G.L. (2001). Pathologic features of *Mycobacterium fortuitum* infections: an emerging pathogen in patients with AIDS. *American Journal of Clinical Pathology*. 116: 225–232.

White V.L.C., Moore-Gillan J. (2000). Resource implications of patients with multi-drug resistant tuberculosis. *Thorax*. 55 (11): 962–963.

World Health Organization (2011). *WHO Report 2011: Global TB Control*. World Health Organization, Geneva.

Zink A.R., Sola C., Reischi U., Grabner W., Rastogi N., Wolf H., *et al.* (2003). Characterisation of *M. tuberculosis* complex DNAs from Egyptian mummies by spoliogotyping. *Journal of Clinical Microbiology*. 41 (1): 35.

Further reading

Ryan F. (1992). *Tuberculosis. The Greatest Story Never Told*. Swift Publishers Ltd. ISBN: 978-1874082006

22

Clostridium difficile

Contents

Fundamentals of Infection Prevention and Control: Theory and Practice, Second Edition. Debbie Weston.
© 2013 John Wiley & Sons, Ltd. Published 2013 by John Wiley & Sons, Ltd. Companion Website: www.wiley.com/go/fundamentalsofinfectionprevention

Introduction

Clostridium difficile was first described in 1935 as 'the difficult Clostridium' (Hall and O'Toole, 1935), a reference to the difficulties experienced in isolating and then culturing the organism under laboratory conditions, but it wasn't until the 1970s that its association with antibiotic administration and pseudomembranous colitis was recognised (Larson *et al.*, 1977). Since the late 1990s, *Clostridium difficile* has become notorious for being the most important cause of hospital-acquired diarrhoea in adults and a significant cause of patient morbidity and mortality. It is a particularly distressing infection for patients and their families and causes a spectrum of illness which ranges from asymptomatic colonisation of the bowel to trivial diarrhoea to life-threatening illness as a result of pseudomembranous colitis and toxic megacolon.

This chapter looks at *C. difficile* in detail, discussing the organism; the pathogenesis of infection, including risk factors for acquisition; clinical features and diagnosis (testing is covered in Chapter 7); antibiotic management and novel treatments such as the use of probiotics and immunoglobulin, and infection control precautions and best practice.

Learning outcomes

After reading this chapter, the reader will be able to:

- Understand and be able to describe the pathogenesis of infection and the risk factors for acquisition.

- Recognise and be able to describe the clinical features of *C. difficile* infection.

- Be able to discuss the infection control precautions that need to be taken when caring for a symptomatic patient, and understand the importance of strict compliance.

- Understand the management of *C. difficile*, including the role of novel treatment.

Background

Fact Box 22.1 Clostridia

Clostridia are the most clinically important of the Gram-positive anaerobic rods (the other significant Gram-positive rods being aerobes). As obligate anaerobes, they colonise oxygen-deficient areas of the body where they co-exist alongside the normal resident flora, but if displaced into a sterile body site they can result in potentially life-threatening conditions (Ryan and Drew, 2010). Out of the 160 species of Clostridia which occur naturally in the environment in soil, water, sewage and also the human and animal gastro-intestinal tract, only a very small minority are pathogenic to humans, such as *Clostridium tetani*, *Clostridium botulinum*, *Clostridium perfringens* and *Clostridium difficile*. They tend to cause opportunistic infections, and their potent toxins (see Chapter 5) can result in invasive and destructive damage to the host. Their ability to form endospores facilitates their survival in extreme environmental conditions for months or years. They have the ability to return to their vegetative state when the environmental conditions are favourable.

C. difficile infection places a significant financial burden on the NHS, costing in the region of £4200 per patient in the United Kingdom and between $9179 and $11456 per patient in the United States (McGlone et al., 2012). It has also had a significant national media focus in recent years, with inquiries into large outbreaks in England and Northern Ireland (Healthcare Commission, 2006, 2007; www.cdiffinquiry.org).

In recognition of the burden of C. difficile infection, and the drive towards no avoidable infections, the Department of Health set national C. difficile reduction targets for the NHS in 2008, whereby NHS organisations were required to achieve a 30% reduction in cases by 2010–2011 based on their 2007–2008 baseline (Department of Health, 2007). In addition, new national guidance on the prevention, management and control of C. difficile was published by the Department of Health in conjunction with the Health Protection Agency in December 2008 (Department of Health and Health Protection Agency, 2008). The reduction targets were achieved in 2009 and then reduced further still; for the financial year 2010–2011, there were 21 695 cases of C. difficile infection, representing a 15% decrease from 2009–2010, and a 40% reduction from 2008–2009 (36 095 cases), demonstrating that C. difficile is an **avoidable** infection and that its incidence can be greatly reduced through stringent infection control measures, including prudent antimicrobial prescribing.

The protective role of resident bowel flora

Fact Box 22.2   Resident bowel flora

Healthy adults carry at least 500 species of bacteria in the colon, of which 90% are anaerobes. A gram of faeces contains up to 10^{12} bacteria (Tonna and Welsby, 2005), and this normal colonic flora inhibits the growth of other bacteria that could proliferate within the bowel if the normal balance of bacterial flora is disrupted.

C. difficile is part of the resident bowel flora in 2–5% of the population. In the 'normal healthy' adult, the flora of the colon is generally resistant to colonisation by C. difficile, and even if the organism is acquired, the risk of the individual progressing to clinical illness is negligible (Shim et al., 1998) due to host defence mechanisms that are considered to be inhibitory to C. difficile (Box 22.1).

Box 22.1   Host defence mechanisms inhibitory to C. difficile

The presence of volatile fatty acids produced by bowel flora as toxic metabolic end products
Competition amongst bacteria for adhesion sites
The stimulation of colonic peristalsis
Immune response mechanisms
The production of gastric acid.

Source: McCracken and Lorenz, 2001; Rastall, 2004; Keel and Songer, 2006.

However, if the normal flora of the large intestine has been disrupted by the administration of antibiotic therapy, it can be readily colonised by *C. difficile*, which does not have to compete with other bacteria for nutrients, and this can predispose the patient to developing diarrhoea.

The pathogenesis of *C. difficile* infection

Four key steps have been identified in the pathogenesis of *C. difficile* infection (Thielman and Wilson, 2009):

Step 1: disruption of the normal colonic flora by the administration of antibiotics

The disruption and subsequent alteration of the bowel flora through the administration of anti-biotics are the main precipitating factors for symptomatic *C. difficile* infection, with overgrowth of *C. difficile* increasingly linked to broad-spectrum agents such as clindamycin, the cephalosporins (with cefotaxime in particular implicated in the onset of symptomatic cases), penicillins and fluo-roquinolones (e.g. ciprofloxacin), although any antibiotic with anti-bacterial activity can induce diarrhoea. The risk is partly dependent upon the antibiotic used and the duration of treatment. Symptoms may occur within 5–10 days of commencing antibiotic therapy or 2–10 weeks after it has been completed (Thielman and Wilson, 2009).

Step 2: colonisation with toxigenic (toxin-producing) strains of *C. difficile*

The main route of acquisition is via the faecal-oral route. As they are not affected by stomach acid (unlike vegetative cells), spores are able to pass through the stomach; they germinate into the vegetative form (from which they replicate and produce *Clostridium difficile* toxins) in the small intestine following exposure to bile acids, before reaching the colon, which they can then colonise. Symptomatic disease will develop only if the strain of *C. difficile* possesses the gene for toxin production, producing enteroxin A and/or cytotokin B.

In addition to antibiotic exposure and alteration of the colonic flora, there are other documented risk factors:

Age over 65 years: Increasing age is generally associated with increased risk of infection and higher mortality rates (see Chapter 8), and older persons are more likely to have co-morbidities.

Environmental reservoirs: Close proximity to a symptomatic patient has been given an attributable risk of 12% (Chang and Nelson, 2000), and the level of contamination on healthcare workers' hands has been found to be proportionate to the level of environmental contamination (Fawley and Wilcox, 2001). Therefore, it is perhaps not surprising that rates of carriage have been reported in hospitalised patients ranging from 13% to 50% depending on their length of stay (Poutanen and Simor, 2004), and as low as 7% and as high as 70% in long-term care facilities (Denève *et al.*, 2009).

Fact Box 22.3   Dispersal of spores through the air

A study by Best et al. (2010) suggests that the air within the patient's immediate environment is contaminated with *C. difficile* spores, which arise either directly from the patient or as a result of movement and activity within the environment, aiding the circulation and dispersal of airborne *C. difficile* and contaminating surfaces.

A large-scale research study undertaken by Walker *et al.* (2012) indicated that approximately 75% of all new cases of *C. difficile* infection included in their dataset could not be explained by transmission from symptomatic patients, particularly where there are well-established infection control practices. They conclude that a greater understanding of other potential routes of transmission and reservoirs are necessary in order that other control measures can be identified.

Proton pump inhibitors (PPIs): The natural acidity of the stomach serves as a 'disinfectant' for the gastro-intestinal tract and is part of the innate immune response. Proton pump inhibitors and histamine H_2 antagonists, used to prevent the development of gastric and duodenal ulcers and reduce the secretion of gastric acid, have been implicated as possible contributing factors in *C. difficile* infection (Brazier, 1998; Cunningham *et al.*, 2003; Dial *et al.*, 2004), as the natural acidity of the stomach declines, and therefore the vegetative forms of *C. difficile*, including the spores, are less likely to be destroyed.

Other documented risk factors: Naso-gastric tube insertion, bowel preparation prior to surgery, gastro-intestinal surgery, altered gut motility, intensive care unit admission, and patients receiving immunosuppressive therapy and cytotoxic agents (Bignardi, 1998; Kyne *et al.*, 2001; Loo *et al.*, 2011).

Step 3: amplification of toxins

Enterotoxin A binds to receptors in the bowel wall and causes extensive tissue damage with injury to the mucosa by activating macrophages and mast cells to release inflammatory mediators, and is responsible for nearly all of the gastro-intestinal symptoms seen (Vaishnavi, 2010). It also facilitates the entry of cytotoxin B into the epithelial cells that line by colon by loosening the tight junctions between them (Starr, 2005). Toxin B has a cytotoxic potency that is 1000 times greater than that of toxin A, and is thought to play a major role in activating the inflammatory response (Tabaqchali and Jumma, 1995).

Fact Box 22.4   Enterotoxin A and cytotoxin B

Enterotoxin A and cytotoxin B are regarded as ranking amongst the most lethal bacterial toxins that have been studied (Thielman and Wilson, 2009) and together they have a synergistic effect, with one toxin enhancing the effects of the other, which incites an inflammatory cascade that causes fluid loss and increased damage to host cells (Keel and Songer, 2006).

Some strains of *C. difficile* such as ribotype 027 contain a third toxin, known as binary toxin (first described in 1988), which contains both toxin A and B, and is generally associated with more severe disease (Vaishnavi, 2010).

Fact Box 22.5   Ribotypes 027 and 332

Ribotype 027 has been associated with large hospital outbreaks in Canada and the United Kingdom, and in 2006 it was the second most common strain isolated by the HPA's national sampling surveillance programme (Healthcare Commission, 2006). The most striking feature of 027 is hypertoxin production (Brazier, 2006). It produces 10–20 times more toxin than other strains as it lacks a gene that regulates how much toxin is produced (Brierly, 2005; Warney *et al.*, 2005). Patients infected with the 027 strain tend to have a more acute illness and increased severity of symptoms (Bartlett and Perl, 2005) (although diarrhoea may not always be present), together with important diagnostic markers – a raised white cell count and elevated C-reactive protein (CRP) (see Chapter 8). Patients may fail to respond to metronidazole and have a higher rate of progression towards developing pseudomembranous colitis. In May 2013 a novel ribotype, 332, was reported by Health Protection Scotland to have killed three patients in two Scottish hospitals. The cases were unrelated, although two were from the same clinical setting and contracted *C. difficile* in December 2012 and January 2013; the third case was confirmed in April 2013. All three patients had severe underlying illness.

Step 4: mucosal injury and inflammation

The resulting inflammation may lead to the development of pseudomembranes, whereby the inflamed mucosa is studded with raised white and yellow plaques, consisting of neutrophils, fibrin, mucin and cellular debris, which range from 2 to 10 mm in diameter and are usually, though not always, confined to the distal colon (Vaishnavi, 2010), although there may be intervening patches of 'normal' mucosa.

Diagnosis of pseudomembranous colitis is made by colonoscopy. In symptomatic but neutropenic patients, colonoscopy may give a false-negative result, as pseudomembranes do not form due to lack of neutrophils (Tabaqchali and Jumma. 1995). If symptoms progress, patients are at increased risk of developing paralytic ileus and toxic megacolon (acute dilation of the colon to a diameter greater than 6 cm, associated with systemic toxicity in the absence of mechanical obstruction) (Thielman and Wilson, 2009).

Diarrhoea will be absent. X-rays will reveal dilated colon and oedema of the mucosa; invasive investigations such as sigmoidoscopy and colonoscopy are contra-indicated here as they can induce perforation.

Fact Box 22.6   *C. difficile* mortality

The mortality rate from *C. difficile* ranges from 6% to 30% in patients with pseudomembranous colitis, and 64% in patients with toxic megacolon.

Clinical features of *C. difficile* infection

- Sudden onset of diarrhoea. Patients may pass unformed or watery diarrhoea more than twice a day and in severe cases the diarrhoea is often profuse and watery, with the patient passing more than 20 stools a day, often accompanied by abdominal pain.

Reporting and managing patients with diarrhoea

It is important that staff understand what is meant by the word 'diarrhoea', as healthcare professionals often rely on their own subjective opinion as to whether or not patients have diarrhoea (Whelan *et al.*, 2004). To simply report cases of 'loose stools' is particularly unhelpful to the Infection Prevention and Control Team (IP&CT). The Royal College of Nursing (RCN) published guidance on the *Management of Diarrhoea in Adults* in March 2013.

Fact Box 22.7   Diarrhoea

The word 'diarrhoea' is Greek in origin, meaning 'flowing through'. It is defined by the World Health Organization (WHO) as '3 or more liquid stools per day, or the passage of more stools than is normal for that person' (www.http://who/int/topics/diarrhoea/en).

The form of the stool is determined by the faecal transit time, and 'true' diarrhoea is the frequent passing of liquid or watery stool with very little, if any, solid contents. The Bristol Stool Chart (Lewis and Heaton, 1997) can be a useful tool in identifying different stool types. Diarrhoea is classed as types 5–7.

While it can, on occasion, be difficult to completely exclude an infectious cause in a patient with diarrhoea, to report *all* patients experiencing diarrhoea can be misleading, particularly if there is an established or suspected cause for the symptoms seen in that individual, and staff do need to exercise a degree of common sense and clinical judgment. Box 22.2 lists some of the common non-infectious causes of diarrhoea.

However, patients presenting with diarrhoea, either on or during the first 72 hours of their admission, should be isolated in a single room unless or until an infectious cause can be **confidently excluded**, and a stool specimen obtained promptly (Department of Health, 2012), ideally on the first episode. If a decision is made that the cause of the diarrhoea is unlikely to be infectious and in the absence of a stool specimen being obtained and/or a negative result being confirmed, there must be clear documentation in the medical notes. In the event of any doubt, the advice of the IP&CT must always be sought.

Box 22.2   Causes of diarrhoea

Post-operative period following bowel surgery
Medication
Laxative or enema administration
Long-standing history of diarrhoea of a chronic nature, as in irritable bowel syndrome or colitis
Anxiety or stress.

Fact Box 22.8   The SIGHT protocol

The Department of Health and Health Protection Agency (2008) recommend the use of the **SIGHT** mnemonic protocol for the management of patients with potentially infectious diarrhoea:

S = Suspect an infective cause if there is no other alternative explanation.
I = Isolate the patient and inform the IP&CT.
G = Wear gloves and aprons appropriately (see Chapter 13).
H = Wash hands with liquid soap and water.
T = Send a stool specimen for testing immediately.

Source: DH/HPA, 2008.

- Characteristic 'farmyard' or 'manure'-type smell

Fact Box 22.9   P-cresols

The distinctive odour associated with *C. difficile* is caused by the production of p-cresols, gaseous by-products of *C. difficile* metabolism, and a major component in pig odour.

- Diarrhoea may be accompanied by mucous or 'jelly' in the stools. Abdominal distension, fever and dehydration may also be present.

Diagnosis

C. difficile definition

'One episode of diarrhoea, defined either as stool loose enough to take the shape of the container used to sample it or as Bristol Stool Chart types 5–7 that is not attributable to any other cause, including medicines, **and** that occurs at the same time as a positive toxin assay **and/or** endoscopic evidence of pseudomembranous colitis' (Department of Health and Health Protection Agency, 2008).

Laboratory testing and interpretation of results are covered in Chapter 7.

- **Note regarding glutamate dehydrogenase antigen-positive results.**

As seen in Chapter 7, glutamate dehydrogenase (GDH) is the common *Clostridium difficile* antigen, and its detection in the absence of toxin indicates carrier status as opposed to overt infection. However, *C. difficile* spores will be shed, and there is a cross-infection risk to other patients if the patient has diarrhoea. Antibiotic treatment is not necessarily indicated unless the patient is clinically unwell and has other symptoms suggestive of *C. difficile* infection and/or the diarrhoea does not spontaneously resolve within 48 hours, although some Trusts may have a policy of treating all patients who are GDH-positive as if they have symptomatic infection. Box 22.3 describes the infection control management of GDH antigen–positive patients.

Box 22.3   Infection control management of patients who are GDH antigen–positive and toxin-negative

- Ensure that the patient is isolated in a single room with the appropriate isolation door sign displayed (see Chapter 11) and dedicated patient equipment until he or she has been asymptomatic for 48 hours. If the room is not en-suite, the patient must be allocated his/her own commode.
- Maintain an accurate stool chart in order to enable assessment of resolution or worsening of diarrhoea. Inform the IP&CT and the patient's Medical Team in the event of any changes.
- Record the patient's vital signs (temperature, pulse and blood pressure) four times hourly, and inform the IP&CT and the Medical Team of any deviations.
- Ensure that the room is cleaned daily, and that a thorough clean is undertaken when isolation is no longer required and/or the patient is discharged.

The significance of community versus hospital-acquired *C. difficile* infection

Determining whether the infection was acquired pre or post admission is important given the national *C. difficile* reduction targets. Only hospital-acquired cases count against the hospital's target and affect their trajectory, but community-acquired cases are monitored by the Clinical Commissioning Groups (CCGs). Hospital-acquired cases are certainly subjected to a root cause analysis (RCA) (see Chapter 2).

Community-acquired *C. difficile* infection: Onset <72 hours of admission to hospital
Hospital-acquired *C. difficile* infection: Onset >72 hours of admission to hospital.

The timing of stool specimen collection is crucial. Obviously, the sooner the specimen is obtained, the sooner laboratory confirmed is made. However, if a patient is admitted with diarrhoea, or develops it within 72 hours of admission, but a stool specimen is not obtained for four days, it will be recorded as a case of hospital-acquired *C. difficile* infection according to the mandatory surveillance guidelines (see Chapter 3).

Clinical considerations regarding the medical management of *C. difficile* infection

For more information, see Department of Health and Health Protection Agency (2008).

- Doctors must consider symptomatic *C. difficile* as a diagnosis in its own right (Healthcare Commission, 2007; Department of Health and Health Protection Agency 2008).
- Each patient must be reviewed daily regarding fluid resuscitation, electrolyte replacement and nutritional status, and this review must be documented in the patient's notes. They must be monitored for signs of increasing severity of disease with early referral to the ITU as patients may deteriorate very rapidly.

Reflection point

Is symptomatic *C. difficile* infection considered as a diagnosis in its own right within your place of work? What documentary evidence can you find in patients' medical notes to support this?

- All antibiotics that are clearly not required should be stopped, along with the pre-disposing antibiotic(s) where possible (it may be necessary to discuss this with the Consultant Microbiologist), and other drugs that may cause diarrhoea.
- All patients should receive oral or intravenous (IV) re-hydration therapy if required.

Fact Box 22.10   Anti-diarrhoeal drugs

Anti-diarrhoeal drugs (e.g. Loperamide and codeine phosphate) must not be prescribed as they will delay faecal transit time and potentially increase toxin retention, leading to increased tissue damage (Thielman and Nelson, 2009).

- If the patient is regularly prescribed proton pump inhibitors, these should not be given unless essential.
- Bloods for white blood count (WBC) and CRP must be taken twice weekly in mild disease and daily in severe disease.
- Vital signs (temperature, pulse and blood pressure) must be recorded four times hourly.
- All patients should be reviewed by the IP&CT and a Dietician once a week to ensure that the infection is optimally treated and that the patient is receiving all necessary supportive care.
- In cases of severe *C. difficile* infection (see Box 22.4), the Consultant Microbiologist should request that the patient is reviewed by a Gastroenterologist or Surgeon.

Box 22.4   Indicators of potential severe disease and poor prognosis

Elderly frail patient
Poor or absent oral intake
Abdominal pain or distension
Diarrhoea may not be present
Unexplained high WBC or CRP
Low serum albumin (<25 g/L)
Radiological or endoscopic confirmation of colitis:
- Acutely rising blood creatinine
- temperature of 38.5°C or above

Treatment

Metronidazole and vancomycin

Treatment is indicated only in patients who are symptomatic, and management therefore depends on the clinical presentation and the inciting agent. The most important first step in treating *C.*

difficile infection is to stop the inciting antibiotic if it is medically appropriate to do so in order that the resident colonic flora can start to recover.

Metronidazole and vancomycin have been the mainstay of *C. difficile* treatment for over 30 years. They do not eradicate spores, but are effective against vegetative cells. Although they are considered to be equally effective, oral metronidazole (400–500 mg) taken eight hourly for 10–14 days is the first line of treatment for mild and moderate infections (Public Health England, 2013), as most *C. difficile* isolates are highly susceptible to it and it is less expensive than vancomycin, which is contra-indicated in women who are pregnant or who are breastfeeding.

Fact Box 22.11   Vancomycin

Vancomycin is bacteriostatic as opposed to bactericidal, inhibiting the growth of *C. difficile* but not killing it, and it is generally not the first drug of choice as it is known to contribute to the spread of vancomycin-resistant bacteria (Cookson *et al.*, 2001), particularly vancomycin or **glycopeptide-resistant enterococci** (GRE) which colonise the bowel. Oral vancomycin 125 mg 6 hourly (qds) for 10–14 days is recommended for the treatment of severe *C. difficile* infection in most patients, including treatment of recurrent infection, where tapering (reduced) doses may be prescribed over four to six weeks to kill viable vegetative cells and allow the resident colonic flora to recover. Vancomycin preparation for injection is now licensed for oral use as an alternative to capsules (Public Health England, 2013). However, new guidance recommends fidaxomicin for the 1st episode of severe *C. difficile* infection in patients with multiple co-morbidities and concomitant antibiotics (other antibiotics that are given at the same time) (Public Health England, 2013).

Stool specimens for clearance

It is not possible to test for *C. difficile* 'clearance' and stools sent for routine 'clearance' will not be tested. Patients are infectious only if they have diarrhoea; therefore, once the diarrhoea has resolved (48 house asymptomatic) and the patient has 'normal' bowel movements (i.e. Bristol stool chart types 1–4), the patient will be non-infectious. In the event that the diarrhoea does not resolve, or it resolves and then recurs, or Bristol stool chart types 5–7 are 'normal' for the patient (e.g. if the patient also has irritable bowel syndrome or colitis), the advice of the IP&CT must be sought.

Treatment of recurrent *C. difficile*

Fact Box 22.12   Recurrence and infection

A recurrence of symptomatic disease occurs in 5–20% of cases, with 12–24% developing a second case of *C. difficile* within two months of the initial infection (Barbut *et al.*, 2000). A relapse has been defined as a recurrence of symptoms within two months of the initial diagnosis whereby treatment has failed to eradicate the organism; re-infection is a recurrence of symptoms after two months due to infection by either a new strain or a cross-infection arising from environmental contamination (Wilcox *et al.*, 1998; Barbut *et al.*, 2000). Patient risk factors for recurrence include increased age, recent abdominal surgery and the survival of *C. difficile* spores in the colon, where they may become trapped within diverticuli and be unaffected by colonic peristalsis, in spite of high intraluminal levels of vancomycin.

New guidance (Public Health England, 2013) recommends that fidaxomicin is prescribed for recurrent mild, moderate or severe infection. Oral vancomycin 125 mg 6 hourly (qds) for 10–14 days can be prescribed as an alternative to fidaxomicin.

Where diarrhoea persists despite 20 days of treatment but frequency of diarrhoea has decreased, and the patient is otherwise stable, with normal inflammatory markers and no evidence of abdominal pain or distension, the cause is likely to be post-infective irritable bowel syndrome, and in this instance an anti-motility drug such as Loperamide can be prescribed, although the therapeutic response must be carefully monitored (Department of Health and Health Protection Agency, 2008).

Probiotics

Much has been written about the value of probiotics, commonly referred to as 'good bacteria', which are live organisms that improve the microbial balance of the host by fighting infections that affect the GI tract and mucosal surfaces. It is thought the administration of bacteria such as *Bifidobacterium* and *Lactobacillus*, along with *Saccharomyces boulardii*, which is a yeast, have a role to play in restoring the equilibrium of the flora within the bowel after antibiotic administration. Although there have been some successes, particularly with the use of *Saccharomyces*, the evidence to support their use generally is not very convincing (Lewis *et al.*, 1998; Starr, 2005). *Saccharomyces* is not licensed for use in the United Kingdom, and the use of probiotics is not a national recommendation (Public Health England, 2013).

Immunoglobulin

There are case reports of successful treatment with intravenous immunoglobulin which contains significant levels of antibodies to *C. difficile* toxins (Salcedo *et al.*, 2000; Murphy *et al.*, 2006). Although, its efficacy has not been established as no clinical trials have been undertaken it could be considered for use in severe or recurrent *C. difficile* infection (Department of Health, 2011).

Other potential treatment options include Fidaxomicin and faecal transplants.

Fact Box 22.13   Fidaxomicin

Fidaxomicin is a new narrow-spectrum bactericidal antibiotic that has been developed for the treatment of *C. difficile* infection. It has been demonstrated on testing to be eight times more potent than vancomycin, achieves high faecal concentrations in the bowel, has a long post-antibiotic effect and has restricted activity against normal bowel flora.

Source: Thielman and Wilson, 2009; Louis *et al.*, 2011; Cornley *et al.*, 2012.

> ## Fact Box 22.14   Faecal transplants
>
> Faecal transplant involves transplanting faecal bacteri from a healthy individual or donor to a recipient via enema, colonoscopy or naso-gastric tube in order to restore colonic flora in an individual with *C. difficile* infection. The donor is usually a relative from the same household as the bacterial flora is likely to be similar (MacConnachie *et al.*, 2009).

Clinical practice points: the infection control management of patients with symptomatic *C. difficile* infection

Isolation (see Chapter 11)

In the event of confirmation of a *C. difficile* toxin–positive result in a patient with diarrhoea who is not already isolated, the patient must be moved to a single room with en-suite facilities (or dedicated commode if en-suite facilities are not available). If isolation is not possible immediately (e.g. due to a general lack of isolation facilities on the ward, unavailability of a single room due to pressure from other competing 'alert' organisms or specific patient-related risk factors), the nurse looking after the patient should inform the IP&CT and ensure that a risk assessment is documented in the notes. If the patient was in an open bay when the positive *C. difficile* result was confirmed, the bay must be deep-cleaned following the patient's transfer to a single room.

An isolation notice must be displayed on the door.

Isolation can be discontinued once the patient has been asymptomatic for 48 hours **and** is passing 'normal' stools.

Equipment and cleaning

Dedicated patient equipment must be used, including disposable blood pressure cuffs and tourniquets. See Chapter 15 for more information.

Floors, commodes, toilets and bed frames are subject to the heaviest faecal contamination. Therefore it is important that the ward environment should not be cluttered in order to facilitate thorough and effective ward cleaning.

Given *C. difficile*'s long persistence in the environment, it is important that a thorough clean of the room is undertaken on discharge or transfer of the patient using 1000 ppm available chlorine and/or a sporicidal agent. This includes laundering curtains and washing all parts of the bed frame and the base mattress. Dynamic mattress systems also need to be decontaminated according to local arrangements.

Hand hygiene

The patient should be assisted with hand hygiene after using the toilet or commode and before eating if unable to wash his or her hands independently. Healthcare workers must wash their hands with soap and water after contact with the patient or his/her environment. See Chapter 12 for more information.

Personal protective equipment (PPE)

See Chapter 13.

Use of bowel management systems (BMSs)

Patients with *C. difficile* who are incontinent with liquid or semi-liquid stool, and who are confined to bed, may benefit from the use of a bowel management system (BMS), which helps to prevent skin damage and also contains liquid or semi-liquid stool, reducing the risk of environmental contamination. Staff require training in their insertion and management.

Waste and Linen

All clinical waste and linen, including bedding and curtains, should be considered to be contaminated and managed appropriately.

Care of the deceased patient

Infection control precautions for handling the deceased patient are the same as those used when the patient is alive. Body bags are not routinely necessary unless there is any leakage of faeces. There is negligible risk to mortuary staff or undertakers provided that standard infection control precautions are used. If there is any faecal soiling in the area around the cadaver, it should be cleaned with a sporicidal agent.

Visitors

Healthy individuals are not at risk of acquiring *C. difficile* infection. Gloves and aprons are not required providing there is no contact with other hospital patients. Visitors must be advised to wash their hands with liquid soap and water on leaving the isolation room.

337

Movement of patients

Patients with *C. difficile* infection should not be transferred to other wards in the hospital, except for isolation purposes, or if they require specialist care on another ward. Where patients need to attend departments for essential investigations, it is the responsibility of the nurse looking after the patient to inform the receiving area in advance of the patient's *C. difficile*–positive status, and arrangements should be put in place to minimise their waiting time and contact with other patients. Whenever possible, symptomatic patients should be seen at the end of the working session and should be sent for only when the department is ready to see them; they should not be left in a waiting area with other patients.

All procedures should be planned in advance to keep equipment and staff to a minimum. Disposable equipment must be used whenever possible. All other equipment must be decontaminated according to manufacturer's instructions or local guidelines.

Patient discharge or transfer

At the discretion of the medical team, patients may be discharged to their own home to complete their course of treatment in the community, but this is largely dependent upon the severity of the infection and the patient's general condition.

If the patient is to be discharged or transferred to a community hospital or a nursing or residential home, the patient must be asymptomatic on discharge for a minimum of 72 hours with 'normal' stools for him or her (no type 5–7 stools as per the Bristol Stool Chart), and have completed a course of the appropriate antibiotics.

It is important the GP is notified of the patient's diagnosis of *C. difficile* and that advice is given on discharge to both the GP and the patient regarding action to be taken if there is a recurrence of symptoms. It is also important that patients and their relatives or carers are informed that no special precautions are required at home beyond 'normal' hygiene measures, and that there is no need to restrict their daily activities or contact with others.

Box 22.5 lists some best-practice recommendations for the prevention of avoidable *C. difficile* infection.

Box 22.5   The prevention of avoidable *C. difficile* infection

- Prescribe antibiotics in accordance with local antimicrobial prescribing guidelines and policies, and ensure that there is an organisation-wide culture of antimicrobial stewardship (see Chapter 10).
- **Isolate patients with diarrhoea in a single room unless or until an infectious cause can be confidently excluded.**
- Patients who are GDH antigen–positive only should be isolated until they have been asymptomatic for 48 hours.
- Ensure that stool specimens are obtained promptly with patients with suspected infectious diarrhoea.
- Ensure that all healthcare workers wash their hands with soap and water following contact with patients with diarrhoea or contact with the patients' equipment or environment.
- Ensure that all healthcare workers wear and dispose of PPE appropriately.
- Ensure that patients in isolation with suspected or confirmed *C. difficile* have their own dedicated patient equipment.
- Ensure that all other equipment in use on the ward is cleaned in between each patient use.
- Ensure that the environment (including bathrooms and toilets) is cleaned thoroughly as per local service-level agreements and that an appropriate hypochlorite or sporicidal agent is used.
- Ensure that all commodes are cleaned in between each patient use at all times using a sporicidal agent. Audit compliance with commode cleanliness (see Chapter 3).
- The provision of a dedicated 'toilet team' for the twice-daily *disinfection* of all commodes and all ward toilets, in addition to the routine cleaning of commodes and toilets, is an additional safeguard and helps to provide additional assurance that attention is being paid to these high-risk items or areas.
- **Note**: A root cause analysis (RCA) should be undertaken for all cases of *C. difficile* infection to determine whether each infection is avoidable or unavoidable, and whether there has been compliance and non-compliance with Trust policy (see Chapter 2). This is particularly important in cases of avoidable infection, where actions need to be put in place and monitored in order to prevent it.

Chapter summary: key points

- *Clostridium difficile* is the most important cause of hospital-acquired diarrhoea in adults and is a significant cause of patient morbidity and mortality.

- It causes a spectrum of illness which ranges from asymptomatic colonisation of the bowel, to trivial diarrhoea to life-threatening pseudomembranous colitis and toxic megacolon.

- Although antibiotics are the main cause of *C. difficile* infection, there are numerous other factors that can increase the risk of *C. difficile* acquisition.

- *C. difficile* produces two potent toxins that cause extensive damage to the bowel mucosa.

- Symptomatic *C. difficile* infection must be regarded as a separate diagnosis in its own right and not simply as an 'add on' to the patient's other illness.

- Recurrent *C. difficile* infection is not uncommon, and more than one course of metronidazole or vancomycin may be required.

- *C. difficile* infection can be prevented.

Further resources are available for this book, including interactive multiple choice questions. Visit the companion website at:

www.wiley.com/go/fundamentalsofinfectionprevention

339

References

Barbut F., Richard A., Hamadi K., Chomette V., Beurghoffer B., *et al.* (2000). Epidemiology of recurrences or re-infections of *Clostridium difficile*-associated diarrhoea. *Journal of Clinical Microbiology*. 38: 2386–2388.

Bartlett J.G., Perl T.M. (2005). The new *Clostridium difficile*. What does it mean? *New England Journal of Medicine*. 353 (23): 2503–2505.

Best E.L., Fawley W.N., Parnell P., Wilcox M.H. (2010). The potential for airborne dispersal of *Clostridium difficile* from symptomatic patients. *Clinical Infectious Disease*. 1 June: 1450–1457.

Bignardi G.E. (1998). Risk factors for *Clostridium difficile* infection. *Journal of Hospital Infection*. 40 (1): 1–15.

Brazier J.S. (1998). The diagnosis of *Clostridium difficile* associated disease. *Journal of Antimicrobial Chemotherapy*. 41 (Suppl. 3): S29–S40.

Brazier J. (2006). *Clostridium difficile*-associated disease: a case of greater virulence and new risk factors. *Health Protection Matters: The Magazine of the Health Protection Agency*. 5 (Summer): 20–22.

Brierly R. (2005). *Clostridium difficile*: a new threat to public health? *The Lancet*. 5: 535.

Chang V.T., Nelson K. (2000). The role of physical proximity in nosocomial diarrhoea. *Clinical Infectious Disease*. 31: 717–722.

Cookson B.D., Macrae M.B., Barrett S.P., Brain D.F.J., Chadwick C. *et al.* (2001). *A Report of a Combined Working Party of the HIS/ICNA/BSAC. Guidelines for the Control of Glycopeptide-resistant Enterococci in Hospitals*. Hospital Infection Society, *Infection Control Nurses Association* and British Society for Antimicrobial Chemotherapy, London.

Cornley O.A., Crook D.W., Esposito R., Poirier A., Somero M.S. *et al.* (2012). Fidaxomicin versus vancomycin for infection with *Clostridium difficile* in Europe, Canada and the USA: a double-blind, non-inferiority, randomized control trial. *The Lancet Infectious Diseases*. 12 (4): 281–289.

Cunningham R., Dale B., Undy B., Gaunt N. (2003). Proton pump inhibitors as a risk factor for *Clostridium difficile* diarrhoea. *Journal of Hospital Infection*. 54 (3): 243–245.

Denève C., Janoir C., Poilane I., Fantinato C., Collignon A. (2009). New trends in *Clostridium difficile* virulence and pathogenesis. *International Journal of Antimicrobial Agents*. 33: S1, S24–S28.

Department of Health (2007). *The Operating Framework for the NHS in England*, 2008/09. Department of Health, London.

Department of Health (2011). *Clinical Guidelines for Immunoglobulin Use*. 2nd edition. Department of Health, London.

Department of Health (2012). *Updated Guidance on the Diagnosis and Reporting of* Clostridium difficile. Department of Health, London.

Department of Health and Health Protection Agency (2008). Clostridium difficile *Infection: How to Deal with the Problem*. Department of Health and Health Protection Agency, London.

Dial S., Alrasadi K., Manoukian C., Huang A., Menzies D. (2004). Risk of *Clostridium difficile* diarrhoea among hospital patients prescribed proton pump inhibitors: cohort and case control studies. *Canadian Medical Association Journal*. 171 (1): 33–38.

Fawley W.N., Wilcox M. (2001). Molecular typing of endemic *Clostridium difficile* infection. *Epidemiology and Infection*. 126: 343–350.

Hall C., O'Toole E. (1935). Intestinal flora in newborn infants with a description of a new pathogenic anaerobe, *Bacillus difficile*. *American Journal Diseases Children*. 49: 390–402.

Healthcare Commission (2006). *Investigation into outbreaks of* Clostridium difficile *at Stoke Mandeville Hospital, Buckinghamshire Hospitals NHS Trust*. July. Healthcare Commission, London.

Healthcare Commission (2007). *Investigation into Outbreaks of* Clostridium difficile *at Maidstone and Tunbridge Wells NHS Trust*. October. Healthcare Commission, London.

Keel M.K., Songer J.G. (2006). The comparative pathology of *Clostridium difficile*-associated Disease. *Veterinary Pathology*. 43: 225–240.

Kyne L., Warny M., Qamar A., Kelly C.P. (2001). Association between antibody response to toxin A and protection against recurring *Clostridium difficile* diarrhoea. *The Lancet*. 357 (9251): 189–193.

Larson H.E., Parry J.B., Price A.B. (1977). Undescribed toxin in pseudomembranous colitis. *British Medical Journal*. 1 (60710): 1246–1248.

Lewis S.J., Heaton K.W. (1997). Stool form scale as a useful guide to intestinal transit time. *Scandinavian Journal of Gastroenterology*. 32 (9): 920–924.

Lewis S.J., Potts L.F., Barry R.E. (1998). The lack of therapeutic effect of *Saccharomyces boulardii* in the prevention of antibiotic-related diarrhoea in elderly patients. *Journal of Infection*. 36: 171–174.

Loo V.G., Bourgault A., Poirier L., Lamothe F., Michaud S. *et al.* (2011). Host and pathogen factors for *Clostridium difficile* infection and colonisation. *New England Journal of Medicine*. 365 (18): 1693–1703.

Louis T.J., Miller M.A., Mullane K.D., Weiss K., Lentnek A. *et al.* (2011). Fidaxomicin versus vancomycin for *Clostridium difficile* infection. *New England Journal of Medicine*. 364 (5): 422–431.

MacConnachie A.A., Fox R., Kennedy D.R., Seaton R.A. (2009). Faecal transplants for recurrent *Clostridium difficile*-associated diarrhoea: a UK case series. *QJM*. 102 (11): 781–784.

McCracken V.J., Lorenz R.G. (2001). The gastrointestinal ecosystem: a precarious alliance among epithelium, immunity and microbiota. *Cell Microbiology*. 3: 1–11.

McGlone S.M., Bailey R.R., Zimmer S.M., Popovich M.J., Ufberg P. *et al.* (2012). The economic burden of *Clostridium difficile*. *Clinical Microbiology and Infection*. March 18 (3): 282–289.

Murphy C., Vernon M., Cullen M. (2006). Intravenous immunoglobulin for resistant *Clostridium difficile* infection. *Age and Ageing*. 35: 85–86.

Poutanen S.M., Simor A.E. (2004). *Clostridium difficile* associated diarrhoea in adults. *Canadian Medical Association Journal*. 171 (1): 51–58.

Public Health England (2013). *Updated guidance on the management and treatment of* Clostridium difficile *infection*. Public Health England, London.

Rastall R.A. (2004). Bacteria in the gut: friends and foes and how to alter the balance. *Journal of Nutrition*. 134: 2022S–2026S.

Royal College of Nursing (2013). *The Management of Diarrhoea in Adults*. Royal College of Nursing guidance for nursing staff. Royal College of Nursing, London.

Ryan K.J., Drew W.L. (2010). *Clostridium, Peptostreptococcus, Bacteroides* and other anaerobes. In: Ryan K.J., Ray, C.G. (Eds.), *Sherris Medical Microbiology*. 5th ed. McGraw-Hill Medical, New York: 525–534.

Salcedo J., Keates S., Pothoulakis C. (2000). IV immunoglobulin therapy for severe *Clostridium difficile* colitis. *Gut*. 41: 366–370.

Shim J.K., Johnson M.D., Samore M.D., Bliss D.Z., Gerding D.N. (1998). Primary symptomless colonisation by *Clostridium difficile* and decreased risk of diarrhoea. *The Lancet*. 351 (9103): 633–636.

Starr J. (2005). *Clostridium difficile* associated diarrhoea: diagnosis and treatment. *British Medical Journal*. 331 (7515): 498–501.

Tabaqchali S., Jumaa P. (1995). Fortnightly review: diagnosis and management of *Clostridium difficile* infection. *British Medical Journal*. 310: 1375–1380.

Thielman N.M., Wilson K.H. (2009). *Clostridium difficile*–associated disease. In: Mandell G.L., Bennett J.E., Dolin R. (Eds.), *Mandell, Douglas and Bennett's Principles and Practice of Infectious Diseases*. 7th ed. http://expertconsult.com (accessed 19 October 2012)

Tonna I., Welsby P.D. (2005). Pathogenesis and treatment of *Clostridium difficile* infection. *Postgraduate Medical Journal*; 81: 367–369.

Vaishnavi C. (2010). Clinical spectrum and pathogenesis of *Clostridium difficile* associated diseases. *Indian Journal of Medical Research*. 131: 487–499.

Walker A.S., Eyre D.W., Wyllie D.H., Dingle K.E., Harding R.M. *et al.* (2012). *Characterisation of Clostridium difficile hospital ward-based transmission using extensive epidemiological data and molecular typing*. http://www.plosmedicine.org/article/info%3Adoi%2F10.1371%2Fjournal.pmed.1001172 (accessed 22 March 2013)

Warney M., Pepin J., Fang A. (2005). Toxin produced by an emerging strain of *Clostridium difficile* associated with outbreaks of severe disease in North America and Europe. *The Lancet*. 366: 1079–1084.

Whelan K., Judd P.A., Preedy V.R., Taylor M.A. (2004). Enteral feeding: the effect on faecal output, the faecal microflora and SCFA concentrations. *Proceedings of the Nutrition Society*. 63: 105–113.

Wilcox M.H., Fawley W.N., Settle C.D., Davidson A. (1998). Recurrence of symptoms in *Clostridium difficile* infection–relapse or re-infection? *Journal of Hospital Infection*. 38 (2): 93–100.

23

Norovirus

Contents

Fundamentals of Infection Prevention and Control: Theory and Practice, Second Edition. Debbie Weston.
© 2013 John Wiley & Sons, Ltd. Published 2013 by John Wiley & Sons, Ltd. Companion Website: www.wiley.com/go/fundamentalsofinfectionprevention

Introduction

Reports of outbreaks of viral gastroenteritis due to norovirus are a common occurrence in the media, with small clusters and large outbreaks affecting hotels, cruise ships, schools, colleges and nursing and residential homes (Patterson *et al.*, 1997; Chadwick *et al.*, 2000; Isakbaeva *et al.*, 2005). The significance of norovirus as an important pathogen cannot be underestimated, and infection with norovirus can be far from trivial. Norovirus is a source of major disruption to the provision of healthcare services within the NHS, often resulting in the closure of wards and sometimes hospitals (Cooper *et al.*, 2011), and managing outbreaks can be a logistical nightmare for Infection Prevention and Control Teams (IP&CTs) in particular, given the impact that ward or hospital closures have on service provision (lost bed days, increased length of stay, staff sickness, and cancellation of admissions and surgery) and the local healthcare economy.

This chapter looks at the epidemiology of norovirus infection, its transmission and the management of periods of increased incidence and outbreaks drawing on the guidelines for the management of norovirus outbreaks in acute and community healthcare and social care settings (Health Protection Agency and Norovirus Working Party, 2011).

Learning outcomes

After reading this chapter, the reader will be able to:

- Understand the significance of norovirus outbreaks.

- Be able to describe the clinical features of norovirus.

- Understand the infection control precautions that need to be taken in order to reduce the risk of spread.

343

The virus

Norovirus belongs to the virus family Caliciviridae, whose name is derived from the Latin word 'calyx', meaning goblet or cup, in reference to the 32 cup-shaped depressions on the surface of the capsid (Dolin and Treanor, 2009; Collier *et al.*, 2011).

They are a group of non-enveloped single-stranded RNA viruses and the causative agents of acute viral gastroenteritis in humans (Cubitt, 2007). They are also known as small round structured viruses (SRSVs). The media often report outbreaks of norovirus infection as winter vomiting disease, which was first described in 1929 (Vipond *et al.*, 1999) and so named because of its seasonal incidence and the dominant symptom of vomiting.

There are now at least five different norovirus genogroups (GI–GV), which are further divided into gene clusters, with most of the strains responsible for causing outbreaks residing in genogroup GII (Dolin and Treanor, 2009), and 80% of infections associated with genotype II.4 in particular.

As with bacteria, mutations can occur during the process of viral replication, giving rise to mutations within the viral genome, which can assist the virus to evade host immune response mechanisms (Harris *et al.*, 2011). This leads to the emergence of new strains which may be associated with increased outbreaks, the severity of which may vary from year to year depending on which strains are in circulation and the immunity of the local population (Dolin and Treanor, 2009).

Fact Box 23.1   SRSVs

SRSVs were first identified following an outbreak of non-bacterial gastroenteritis in the town of Norwalk, Ohio, in the United States in 1968 (Ahmad *et al.*, 2010), where a range of morphologically identical viruses were later detected in 1972 by electron microscopy from saved stool samples (Dolin and Treanor, 2009). Additional SRSVs have since been identified and named for the geographical region in which they were first identified (Collier *et al.*, 2011), but they are often reported as Norwalk-like viruses (NLVs), which is the term adopted by the International Committee on the Taxonomy of Viruses, and they are now more commonly known as noroviruses.

Fact Box 23.2   Peaks in incidence

Peaks in incidence have been seen globally with the emergence of new variant genotypes in 1995, 2002 and 2004 (Bull *et al.*, 2006). In the United States, where norovirus is estimated to be responsible for approximately 60% of all cases of acute gastroenteritis (Atmar and Estes, 2006), 21 million people are affected annually, with 70 000 requiring admission to hospital (http://www.cdc.gov/norovirus/about/overview.htm). In periods of high incidence in the United Kingdom, outbreaks are estimated to cost in excess of £100 million per annum (Lopman *et al.*, 2004). The burden of norovirus infection in England and Wales was particularly heavy in 2009 and 2010, with 19 483 positive cases confirmed by laboratories in total; over 11 000 of these were confirmed in 2010 alone. As of 23 December 2012, the Health Protection Agency reported an 83% increase in confirmed laboratory reports to date compared to the same time in 2011, with 61 hospital outbreaks reported in the first two weeks of December (www.hpa.org.uk). There are often several different strains in circulation during outbreaks, but the increase in cases seen in the United Kingdom during the 2011–2012 norovirus season has been attributed to the emergence of a new strain called Sydney 2012, which has become the dominant strain and is a variant of genotype II.4, first reported in Australia in March 2012 (van Beek *et al.*, 2013).

Incubation period, transmission and clinical features

Norovirus is highly contagious. The incubation period is relatively short, ranging from 12 to 48 hours, and the attack rate is often more than 50%, affecting both patients and staff. Box 23.1 describes the clinical features of norovirus.

Box 23.1   Clinical features

Profuse, watery diarrhoea and/or forceful (projectile) vomiting are the presenting clinical features. Other symptoms, including nausea, abdominal cramps, headache and myalgia, are commonly reported following onset of the initial symptoms.

Within the healthcare setting, outbreaks arise as a result of faecal-oral spread and person-to-person spread following the dissemination of virus particles through the air, which leads to widespread environmental contamination. Hard surfaces, equipment and soft furnishings readily become contaminated, along with food (see Box 23.2), particularly if handled by a contaminated or infected food handler, and water jugs.

Box 23.2   Foods implicated in community outbreaks

Cold foods (e.g. sandwiches and salads)
Bakery items
Liquids (including salad dressing and icing)
Food contaminated at source (e.g. oysters harvested from contaminated waters, and other shell-fish)

Source: Stevenson et al., 1994; Chadwick et al., 2000; Clarke and Lambden, 2000; Dolin and Treanor, 2009; Health Protection Agency, 2009.

Fact Box 23.3   Norovirus – infecting dose and transmission

It has been estimated that more than 30 million virus particles are released during vomiting (Patterson et al., 1997) and the infecting dose necessary to induce symptoms is astonishingly small, at only 10–100 virus particles (Caul, 1994; Vipond et al., 1999).

Up to 5 billion infectious doses of norovirus may be shed by an infected person in each gram of faeces (Hall, 2012).

In the United States, the source of a norovirus outbreak was traced to a re-usable grocery bag and its contents, which were stored in a hotel bathroom used before the outbreak by a person with symptoms of norovirus, and contaminated with aerosolized virus particles (Repp and Keene, 2012).

Contaminated fingers can transfer norovirus onto as many as seven clean surfaces (Baker et al., 2004), and the virus can remain viable within the environment for up to 12 days (Cheesbrough et al., 1997).

Box 23.3 describes the numerous problems with norovirus that make its control so challenging within healthcare settings.

Box 23.3   Problems with norovirus

There is no prodromal illness before the onset of symptoms, which are typically explosive.

While vomiting appears to result in greater numbers of individuals becoming infected because of airborne spread, infectious diarrhoea can also be problematic.

Norovirus can continue to be excreted in faeces after the symptoms have resolved, but it is also thought that virus excretion can occur before the onset of symptoms (Goller *et al.*, 2004), giving rise to the possibility of norovirus being transmissible prior to the onset of clinical symptoms and after resolution, potentially prolonging outbreaks.

Although the duration of illness is generally short, lasting between 12 and 60 hours, and symptoms may be mild in some, the elderly often bear the brunt of norovirus infections with prolonged duration of symptoms, and may be more severely affected than younger 'healthy' individuals (Chadwick *et al.*, 2000; Goller *et al.*, 2004).

There is no specific treatment, other than to rest and remain hydrated.

Immunity to noroviruses is thought to be strain specific and may last only 4–6 months (Dolin and Treanor, 2009). It is possible for individuals to be affected several times during their lifetime, and during the course of an outbreak some may be affected on more than one occasion if there is more than one strain of norovirus in circulation.

Reporting patients with 'diarrhoea and vomiting'

As discussed in Chapter 22, it is important that staff understand what is meant by the word 'diarrhoea', and that they realise the potential implications of reporting all cases of 'diarrhoea' and/ or vomiting without using sound clinical judgment or common sense. The Infection Prevention and Control Team (IP&CT) have to make decisions with regard to ward closures based on the information that they are given by ward staff. It may be 2 a.m. when the on-call Infection Control Nurse Specialist or on-call Consultant Medical Microbiologist is contacted, and a decision to either close a ward to new admissions or keep it open until it can be formally assessed can have implications for patient care. It is absolutely crucial that the information given to the IP&CT is accurate and reliable, and it is the responsibility of the Nurse in Charge at the time that the IP&CT is contacted to make sure that this is the case. Box 23.4 summarises the information that the IP&CT will require, and Box 23.5 gives a case definition for suspected norovirus cases.

Box 23.4   Information to be given to the IP&CT regarding each symptomatic patient

- Full name, date of birth and hospital number
- Date of admission
- Reason for admission and diagnosis

- Any significant past medical history that may account for symptoms (e.g. post-operative or recent surgery; history of or suspected diverticulitis, Crohn's disease or irritable bowel syndrome [IBS])
- Any medication of note, such as antibiotics, laxatives or enemas, or other drugs that can cause diarrhoea
- A full description of the symptoms (diarrhoea must be described as per the Bristol Stool Scale; although types 5–7 are diarrhoea, norovirus is typically types 6 and 7), and their frequency
- Date and time of onset
- Bay and bed number.

Box 23.5   Norovirus case definition

Sudden onset of profuse and watery diarrhoea (types 6–7 on the Bristol Stool Chart) and/or vomiting (may be projectile) in a patient with no other explanation for their symptoms.

Laboratory diagnosis

The IP&CT will advise on the collection of faecal specimens, which ideally must be obtained as soon as possible and no longer than 48 hours after the onset of the symptoms and sent to the laboratory immediately for enzyme-linked immunosorbent assays to detect norovirus antigens or polymerase chain reaction (PCR) to detect norovirus nucleic acid (see Chapter 7). However, they may yield a negative result as a positive result is dependent upon the viral load and the timing of the specimen. Whilst a positive result is useful for epidemiological and surveillance purposes, and can reassure hospital managers in the event of ward closures, IP&CTs generally make a diagnosis of norovirus infection based on the clinical features and the attack rate.

The management of outbreaks in hospitals

In 2000, the PHLS Viral Gastroenteritis Working Group (Chadwick *et al.*, 2000) issued guidance on the management of SRSV outbreaks, which were generally regarded as the UK standard for management of outbreaks. They were superseded in December 2011 by guidelines for the management of norovirus outbreaks in acute and community health and social care settings (Health Protection Agency and Norovirus Working Party, 2011).

Boxes 23.6, 23.7, 23.8, 23.9, 23.10 and 23.11 summarise the key points and considerations regarding the management of norovirus, and most can be applied to care homes as well as hospital wards (the 2011 guidance contains a section on 'The Management and Control of Outbreaks in Care Homes').

Box 23.6 Symptomatic patients in the community and admission avoidance

Patients presenting in the emergency department or contacting their GP for advice should not be admitted to hospital unless the diagnosis is uncertain or they are at significant risk of complications that cannot be rectified through rehydration. The admission of symptomatic patients, even when admitted to a single room, means that there is the possibility of an outbreak igniting on that ward given the nature of the virus.

Where symptomatic patients attend the emergency department, they must be triaged immediately, segregated from other patients and assessed quickly by an experienced member of the Medical team (not a Junior Doctor).

Where care homes and community hospitals are known to be affected by norovirus, this information should be cascaded to local hospitals, specifically to the IP&CT and emergency departments and admissions wards.

Symptomatic residents from care homes should be managed in the home and admission to hospital avoided unless the resident is at risk of serious complications. Prevention of dehydration is essential, and if this is managed appropriately then admission to hospital should be successfully avoided.

If an asymptomatic resident from a care home affected by norovirus requires admission to hospital, it is imperative that the ambulance crew, the IP&CT and the receiving ward or emergency department are informed by the home prior to admission or transfer. The resident may be incubating norovirus and will need to be admitted to a cubicle in the ED or a single room on a ward until he or she has been asymptomatic for at least 48 hours.

348

Reflection point

How are norovirus outbreaks within your organisation communicated to staff generally? Are any strategies employed to inform the general public not to attend the emergency department or visit wards or departments if symptomatic?

Box 23.7 Bay versus ward closures

A risk assessment approach regarding the placement of symptomatic patients and the closing of wards is essential. Whereas the 2000 Guidelines advocated complete ward closure at the earliest opportunity, the 2011 Guidelines advocate closing affected bays, physically segregating symptomatic patients from those who are not symptomatic and considering ward closure only when there is evidence of failure of containment within single rooms and bays.

While bay closure has the advantage of allowing part of the ward area to function in a relatively normal fashion and may shorten the duration of an outbreak, it is largely dependent upon whether or not the bays can be effectively sealed off (e.g. whether or not they have doors, or whether doors can be installed), and also if there is sufficient staffing to enable staff segregation (Illingworth et al., 2011).

Given the low infectious dose and widespread environmental contamination that arises once patients become symptomatic, several cases may be seen within the ward within a matter of hours. Although a patient who is symptomatic on admission can be immediately isolated, there is probably little to be gained from moving a symptomatic patient in an open bay or ward into a side room, unless it takes place immediately after the onset of symptoms and stringent cleaning measures are initiated. The new guidelines recommend leaving the affected patient within the bay and closing it to admissions, treating the other patients within it as exposed contacts.

Where single-room bed occupancy is exceeded, patients are nursed in cohort bays and the bays are closed to admissions and managed as separate isolation units. However, there may be multiple cases spread amongst multiple bays, there are likely to be difficulties segregating staff if staffing is compromised through sickness and therefore ward closure may be the best solution.

Source: Data from HPA, 2011.

Box 23.8   Norovirus and risk management

Risk management is a recurring theme during outbreaks, with IP&CTs continually having to assess the risk to patients of being admitted and acquiring norovirus, against the risks of not receiving medical treatment because the ward or hospital is closed.

Just a single ward closure will have an impact on the activity of the emergency department and the smooth running of the rest of the hospital; multiple ward closures have an even bigger impact. Closure of the hospital, however (a decision that must be approved by the Strategic Health Authority), has massive resource implications for neighbouring Trusts. As outbreaks inconveniently tend to occur during the winter months when bed occupancy is at its height and the turnover of patients is slower, there is increasing pressure to admit patients, and the threat of a major hospital outbreak can loom large.

Symptomatic patients in the emergency department can be admitted to closed wards, as can a symptomatic patient from an unaffected ward who is being transferred out of the ward swiftly in the hope that problems there can be averted, as long as they meet the norovirus case definition. Obviously the admission of symptomatic patients into a closed ward will prolong its closure, but that is preferable to infecting the patients and staff on an unaffected ward.

Complications arise whereby a symptomatic patient may require the specialist services provided by intensive care and cardiac care units, renal units and specialist respiratory or cardiac support wards. Unlike general wards, these specialist areas cannot be closed if they become affected and they will have to remain open to admissions requiring specialist care.

Continued

Under no circumstances should a symptomatic patient be admitted into the middle of an unaffected ward, unless it is either into a side room or the patient requires specialist care.

Asymptomatic patients should never be admitted to closed wards unless their medical condition warrants admission and the only bed available is on a closed ward. In these circumstances, the IP&CT should be contacted as soon as possible (most Trusts now provide infection control advice out of hours), and the patient and relatives should be informed by the medical team that they are being admitted to a closed ward where there is a significant risk that they could contract norovirus, and the reason why they are being admitted there. This should be documented in the nursing and medical notes.

It should be remembered that if a symptomatic patient is admitted into an unaffected ward, other patients are likely to contract norovirus and the worst-case scenario is that a patient could die as a result.

Box 23.9   Duration of ward closure

The new guidance states that declaration of the end of an outbreak, and completion of deep cleaning, is 48 hours after the resolution of symptoms in the last known case, and at least 72 hours after the onset of the last known case.

Some Trusts will keep bays and wards closed until 72 hours after the last symptomatic patient has resolved. Others may keep bays and wards closed until 72 hours after the onset of the last new case, and any remaining symptomatic patients are recovering. Ideally, anyone remaining symptomatic at the time the ward is due to re-open should be moved into a single room or the bay closed to admissions while they recover.

Source: Data from HPA, 2011.

Box 23.10   Summary of infection control precautions and ward management during a norovirus outbreak

Contact the IP&CT without delay.

If one or more patients develops symptoms that meet the norovirus case definition, the IP&CT will advise regarding bay and ward closure and the collection of stool specimens.

Infection control precautions

- Hands must be washed with liquid soap and water (in place of routine hand decontamination with alcohol hand rub or gel) in between each episode of patient contact, task or contact with the environment, and after removing PPE. **Note**: Some Trusts or organisations may have an alcohol hand rub or gel that has been tested and proven to be effective against norovirus. If this is the case, the IP&CT may recommend its use on the ward for routine hand decontamination after contact with symptomatic patients as long as hands are visibly clean. Otherwise, handwashing must be undertaken.

- Gloves and aprons must be worn appropriately (see Chapter 13).
- Equipment should be dedicated to symptomatic patients where possible. Where this is not possible (e.g. all bays on a ward affected and insufficient equipment), it must be cleaned in between patients to help reduce contamination and spread via healthcare workers' hands.
- Ensure that patient water jugs are covered and changed frequently throughout the day; bowls of fruit and opened packets of food (e.g. biscuits) on bedside lockers and tables must be removed.
- Closed wards must not be used as short-cuts or thoroughfares to other wards and departments. Appropriate signage must be displayed on the doors, and staff must challenge inappropriate access.
- Visits from 'non-essential' staff (e.g. hairdressers, menu clerks, the volunteer trolley or volunteers) must be cancelled.
- Healthcare staff must not consume food or drinks on the ward (but they can attend the hospital canteen; there is no indication for segregating staff).

Documentation

- Ensure that records regarding symptomatic patients are accurately maintained (e.g. 'Daily Diarrhoea and Vomiting Record Sheet' or something similar).
- Maintain accurate stool and fluid balance charts.
- Ensure that there is accurate documentation in the patients' notes regarding their symptoms, bowel actions, fluid intake and output and vital signs.

Care of symptomatic patients

- The trained Nurse looking after the patient is responsible for ensuring that:
- Accurate stool and fluid balance charts are maintained.
- Vital signs are recorded four times hourly.
- The patient is reviewed daily by the Medical Team. Any concerns, such as worsening symptoms or vital signs outside of normal limits, must be escalated promptly and appropriately.
- No anti-motility agents (e.g. loperamide) or laxatives are prescribed or administered.
- The patient is assisted with hand hygiene.

Patient care (all patients)

- Patient care within a closed bay or on a closed ward must not be compromised. Not all patients will be symptomatic, and delays in seeing and reviewing patients where appropriate may delay patient discharges by several days once the ward has re-opened. Where possible, affected wards should be visited last.

Continued

- Investigations cannot be cancelled without the direct authorisation of the Medical Team (e.g. the Registrar or Consultant).
- Non-urgent investigations (e.g. routine non-urgent visits to X-ray) should be cancelled or postponed until the ward has reopened.
- Urgent investigations should still go ahead. It is the responsibility of the Nurse in Charge to inform the receiving department in order that the appropriate arrangements can be made.

Healthcare staff

- Members of staff who become symptomatic on duty must go home and remain off duty until they have been asymptomatic for 48 hours. Similarly, staff who become ill at home must not come into work until they have been asymptomatic for 48 hours.
- Where Bank or Agency staff are employed, the Ward Manager or Matron must liaise with the appropriate agencies. Ideally, staff should be block-booked to an affected area, and staff working on an affected ward should not work on an unaffected ward until 48 hours after the shift has ended.

Visitors

- Visitors (relatives or friends) should be contacted and asked not to visit while the ward is closed. However, it is difficult to place an outright 'ban' on visitors who may, of course, wish to visit family members in hospital who may be seriously ill or dying. In this situation, common sense must prevail.
- Visitors who are symptomatic should not visit until they have been asymptomatic for 48 hours. Symptomatic visitors can ignite ward outbreaks, particularly if they are actually 'ill' whilst visiting.
- Visits by children should be discouraged, particularly those of school age, and adult visitors should be informed of the risk of contracting norovirus and the possible implications.
- There may be extenuating circumstances, such as those described above, or visitors who travelled many miles and are unaware of the ward closure, and these need to be assessed and managed by the Nurse in Charge at his or her discretion.

Patient transfers and discharges

- Patients must not be transferred from an affected or closed ward to a non-affected ward unless it is for isolation purposes at the request of the IP&CT, or the patient requires specialist care that can be given only on another ward.
- Patients can be discharged to their own home from affected bays or wards when they are medically fit. The longer asymptomatic patients remain on the ward, the greater the possibility that they will become infected. Even if patients are symptomatic, they may still be discharged as long as they are able to manage their symptoms and/or there is someone to care for them.
- Patients cannot be discharged or transferred to community hospitals or care homes from closed bays or wards until the ward has re-opened unless there is an agreement between

Managers. Generally, symptomatic patients will not be accepted until they have been asymptomatic for 48 hours, and asymptomatic patients will not be accepted until the ward has re-opened.

Environmental cleanliness (see Chapter 15)

- Frequent cleaning of toilets, bathrooms and 'critical touch points' is necessary throughout the day.
- Clutter on bedside tables, lockers and surfaces should be moved to facilitate cleaning.
- All areas of the ward must be cleaned daily using a hypochlorite/chlorine dioxide. Empty beds must be stripped of linen and left unmade, and the bed frames cleaned daily.
- Once the IP&CT have declared that the outbreak is over and that the ward can re-open, the ward must be deep-cleaned before new admissions can be accepted.

Box 23.11 Preventing norovirus outbreaks in clinical settings

- Avoid admitting patients with norovirus to hospital unless admission can be justified on clinical grounds (e.g. for correction of dehydration and electrolyte imbalance, or for a frail, elderly patient with complications).
- Prompt isolation of patients either admitted with, or who develop after admission, symptoms suggestive of viral gastroenteritis.
- Patients attending hospital (e.g. for outpatient appointments or elective admissions), or relatives or friends visiting in-patients, should be discouraged from attending the hospital (in the event of patients due to come in for investigations or surgery, the Medical Team must be contacted and advice sought in the first instance).
- Inform the IP&CT promptly of all patients with vomiting and/or diarrhoea.
- Healthcare staff with vomiting and/or diarrhoea must go off duty and not come to work until they have been asymptomatic for 48 hours.
- Infection control standard precautions must be adhered to at all times.
- Toilets and bathrooms must be cleaned frequently throughout the day; commodes must be cleaned in between each patient use.

Chapter summary: key points

- Although norovirus outbreaks are now a fact of life for the NHS, they are a source of immense disruption, and norovirus infection is highly unpleasant and distressing.
- Mutations during viral replication can result in mutations within the viral genome, giving rise to new strains which may be hyper-virulent and lead to increased outbreaks.

Continued

- Although outbreaks are most common in winter months, they can occur throughout the year, and healthcare staff should always be vigilant.

- Norovirus is highly infectious – as few as 10–100 virus particles will initiate infection.

- The admission of symptomatic patients should be avoided unless admission is clearly required on clinical grounds.

- Patients with diarrhoea and/or vomiting should be isolated promptly unless an infectious cause can be confidently excluded. The IP&CT must be alerted promptly to any patients who cannot be isolated and to patients who meet the norovirus case definition.

- Healthcare staff with diarrhoea and/or vomiting must not come into work until they have been asymptomatic for 48 hours.

- Closed bays or wards will be re-opened only on the advice of the Infection Prevention and Control Team.

 Further resources are available for this book, including interactive multiple choice questions. Visit the companion website at:

www.wiley.com/go/fundamentalsofinfectionprevention

References

Ahmad N., Ray C.G., Drew W.L. (2010). Viruses of diarrhoea. In: Ryan K.J., Ray C.G. (Eds.), *Sherris Medical Microbiology*. 5th ed. McGraw-Hill Medical, New York: 271–278.

Atmar R.L., Estes M.K. (2006). The epidemiological and clinical importance of norovirus infection. *Gastroenterology Clinics of North America*. 35 (2): 275–290.

Baker J., Vipond I.B., Bloomfield S.F. (2004). Effects of cleaning and disinfection in reducing the spread of norovirus contamination via environmental surfaces. *Journal of Hospital Infection*. 58 (1): 42–49.

Bull R.A., Tu E.T., McIver C.J., Rawlinson W.D., White P.A. (2006).Emergence of a new norovirus genotype II.4 variant associated with global outbreaks of gastroenteritis. *Journal of Clinical Microbiology*. 44 (2): 327–333.

Caul E.D. (1994). Small round structured viruses – airborne transmission and hospital control. *The Lancet*. 343 (8098): 1240–1242.

Chadwick P.R., Beards G., Brown D., Caul E.O., Cheesbrough J. *et al.* (2000). Report of the Public Health Laboratory Service Viral Gastro Enteritis Working Group: management of hospital outbreaks of gastro-enteritis due to small round structured viruses. *Journal of Hospital Infection*. 45 (1): 1–10.

Cheesbrough J.S., Barkess-Jones L., Brown D.W. (1997). Possible prolonged environmental contamination survival of small round structured viruses. *Journal of Hospital Infection*. 35 (4): 325–326.

Clarke I.N., Lambden P.R. (2000). Viral gastroenteritis: the human caliciviruses. *CPD Infection*. 2: 14–17.

Collier L., Kellam P., Oxford J. (2011). Gastroenteritis viruses. In: *Human Virology*. 4th ed. Oxford University Press, Oxford: 110–120.

Cooper T., Atta M., Mackay A., Roberts H., Clement A. (2011). A major outbreak of norovirus in an acute NHS hospital in 2010: a practical management approach. *Journal of Infection Prevention*. 12 (3): 111–118.

Cubitt W.D. (2007). Caliciviruses and astroviruses. In: Greenwood D., Slack R., Peutherer J., Barer M. (Eds.), *Medical Microbiology. A Guide to Microbial Infections: Pathogenesis, Immunity, Laboratory Diagnosis and Control*. 17th ed. Churchill Livingstone Elsevier, London: 565–572.

Dolin R., Treanor J.J. (2009). Noroviruses and other caliciviruses. In: Mandell G.L., Bennett J.E., Dolin R. (Eds.), *Mandell, Douglas and Bennett's Principles and Practice of Infectious Diseases*. 7th ed. Churchill Livingstone Elsevier, London.

Goller J.L., Dimitriadis A., Tan A., Kelly H., Marshall J.A. (2004). Long-term features of norovirus gastroenteritis in the elderly. *Journal of Hospital Infection*. 58 (4): 286–291.

Hall A.J. (2012). Norovirus: the perfect human pathogen? *Journal of Infectious Diseases*. http://www.oxfordjournals.or/our_journals/jid/preditorial.pdf (accessed 10 June 2012)

Harris J.P., Allen D.J., Ituriza-Gomara M. (2011). Norovirus: changing epidemiology, changing virology: the challenges for infection control. *Journal of Infection Prevention*. 12 (3): 102–106.

Health Protection Agency (2009). *Foodborne Illness at 'The Fat Duck' Restaurant*. Report of an investigation of a foodborne outbreak of norovirus among diners at *The Fat Duck* Restaurant, Bray, Berkshire, in January and February 2009. Health Protection Agency, London.

Health Protection Agency and Norovirus Working Party (2011). *Guidelines for the Management of Norovirus Outbreaks in Acute and Community Health and Social Care Settings*. Health Protection Agency, London.

Illingworth E., Taborn E., Fielding D., Cheesbrough J., Diggle P.J. *et al.* (2011). Is closure of entire wards necessary to control norovirus outbreaks in hospital? Comparing the effectiveness of two infection control strategies. *Journal of Hospital Infection*. 79: 32–37.

Isakbaeva E.T., Widdowson M.A., Beard R.S., Bulens S.N., Mullens J. *et al.* (2005). Norovirus transmission on a cruise ship. *Emerging Infectious Diseases*. 11 (1). http://wwwnc.cdc.gov/eid/article/11/1/04-0434.htm (accessed 22 March 2013)

Lopman B.A., Reacher M.H., Vipond I.B., Hill D.I., Perry C. *et al.* (2004). Epidemiology and cost of nosocomial gastroenteritis, Avon, England, 2002–2003. *Emerging Infectious Diseases*. 10: 1827–1834.

Patterson W., Haswell P., Fryers P.T., Green J. (1997). Outbreak of small round structured virus gastroenteritis arose after kitchen assistant vomited. *Communicable Disease Report*. 7 (Review 7): R101–R103.

Repp K.K., Keene W.E. (2012). A point-source norovirus outbreak caused by exposure to fomites. *Journal of Infectious Diseases*. http://www.oxfordjournals.org/our_journals/jid/prpaper.pdf (accessed 10 June 2012)

Stevenson P., McCann R., Duthie R., Glew E., Ganguli L. (1994). A hospital outbreak due to Norwalk virus. *Journal of Hospital Infection*. 26 (4): 261–272.

van Beek J., Ambert-Balay AK., Botteldorn N., Eden J.S., Hewitt J. *et al.* on behalf of Noronet (2013). Indications for worldwide increased norovirus activity associated with the emergence of a new variant of genotype II.4 late 2012. *Eurosurveillance 2013*. http://www.eurosurveillance.org.ViewArtcile.aspx?Articleid=20345 (accessed 13 January 2013)

Vipond I.B., Caul E.O., Lambden P.R., Clarke I.N. (1999). 'Hyperemesis hiemis': new light on an old symptom. *Microbiology Today*. 26 (August): 110–111.

24

Blood-borne viruses

Contents

Introduction

Blood-borne viruses (BBVs) are carried in the bloodstream and, unlike most other infections which can be transmitted by normal, everyday social contact, they are spread via direct contact with contaminated blood or high-risk body fluids. The human immunodeficiency virus (HIV), hepatitis B virus (HBV) and hepatitis C virus (HCV) pose a significant threat to public health as many people with BBV infections are undiagnosed, and healthcare workers are exposed to BBVs every day through the handling of clinical waste, contact with blood and high-risk body fluids, procedures such as cannulation and venepuncture, and surgery. This chapter looks at the risks posed by BBVs and the importance of safe working to minimise the risks of occupational exposure and potential transmission to both patients and staff in the workplace. The pathogenesis of infection with HIV, HBV and HCV is discussed, along with diagnosis and treatment, the management of healthcare workers exposed to and infected with BBVs, and the management of infected patients. The safe handling and disposal of sharps are discussed separately in Chapter 14.

Note: Revised guidance on the management of HIV-infected healthcare workers was re-issued by the Department of Health in 2011, and on the management of HBV-infected healthcare workers in 2007, in order to protect patients and also to ensure that infected healthcare workers receive the appropriate support and treatment.

Learning outcomes

After reading this chapter, the reader will be able to:

- Understand the risk factors for the acquisition and transmission of blood-borne viruses.

- Understand the pathogenesis of HIV, HBV and HCV infection.

- Understand the importance of the application of standard precautions to prevent the transmission of BBVs in the healthcare setting.

357

Exposure to blood-borne viruses

A significant exposure to a blood-borne virus (BBV) is classed as a percutaneous exposure to blood and body fluids from a source that is known to be, or as a result of the incident found to be, positive for hepatitis B virus (HBV) surface antigen (HBsAg), hepatitis C virus (HCV) or HIV(Health Protection Agency [HPA], 2008). Within the healthcare setting, percutaneous (exposure via skin puncture) and mucotaneous (exposure via mucous membranes) exposures commonly occur as a result of:

- A skin puncture or scratch with a used needle or other sharp instrument, glassware or an item which may be contaminated with blood or body fluids
- A splash of blood or body fluids onto non-intact skin or the mucous membranes of the eyes and mouth
- Contamination of a cut, graze or break in the skin with blood or body fluids
- A human bite which breaks the skin (UK Health Departments, 1998).

Table 24.1   High and low-risk body fluids

High risk	Low risk
Blood	Urine
Semen	Faeces
Vaginal secretions	Saliva (unless blood stained or
Saliva (only if blood stained or if exposure occurs during	exposure occurs during dental work)
dental work)	Vomit
Cerebral spinal fluid	
Synovial fluid	
Amniotic fluid	
Breast milk	
Pleural fluid	
Pericardial fluid	

Healthcare workers should be aware of the types of body fluids that are classed as 'high' and 'low' risk with regard to BBVs (Table 24.1).

The risk of transmission of BBVs is greater from patient to healthcare worker than from healthcare worker to patient, and non-compliance with local protocols and procedures is one of the most common contributing factors leading to accidental exposure (HPA, 2008).

HIV and AIDS

Table 24.2 describes the global burden of HIV infection.

History

The greatest threat to public health seen so far, which heralded the onset of a worldwide pandemic, silently emerged between 1979 and 1981 and almost came out of nowhere, when the Centers for Disease Prevention and Control (CDC), Atlanta, United States, was alerted to an unusual number of opportunistic infections and rare skin cancers occurring among homosexuals in Los Angeles and New York (Durack, 1981). These infections were notable in that they were normally seen in individuals who were immunocompromised. It was clear that these men, who had previously been fit and healthy, were all suffering from a common syndrome, and on investigation they were found to have profound immunodeficiency with no underlying cause. Cases were subsequently identified at an alarming rate across the United States, Africa and other parts of the world, including the United Kingdom, from 1981 to 1983, and it was becoming evident that this was both a blood-borne and a sexually transmitted disease, affecting not only the homosexual population but also injecting drug users and those who had received blood transfusions.

Fact Box 24.1   AIDS

The term AIDS, or acquired immune deficiency syndrome, was first used by the CDC in 1982 to describe the collection of opportunistic infections that had been seen in these cases. AIDS was defined as 'a disease at least moderately predictive of a defect in cell-mediated immunity, occurring with no known cause for diminished resistance to that disease' (CDC, 1982).

Table 24.2   The burden of HIV – the United Kingdom, the United States and a global perspective

United Kingdom (HPA, 2011a)	United States (Centers for Disease Prevention and Control; www.cdc.gov)	Global (World Health Organization, 2011)
120 000 people have been diagnosed with HIV since 1981; 27 000 developed AIDS; >20 000 have died. At the end of 2009, 86 500 people were living with HIV in the United Kingdom. There were 6660 new cases of HIV diagnosed in 2010 that were probably acquired in the United Kingdom via sexual transmission (as opposed to 3020 cases acquired abroad). At the end of 2010, it was estimated that there were 91 500 people living with HIV in the United Kingdom, of whom approximately 24% were believed to be undiagnosed. By the end of 2012, approximately 100 000 people were living with HIV in the United Kingdom.	Currently 1.2 million people are living with HIV, of whom 20% are unaware of their status. Approximately 500 000 new infections per year. In 2009, 17 714 were estimated to have died. In 2010, it was estimated that there were 47 129 new infections diagnosed in 46 states; 33 015 people were diagnosed with AIDS. Since the AIDS epidemic began in 1981, it is estimated that 1 129 127 people in the United States have been diagnosed with AIDS, and 61 400 have died.	There has been a 19% global decline over the last decade, with a 19% decline in AIDS-related deaths between 2004 and 2009. In 15 high-burden countries, HIV prevalence has fallen by >25% in the 15–24 years age group, largely due to expanded HIV programmes. *But* the global prevalence of HIV infection stands at 33.3 million, and the incidence of HIV is increasing in some countries. There were 2.6 million new infections in 2009 – new infections have been out-pacing the number of people started on treatment. Sub-Saharan Africa accounts for 68% of the global prevalence of HIV; 60% of cases are in women, and HIV infections in women account for nearly 62% of the global number of people with HIV.

In 1983, at the Pasteur Institute in France, a new virus associated with AIDS was discovered by Luc Montagnier and Françoise Barre-Sinoussi (who went on to be awarded the Nobel Prize in Medicine in 2008 for their work), and research undertaken at the National Cancer Institute in Washington, DC, by Robert Gallo the following year established it as the causative agent (Gallo and Montagnier, 2003; Pratt, 2003a; Collier *et al.*, 2011a). It was not until 1986 that the AIDS-associated virus was named the human immunodeficiency virus (HIV).

The virus

HIV, of which there are two subtypes, belongs to the group of retroviruses known as lentiviruses ('lenti' = slow), so named because they cause slow, progressive disease and can persist for long periods of time in a latent state before there are any clinical manifestations (Ahmad *et al.*, 2010a).

HIV-1 is largely responsible for the AIDS pandemic.

HIV-2, discovered in 1986, is prevalent in West Africa, and although also associated with oppor-tunistic infections and progression to AIDS, it is less pathogenic (CDC, 1992).

Fact Box 24.2   Origins of the HIV retrovirus

The HIV retrovirus is believed to be linked to the simian immunodeficiency virus (SIV-1) which causes disease in chimpanzees. HIV-1 has specifically been linked to a species of chimpanzee residing in Africa known as *Pan troglodytes troglodytes*, which is 98% related to humans and whose natural habitat directly corresponds to the HIV epidemic in that part of the country (Gao *et al.*, 1999). Human retroviral infections are believed to have originated as a result of the virus jumping the species barrier (Reitz and Gallo, 2010).

Retroviruses differ from other viruses in that they are not transmissible by ordinary routes, instead requiring contact with blood and body fluids in order to infect the host.

Another distinguishing feature is that they are encoded for an enzyme called reverse transcriptase, which converts viral RNA into a DNA copy which becomes integrated into the DNA of the host cell (Ahmad *et al.*, 2010a).

The HIV virus consists of a viral envelope made out of host cell membrane, which is studded with 72 spikes consisting of transmembrane and surface proteins (Collier *et al.*, 2011a). These proteins aid the binding of the virus to CD4 T lymphocytes. Within the icosahedral capsid, there are three viral proteins which are essential for the process of viral replication: reverse transcriptase, integrase (which splices the DNA into the host cell gene) and protease (which facilitates the processing of virus particles). Also contained within the capsid are genes, which assist in the formation of new virus particles and produce 'copies' of the virus, and are believed to play regulatory or accessory roles during infection (Champoux and Drew, 2004).

HIV-1 is inactivated by heat, hypochlorite (bleach) 10 000 ppm and alcohol, and can survive in the environment for up to 15 days at room temperature (Simmonds and Peutherer, 2003a).

The pathogenesis of HIV infection

HIV specifically targets the CD4 T helper cells, which aid the T lymphocytes with antibody responses, and assist in the overall immune response (see Chapter 8). The CD4 cells carry surface receptors for antigens, and the transmembrane and surface proteins on the HIV cell membrane enable the virus to adhere to CD4 cell membrane. The viral envelope fuses with the CD4 cell, releasing its contents, and reverse transcriptase begins the process of converting viral RNA into DNA (Ahmad *et al.*, 2010a; Collier *et al.*, 2011a).

Within 24–48 hours of the virus entering the body, a period of intense viral replication takes place within the regional lymph nodes and the blood.

It has been estimated that up to 10 billion HIV particles are produced every day and that 1 billion CD4 cells are produced in each day in response, which have a very rapid turnover (Ahmad *et al.*, 2010a).

During this phase of primary infection and intense viral replication and dissemination, which occurs 2–12 weeks after infection and is known as seroconversion, 50–70% of infected individuals may experience what is known as an acute seroconversion illness lasting 2–4 weeks (Pratt, 2003b). This can manifest as a non-specific flu-like illness with symptoms which may include a generalised rash and lymphadenopathy, hepatosplenomegaly, arthralgia, fatigue, sore throat, nausea, weight loss, diarrhoea and mouth ulcers and is generally self-limiting (Pratt, 2003b; Ahmad *et al.*, 2010a). If symptoms are severe and significant illness is experienced during this time, it is associated with a more rapid progression to end-stage AIDS (Pratt, 2003b; Strohl *et al.*, 2001).

In the majority of people though, the CD4 count increases after this episode of primary infection, although the damage has been done and it does not return to baseline values (Pratt, 2003b).

The individual then enters a long asymptomatic period often referred to as clinical latency which can last 9–10 years, and during this time the immune system very slowly deteriorates. When an individual is first infected, the viral load increases and the CD4 T lymphocyte count falls as the immune system tries to fight the infection by producing antibodies.

As the infection progresses, the proportion of infected CD4 cells increases, as does the circulating viral load; immune function decreases, and the individual eventually develops signs of early symptomatic disease. These include malaise, weight loss, fever, night sweats and chronic diarrhoea (Strohl *et al.*, 2001) and may also include minor opportunistic infections such as oral thrush (candida), shingles (varicella zoster virus [VZV]), herpes simplex virus (HSV-1 or 2) and listeria (Pratt, 2003b).

Fact Box 24.3 CD4 counts and the significance of viral load explained

After diagnosis of HIV, the CD4 count (the number of CD4 T lymphocytes in a cubic mm of blood) is initially checked at 3–6 monthly intervals to monitor the immune response and determine when to start antiretroviral therapy.

A typical CD4 count in a healthy adult ranges from 400 to 1600 cells mm^3 and can fluctuate for a variety of reasons, none of which affect the competence of the immune system.

A count of 200–500 indicates that damage has occurred to the immune system. In someone infected with HIV, it is estimated that the CD4 count can decrease by 45 cells per month, and although thousands more are produced every day as the immune system is very resilient, there comes a point where the immune system is unable to keep up with the rate of destruction.

Viral load measures the number of copies of HIV RNA per ml of blood, and viral replication can exceed 10 000 new viral copies a day.

More than 100 000 viral copies per ml per blood is considered to be a high viral load, and fewer than 10 000 copies is considered to be low.

Ideally, the viral load should be undetectable (fewer than 50 copies), as the higher the viral load, the faster CD4 cells are likely to be destroyed and the faster the progression to the onset of AIDS.

Once antiretroviral therapy begins, the aim of treatment is to get the viral load down to an undetectable level within six months.

Progression to AIDS

Approximately 50% of individuals infected with HIV develop significant disease within 10 years of infection (Ahmad *et al.*, 2010a).

As the immune system starts to fail, the viral load increases and the CD4 count decreases; the end stage of the disease begins, with the development of opportunistic infections known as AIDS-defining illnesses (see Box 24.1), as defined by the CDC (1992).

Box 24.1   Some AIDS-defining illnesses

Lymphocytopenia – CD4 count <200/mm3
Recurrent pneumonia
Toxoplasmosis (http://hpa.org.uk/InfectiousDiseases/InfectionsAZ/Toxoplasmosis)
Cryptosporidiosis (http://www.hpa.org.uk/InfectiousDiseases/InfectionsAZ/Cryptosporidium)
Pnemocystis jiroveci pneumonia
Kaposi's sarcoma
HIV encephalopathy
HIV wasting syndrome
Histoplasmosis (http://www.cdc.gov/fungal/histoplasmosis)
Invasive cervical cancer
Lymphoma of the brain
Salmonella septicaemia (see Fact Sheet 3.5 on the companion website)
Disseminated or extra-pulmonary *Mycobacterium* avian complex or *Mycobacterium kansasii* disease (see Chapter 21)
Respiratory tuberculosis (see Chapter 21)
Other mycobacterial infections.

The treatment of HIV

Antiretroviral therapy

The aim of antiretroviral therapy is to reduce the viral load to non-detectable levels as quickly as possible and for as long as possible, and the British HIV Association recommends that antiretroviral therapy should be commenced before the CD4 count has fallen below 200 cells/mm^3 because of the increased risk of death or rapid progression to AIDS (British HIV Association, 2012). The recommendation is that the decision to start treatment should be based on an assessment of the risk of disease progression over the medium term if it is not started, versus the potential risk of toxicity and drug resistance if the treatment is commenced too soon; the risk of disease progression is largely determined by the CD4 count, the viral load and the age of the person infected.

The first drug used in the treatment of HIV was zidovudine (AZT or ZDV), but by the mid-1990s other drugs had been developed and highly active antiretroviral therapy, or HAART, was introduced (Pratt, 2003c).

How antiretroviral therapy works

Antiretroviral therapy works by targeting the viral enzymes which are responsible for HIV replication, and drugs are classed as reverse transcriptase inhibitors, which include AZT, lamivudine (3TC), didanosine (ddl) and stavudine (d4T), or protease inhibitors such as indinavir, ritonavir and nelfinavir. There are numerous drug combinations, and also clinical trials, and it is not yet clear which combination is the most effective. Treatment may need to be changed because of treatment side effects or treatment failure, which may be attributable to drug resistance.

HIV drug resistance

HIV drug resistance has numerous serious consequences which aside from treatment failure include direct and indirect healthcare costs associated with the need to start more costly second-line treatment, the spread of drug-resistant strains of HIV and the need for new drugs to be developed (see http://www/who.int/hiv/facts/drug_resistance/en/index.html and http://www.hpa.org.uk/hiv).

If compliance and adherence to antiretroviral therapy are monitored carefully, poor compliance will be detected early on and could be addressed.

Hepatitis B

Fact Box 24.4   HBV

Hepatitis B is 50–100 times more infectious than HIV.
Up to one-third of individuals with HBV infection will not know how they acquired it.
It can remain viable in dried blood for up to seven days.
HBV infection is preventable through vaccination.

Source: CDC, 2001; Alter, 2005; British Liver Trust, 2009.

Hepatitis is a general term meaning inflammation of the liver which can be caused by a variety of different forms of viral hepatitis. Hepatitis B is of huge global significance, and like HIV it is a sexually transmitted and blood-borne disease and represents a risk to public health. It has infected two billion people worldwide, with more than 350 million who experience chronic, or lifelong, infection and are at high risk of death from cirrhosis and primary liver cancer (http://www.who.int/topics/hepatitis/en).

Important note: The highly infectious virus particles in the blood of symptomatic and asymptomatic infected individuals pose a serious health risk, with healthy asymptomatic carriers the main reservoir of infection.

The hepatitis B virus explained

Hepatitis B belongs to a group of viruses known as Hepadnaviruses which, although unrelated to other human hepatitis viruses, also include the woodchuck, ground squirrel and Peking duck viruses (Simmonds and Peutherer, 2003b; Drew, 2004; Collier *et al.*, 2011b). It is a small-enveloped, double-stranded DNA virus, and it is the smallest known DNA virus (Drew, 2004). The intact virus is known as the Dane particle.

The hepatitis B viral antigens and antibodies, known as 'markers', can be detected in the blood and indicate both the course of the infection and the individual's degree of infectivity to others.

Hepatitis B surface antigen (HBsAg) and antibody (anti-HBs)

HBsAg is the first antigen to be produced and the first marker to be detected, although in 10% of infected individuals it may be cleared early by the immune response and therefore not be detectable on testing (British Liver Trust, 2009). Generally, though, it is produced in excessive quantities, and can be detected before and after the onset of symptoms. It is at maximum titre in the blood at the height of liver damage (Simmonds and Peutherer, 2003b), and its presence indicates that the person is infectious.

Detection of HBsAg for longer than six months indicates chronic infection.

The specific antibody, anti-HBs, does not appear until 1–4 months after the onset of symptoms; the disappearance of HBsAg from the blood and the presence of antibody indicate clinical recovery and immunity (British Liver Trust, 2009; Ahmad *et al.*, 2010b). Anti-HBs also develops in individuals in response to HBV vaccination.

Hepatitis B e antigen (HBeAg), HBV-DNA and antibody (anti-HBe)

HBeAg is the soluble component of the nucleocapsid core. Produced when the virus is replicating, it is indicative of high infectivity, and is detected in the bloodstream along with HBV-DNA. It can appear concurrently with, or shortly after, HBsAg (British Liver Trust, 2009).

When HBeAg disappears from the bloodstream and HBV-DNA declines, the presence of anti-HBe, which can continue to be detected for one or more years, indicates resolution of both viral replication and acute hepatitis B infection.

Hepatitis B core antigen (HBcAg) and antibody (anti-HBc)

HBcAg is produced when the virus replicates in the liver but is not detectable in serum and is not used as a serological marker (Ahmad *et al.*, 2010b).

Core antibodies usually appear in the bloodstream within weeks of the infection occurring and are present in individuals with acute or chronic infection.

HBcAg stimulates the production of IgG (which indicates that infection occurred >6 months previously and is indicative of chronic infection) and IgM (HBV infection occurred within the past 6 months; this indicates acute infection).

Fact Box 24.5   HBV: infection and immunity

Acute infection and infectiousness: detection of HBsAg, HBeAg and anti-HBc (IgM)
Chronic infection: detection of HBeAg for longer than 6 months; anti-HBc (IgG)
Clinical recovery and immunity: detection of anti-HBs and anti-HBe.

The clinical features of HBV infection and routes of transmission are described in Boxes 24.2 and 24.3.

Box 24.2   Clinical features of HBV infection

- Long incubation period of between 45 and 120 days (the duration of which is affected by the size of the inoculum and the route of infection), and it is during this time that HBsAg and HBeAg may be detected in the blood.
- Pre-jaundice or pre-icteric phase (days to weeks), characterised by malaise, anorexia, nausea, mild fever and right-sided upper abdominal discomfort.
- Jaundice or icteric phase – bilirubinuria (dark urine caused by the jaundice) and an enlarged tender liver, as well as jaundice of the skin, mucous membranes and conjunctivae.
- Recovery usually takes several months.

Box 24.3   Transmission of hepatitis B

Percutaneous exposure

Transfusion of unscreened blood or blood products
Sharing drug-injecting equipment
Haemodialysis
Acupuncture
Tattooing
Inoculation from needlestick injuries
Blood glucose monitoring – injuries from lancer devices.

Mucous membrane exposure

Sexual and perinatal transmission as a result of exposure to high-risk body fluids.

Indirect exposure

Via inanimate objects such as toothbrushes, razors and eating utensils that are contaminated with blood, and hospital equipment.

Source: UK Health Departments, 1998; British Liver Trust, 2009; HPA, 2009.

Immunisation against hepatitis B

Protection against hepatitis B infection can be given by the administration of a vaccine containing HBsAg, which confers active immunity, and it can be administered as pre-exposure prophylaxis in high-risk groups, or as post-exposure prophylaxis. It is given as an accelerated course at zero, one and two months followed by a fourth dose at 12 months for those who remain at continued risk.

Vaccination should be given to the following categories of people (Box 24.4) who are at high risk of exposure to HBV:

Box 24.4   HBV vaccination

Injecting drug users (IDUs), including all current IDUs, those who inject intermittently, those likely to progress to injecting, non-injectors living with injecting partners, sexual partners of injectors, children of injectors and those with frequent sexual partners

Close family contacts of a case or individual with chronic HBV infection

Families adopting children from countries where there is a high prevalence of HBV

Foster carers

Those receiving regular blood transfusions or blood products

Patients with chronic renal failure

Patients with chronic liver disease

Those planning travel to or residence in areas of high or intermediate prevalence

Prisoners in the United Kingdom

Those at risk of occupational exposure to BBV (e.g. all healthcare workers who may have contact with blood, blood-stained body fluids and tissue; laboratory staff; staff of residential accommodation for people with learning difficulties; and other occupational at-risk groups, such as the police, fire and rescue services as well as morticians and embalmers)

Post exposure – accidental inoculation and contamination

Sexual partners of infected individuals

Babies born to mothers who are chronically infected or who had acute infection during pregnancy

Source: Data from DH, 2006.

Where exposure to HBV has occurred following an inoculation or contamination incident, specific immunoglobulin (hepatitis B immunoglobulin, or HBIG) is given at the same time as the vaccination to provide immediate but temporary protection against HBV while the vaccine takes effect. It is also used to give protection to those who have a failed response to the vaccine but who have been exposed to HBV.

Antibody responses to the vaccine are variable and should be checked one to four months after the primary course has been given in order to confirm that the recipient is adequately protected against HBV. Ideally, anti-HBs levels should be above 100 IU/ml, and if the anti-HBs level is between 1 and 100 IU/ml, an additional dose should be administered. Non-responders have antibody levels of below 10 IU/ml and a further course of vaccine should be given, followed by further checking of the antibody titre at one to four months (DH, 2006).

Hepatitis C

Fact Box 24.7   HCV incidence

Approximately 216 000 people in the United Kingdom have chronic hepatitis C infection (HPA, 2011b), whilst in the United States, it is the most common blood-borne infection, and 3.2 million people are estimated to be infected (www.cdc.gov).

The virus and clinical features

HCV belongs to the genus *Hepacivirus* (a member of the virus family Flaviviridae) and is a small, enveloped, single-stranded RNA virus that is 55–65 nm in diameter (Ahmad *et al.*, 2010b; Collier *et al.*, 2011c).

It has an incubation period of 6–12 weeks, and while fatigue and jaundice have been reported, most infected individuals are completely asymptomatic.

Although disease progression can be variable, infected individuals may be asymptomatic for anything from 20 to 50 years, and it is not until the liver has been extensively damaged that symptoms become apparent.

Of those infected, 80% will develop chronic hepatitis C, of whom 30% will develop cirrhosis within 30 years of infection, and chronic infection and hepatocellular cancer are the leading indicators for liver transplantation (Patel *et al.*, 2006).

During this long period of undiagnosed and asymptomatic infection, countless other people may become infected through certain high-risk behaviours and practices.

Acquisition and transmission of HCV

See Box 24.5.

Diagnosis and treatment

Clinically, infection with HCV is indistinguishable from other hepatitis viruses, and diagnosis is dependent upon the detection of antibodies through serological assays, and molecular techniques

Box 24.5 High-risk groups for acquisition and transmission of HCV

- Recipients of unscreened blood donations prior to 1991
- Anyone who may have received blood products such as factor VIII, anti-D and immunoglobulin which were manufactured before virus inactivation procedures were implemented in 1986
- Injecting drug users
- Dialysis patients
- Men and women with multiple sexual partners who have unprotected sex
- People who share toothbrushes and razors that are contaminated with blood
- Tattooing and skin piercing
- Healthcare workers – exposure through poor infection control practices.

Source: Data from DH, 2002; Morgan-Capner and Simmonds, 2004; Collier *et al.*, 2011c; HPA, 2011b.

such as PCR for the detection of viral RNA (see Chapter 7). HCV-RNA can be detected in the blood 1–3 weeks following exposure; the specific antibody, anti-HBC, can be detected within 8–9 weeks.

The aim of treatment is to eradicate HCV-RNA in order to prevent progressive viral fibrosis occurring, and the duration of treatment varies according to the serotype and the viral load (Patel *et al.*, 2006).

For mild chronic hepatitis C in adults over the age of 18, combination therapy with weekly subcutaneous injections of peginterferon alpha and daily oral ribavirin is the recommended regimen; in moderate to severe chronic disease, peginterferon alfa-2a or peginterferon alfa-2b in conjunction with ribavirin is prescribed (National Institute of Clinical Excellence, 2006).

Clinical practice

Protection against BBVs in the healthcare setting

In 1985, in response to the mounting problems with HIV and growing concerns over the risks that occupational exposure to HIV posed to healthcare workers, the CDC introduced the term 'universal precautions'. This was in recognition of the fact that not all patients with a blood-borne virus have their infection diagnosed, and included within universal precautions were blood and body fluid precautions which incorporated the use of masks and face protection in order to protect healthcare workers against mucous membrane exposures. In 1987 (Garner *et al.*, 1996), another category of precautions called body substance isolation was developed; this latest set of precautions high-lighted the need to protect healthcare workers, and other patients, from the cross-infection risks potentially posed from other pathogens apart from blood-borne viruses, isolated from moist body sites such as faeces, urine, sputum and other body fluids and secretions. Then, in 1996, the CDC replaced universal precautions with standard principles, incorporating infection control measures to protect against blood-borne viruses as well as other pathogens, and transmission-based precautions focusing on preventing the spread of infection from airborne, droplet and direct contact.

The DH commissioned the development of national evidence-based guidelines for the prevention of healthcare-associated infections (HCAIs) (known as the EPIC Guidelines) which were published in 2001 and revised in 2006 (Pratt *et al.*, 2001, 2007). These guidelines on the standard principles for preventing HCAIs aim to inform best practice in relation to preventing the spread of HCAIs based on the best evidence currently available.

Standard precautions are discussed elsewhere in this book and include in particular:

- Hand hygiene (Chapter 12)
- The use of personal protective equipment (PPE) (Chapter 13)
- The safe use and disposal of sharps (Chapter 14)
- Environmental cleanliness and decontamination (Chapter 15).

Measures to reduce eye and other facial exposure

- Protect the mucous membrane of eyes with protective eyewear. This should prevent splash injuries (including lateral splashes) without loss of visual acuity and without discomfort. Face shields should be considered appropriate for procedures which involve a risk of splatter of blood, including aerosols or other potentially infectious material.
- Eye wash should be available in case of accidental exposure. Contact lenses should be removed prior to eye washing.

The management of BBV-exposed healthcare workers

1. Immediate first aid:
    - For wounds:
        - Encourage bleeding by gently squeezing the site of injury.
        - Wash the site of injury thoroughly with soap and water.
        - Cover with a waterproof plaster.
    - For mucous membranes:
        - Irrigate contaminated areas thoroughly with normal saline or tap water.
2. Inform Person in Charge: record and report – report to Person in Charge or Line Manager; complete risk assessment/clinical incident reporting proforma as per local policy.
3. Attend the Occupational Health Department or Emergency Department, where the following assessments and actions should be implemented:
    - The source patient (if known). Is the patient suspected or known to have HBV, HBC or HIV? Is the source patient septicaemic and not on antibiotic therapy?
    - The severity of the exposure
    - The type of sharp (if any) causing the injury
    - The depth of the injury
    - Was there a splash to the mucous membranes or eyes?
    - The type of body fluid involved
    - If a needlestick injury, was the recipient wearing gloves?
    - The recipient's vaccination history: Has the recipient been vaccinated against HBV? Was he or she a good responder or a non-responder?
    - Is HBV vaccine needed? If the source patient is suspected or known to be a HBV carrier, and the exposed recipient is not immune to HBV, an accelerated course of hepatitis B vaccine is needed.

- Is hepatitis B immunoglobulin needed? HBIG may be required if the source is a high risk of hepatitis B (HBsAg-positive) and the recipient has no documented immunity to hepatitis B.
- Is HIV post-exposure prophylaxis (PEP) appropriate? If the source patient is suspected or known to be HIV-positive, PEP treatment should be commenced as soon as possible after the incident (preferably within the hour), but up to 72 hours after the incident it may still be effective. Therefore, a decision needs to be made about whether PEP is needed before the source blood results are available from the laboratory. The risk assessment informs these decisions.

Clinical practice points: the infection control management of patients

As discussed in this chapter, not all patients with a BBV have their infection diagnosed, and therefore the application of standard precautions must apply to **all** patients in **all** settings at **all** times when dealing with blood and body fluids.

Reflection point

- What is the policy for dealing with blood or body fluid spillages within your place of work?
- Who is responsible for dealing with the spillage or cleaning the area?
- Do your colleagues know the correct procedure for dealing with blood or body fluid spills? How compliant are staff with the policy?

Patients with a confirmed or suspected BBV infection do **not** need to be nursed in a single room **or** be placed last on the theatre or clinic list. They can be nursed in the open ward with the application of standard precautions. With regard to theatre, the Consultant and the Theatre Co-ordinator should be informed of the patients' BBV status beforehand.

Within the operating theatre environment, there are additional precautions that can be implemented if a patient is suspected or known to have a BBV (see Chapter 14). These include:

- Adjusting the operating technique or approach, and the instruments used, in order to reduce the use or passage of sharp instruments
- Heightened 'sharps awareness'
- Using retractors rather than the hands of scrub staff to hold open wound edges.

All blood or body fluid spillages (even minute blood splatters) must be dealt with promptly in accordance with local policy to reduce environmental contamination and potential BBV exposure to healthcare staff and patients. Some blood spills can be large (e.g. within the Emergency Department, Theatres and the Delivery and Labour Ward).

When obtaining clinical specimens from patients with a suspected or confirmed BBV infection, 'danger of infection' labels should be applied to both the specimen and the specimen request form (see Chapter 6).

Whenever a person who is known or suspected to be infected with a BBV dies, it is the duty of those with knowledge of the case to ensure that those who need to handle the body, including funeral personnel and mortuary and post-mortem room staff, are aware that there is a potential risk of infection. Making those who may be at risk aware of a known or suspected hazard is a statutory duty under the Health and Safety at Work Act. Although the diagnosis should be kept confidential, the discreet use of 'danger of infection' or similar labelling is appropriate, always making clear what type of precautions are needed. Any deceased body that is externally contaminated with blood, or known or suspected to be infected with a BBV, should be placed in a disposable plastic body bag as soon as possible. Absorbent material may be needed when there is leakage (e.g. from surgical incisions or wounds). Mortuary staff should ensure that good liaison is maintained between themselves and those who submit bodies for post-mortem examination or storage and those who collect bodies for disposal.

Chapter summary: key points

- BBVs pose a significant public health threat as many people have their infection undiagnosed.

- Healthcare workers are exposed to BBVs every day through the handling of clinical waste, contact with blood and high-risk body fluids, procedures such as cannulation and venepuncture, and surgery.

- The risk of transmission of BBVs is greater from patient to healthcare worker than from healthcare worker to patient.

- Non-compliance with Infection Control protocols, policies and procedures is one of the most common contributing factors leading to accidental exposure.

- There is no vaccination against HIV infection, but it can be treated with antiretroviral therapy, which may be given as post-exposure prophylaxis (PEP) in the event of HIV exposure in the workplace.

- Protection against HBV is available via vaccine.

- There is no vaccination against HCV.

- Standard precautions must apply to all patients in all settings at all times when dealing with blood and body fluids.

Resources

The Terence Higgins Trust: www.tht.org.uk
www.aidsmap.com
www.hivaware.org.uk

www.thebritishlivertrust.org.uk
http://hepbadvocate.org
www.hepb.org.uk
www.hepcsupport.org
www.worldhepatitisalliance.org
Health Protection Agency (Public Health England): www.hpa.org.uk
World Health Organization: www.who.int
Centers for Disease Control and Prevention: www.cdc.gov

See also the 'Further reading' section at the end of this chapter.

Further resources are available for this book, including interactive multiple choice questions. Visit the companion website at:

www.wiley.com/go/fundamentalsofinfectionprevention

References

Ahmad N., Ray C.G., Drew W.L. (2010a). Retroviruses: human T-lymphotropic virus, human immunodeficiency virus, and acquired immune deficiency syndrome. In: Ryan K., Ray C.G. (Eds.), *Sherris Medical Microbiology*. 5th ed. McGraw-Hill Medical, New York: 305–326.

Ahmad N., Ray C.G., Drew W.L. (2010b). Hepatitis viruses. In: Ryan K., Ray C.G. (Eds.), *Sherris Medical Microbiology*. 5th ed. McGraw-Hill Medical, New York: 225–246.

Alter M.J. (2005). The epidemiology of hepatitis B infection in healthcare workers in the West and Asia. *Hepatitis B Annual*. 2: 186–192.

British HIV Association (2012). *BHIVA Guidelines for the Treatment of HIV-1 Infected Adults with Antiretroviral Therapy 2012*. British HIV Association, London.

British Liver Trust (2009). *Fighting Liver Disease: A Guide for Health Professionals*. www.britishlivertrust.org.uk (accessed 23 December 2012)

Centers for Disease Control and Prevention (CDC) (1982). Update on acquired immune deficiency syndrome – United States. *Morbidity Mortality Weekly Review*. 31: 507–514.

Centers for Disease Control and Prevention (CDC) (1992). Revised classification system for HIV infection and expanded surveillance case definition for AIDS among adolescents and adults. *Morbidity Mortality Weekly Review*. 41 (RR-17): http://www.cdc.gov/mmwR/preview/mmwrhtml/00018871.htm (accessed 22 March 2013)

Centers for Disease Control and Prevention (CDC) (2001). Updated United States public health service guidelines for the management of occupational exposures to HBV, HCV and HIV and recommendations for postexposure prophylaxis. *Morbidity Mortality Weekly Review*. 50 (RR-11): 1–42.

Champoux J.J., Drew W.L. (2004). Retroviruses, human immunodeficiency virus and acquired immune deficiency syndrome. In: Sherris J.C., Ryan K.J., Ray G.C. (Eds.), *Medical Microbiology: An Introduction to Infectious Diseases*. 4th ed. McGraw-Hill, London: 601–616.

Collier L., Kellam P., Oxford J. (2011a).Retroviruses and HIV. In: *Human Virology*. 4th ed. Oxford University Press, London: 223–236.

Collier L., Kellam P., Oxford J. (2011b).The blood-borne hepatitis viruses B and D. In: *Human Virology*. 4th ed. Oxford University Press, Oxford: 119–209.

Collier L., Kellam P., Oxford J. (2011c). The blood-borne hepatitis C. In: *Human Virology*. 4th ed. Oxford University Press, Oxford: 210–217.

Department of Health (DH) (2002). *Hepatitis C Strategy for England: Implementing 'Getting Ahead of the Curve' Action on Blood Borne Viruses*. Department of Health, London.

Department of Health (DH) (2006). Hepatitis B. *Immunisation against Infectious Disease*. Department of Health, London. http://www.dh.gov.uk/greenbook (accessed 23 December 2012)

Department of Health (DH) (2007). *Hepatitis B Infected Healthcare Workers and Anti-viral Therapy*. Department of Health, London.

Department of Health (DH) (2011). *Management of HIV-infected Healthcare Workers: The Report of the Tripartite Working Group*. Department of Health, London.

Drew W.L. (2004). Hepatitis viruses. In: Sherris. J.C., Ryan K.J., Ray G.C. (Eds.), *Medical Microbiology: An Introduction to Infectious Diseases*, 4th ed. McGraw-Hill, London: 541–553.

Durack D.T. (1981). Opportunistic infections and Kaposi's sarcoma in homosexual men. *New England Journal of Medicine*. 305 (24): 1465–1467.

Gallo R., Montagnier L. (2003). The discovery of HIV as the cause of AIDS. *New England Journal of Medicine*. 349: 2283–2285.

Gao F., Bailes E., Robertson D.L., Chen Y., Rodenburg C.M. *et al.* (1999). Origin of HIV-1 in the chimpanzee *Pan troglodytes troglodytes*. *Nature*. 397: 436–441.

Garner J.S. and the Hospital Infection Control Practices Advisory Committee (1996). Guideline for isolation precautions in hospitals. *Infection Control Hospital Epidemiology*. 15 (53): 53–80.

Health Protection Agency (HPA) (2008). *Eye of the Needle. United Kingdom Surveillance of Significant Occupational Exposures to Blood Bourne Viruses in Healthcare Workers*. Health Protection Agency, London.

Health Protection Agency (HPA) (2009). *Infection Prevention and Control Guidelines for Blood Glucose Monitoring in Care Homes*. Health Protection Agency, London.

Health Protection Agency (HPA) (2011a). *HIV in the United Kingdom: 2011 Report*. Health Protection Agency, London.

Health Protection Agency (HPA) (2011b). *Hepatitis C in the UK: 2011 Report*. Health Protection Agency, London.

Morgan-Capner P., Simmonds P.N. (2004). Togaviruses and hepaciviruses. In: Greenwood D., Slack R.C.B., Peutherer J.F. (Eds.), *Medical Microbiology: A Guide to Microbial Infections: Pathogenesis, Immunity, Laboratory Diagnosis and Control*. 16th ed. Churchill Livingstone, London: 501–512.

National Institute of Clinical Excellence (2006). *Peginterferon Alfa and Ribavirin for Treatment of Mild Chronic Hepatitis C*. National Institute of Clinical Excellence, London.

Patel K., Muir A.J., McHutchinson J.G. (2006). Diagnosis and treatment of chronic hepatitis C infection. *British Medical Journal*. 332 (7548): 1013–1017.

Pratt R.J. (2003a). The evolution of a pandemic. In: *HIV and AIDS: A Foundation for Nursing and Healthcare Practice*. 5th ed. Hodder Arnold, London: 1–14.

Pratt R.J. (2003b). The clinical spectrum of HIV disease. In: *HIV and AIDS: A Foundation for Nursing and Healthcare Practice*. 5th ed. Hodder Arnold, London: 80–122.

Pratt R.J. (2003c). Understanding antiretroviral therapy. In: *HIV and AIDS: A Foundation for Nursing and Healthcare Practice*. 5th ed. Hodder Arnold, London: 362–379.

Pratt R.J., Pellowe C.M., Loveday H.B., Robinson M., Smith G.W. and the EPIC Guidelines Development Team (2001). The EPIC project: developing national evidence-based guidelines for preventing healthcare associated infections. *Journal of Hospital Infection.* 47 (Suppl.): S1–S82.

Pratt R.J., Pellowe C.M., Wilson J.A., Loveday H.P., Harper P.J. *et al.* (2007). EPIC2: national evidenced-based guidelines for preventing healthcare-associated infections in NHS hospitals in England. *Journal of Hospital Infection.* 65 (Suppl. 1): S1–S64.

Reitz J.R., Gallo R.C. (2010). Human deficiency viruses. In: Mandell G.L., Bennett J.E., Dolin R.D. (Eds.), *Mandell's Principles and Practices of Infectious Diseases.* 6th ed. Churchill Livingstone Elsevier, London. www.expertconsult.com (accessed 23 December 2012)

Simmonds P., Peutherer J.F. (2003a). Retroviruses. In: Greenwood D., Slack R.C.B., Peutherer J.F. (Eds.), *Medical Microbiology: A Guide to Microbial Infections: Pathogenesis, Immunity, Laboratory Diagnosis and Control.* 16th ed. Churchill Livingstone, London: 527–538.

Simmonds P., Peutherer J.F. (2003b). Hepadnaviruses. In: Greenwood D., Slack R.C.B., Peutherer J.F. (Eds.), *Medical Microbiology: A Guide to Microbial Infections: Pathogenesis, Immunity, Laboratory Diagnosis and Control.* 16th ed. Churchill Livingstone, London: 438–447.

Strohl W.A., Rouse H., Fisher B.D. (2001). Retroviruses and AIDS. In: *Lippincott's Illustrated Reviews: Microbiology.* Lippincott, Williams and Wilkins, Philadelphia: 359–378.

UK Health Departments (1998). *Guidance for Clinical Health Care Workers: Protection against Infection with Blood-borne Viruses: Recommendations of the Expert Advisory Group on AIDS and the Advisory Group on Hepatitis.* UK Health Departments, London.

World Health Organization (2011). *Global Health Sector Strategy on HIV/AIDS, 2011–2015.* World Health Organization, Geneva.

Further reading

Department of Health (2002). *Good Practice Guidelines for Renal Dialysis / Transplantation Units: Prevention and Control of Blood-borne Virus Infections.* Department of Health, London.

Department of Health (2005). *Hepatitis C Infected Healthcare Workers.* Department of Health, London.

Department of Health (2005). *HIV Infected Healthcare Workers: Guidance on Management and Patient Notification.* Department of Health, London.

Department of Health (2009). *Hepatitis C: Quick Reference Guide for Primary Care.* Department of Health, London.

Department of Health (2009). *Infection Prevention and Control Guidelines for Blood Glucose Monitoring in Care Homes.* Department of Health, London.

Department of Health (2010). *Good Practice Guidelines for Renal Dialysis Transplantation Units. Prevention and Control of Blood-borne Virus Infections.* Department of Health, London.

Department of Health (2010). *Good Practice Guidelines for Renal Dialysis Transplantation Units. Prevention and Control of Blood-borne Virus Infections. Addendum: Guidelines for Dialysis away from Base (DAFB). Recommendations of a Working Group Convened by the Department of Health.* October. Department of Health, London.

Glossary

Acidosis	Disruption of the acid–base balance (pH) of the body, detected by taking an arterial blood sample (pH < 7).
Alveoli	Small air sacs within the lungs where gaseous exchange (oxygen and carbon dioxide) occurs.
Amniotic (fluid)	The protective fluid (liquor amnii) within the amniotic sac (membranes) surrounding the foetus in utero.
Anaemia	A condition in which there are fewer red blood cells, or the haemoglobin (iron) content of red blood cells is lower than normal.
Anti-D	Immunoglobulin to prevent the formation of antibodies in rhesus positive women with a rhesus negative baby (rhesus – antigen found on the surface of red blood cells in some people).
Anti–tumour necrosis factor	Drugs that block the action of tumour necrosis infector (TNF), an inflammatory cytokine produced by monocytes and macrophages.
Arteriovenous fistula	A surgically created connection between an artery and a vein. Increased blood flow and arterial pressure cause the vein to enlarge, making repeated insertions of haemodialysis needles easier.
Arteriovenous graft	The insertion of an artificial or synthetic graft (tube) connecting an artery and a vein. Used when the creation of an arteriovenous fistula is not possible.
Arthralgia	Joint pain.
Asepsis, aseptic technique	The technique used to minimise the possibility of contamination.
Autoclaving	Sterilisation (the complete destruction of vegetative bacteria, bacterial spores and viruses, but not prions) using high-pressure saturated steam at 121 °C for 15–20 minutes.
Bacteroides	Gram-negative bacilli; part of the resident colonic flora.
Blood gas	Measurement of oxygen, carbon dioxide and acidity in the blood.

Fundamentals of Infection Prevention and Control: Theory and Practice, Second Edition. Debbie Weston.
© 2013 John Wiley & Sons, Ltd. Published 2013 by John Wiley & Sons, Ltd. Companion Website: www.wiley.com/go/fundamentalsofinfectionprevention

Bone marrow suppression, myelosuppression	Short-term suppression of the bone marrow leading to reduced production of red and white blood cells and platelets.
Cellulitis	Infection of the dermis and subcutaneous tissue; characterised by spreading inflammation, swelling and tenderness.
Clinical governance	A system through which health care services and the individuals working within them are held accountable for the safety, quality and effectiveness of clinical care given to patients.
Clinical risk management	A key component of clinical governance, essentially concerned with reducing the risk of harm to patients, the public and staff.
Coagulopathy	Clotting and bleeding disorder; the blood's ability to clot is impaired.
Colonoscopy	An endoscopic examination of the large bowel (colon) and distal (lower) part of the small bowel using a flexible fibre-optic scope (colonoscope) with a light source, which is passed into the colon via the anus.
Conjunctivitis	Inflammation of the mucous membrane that covers the white of the eye and also the inner eyelid; can be caused by bacteria or viruses, or may be caused by an allergy.
Consolidation	Lung tissue, which is normally 'elastic' and able to expand, becomes solid and compressed due to inflammation or infection.
Crohn's disease	An inflammatory bowel disease typically affecting the ileum or the colon.
Cytotoxic	Damaging to cells; for example, drugs that are administered to destroy cancer cells as part of chemotherapy treatment.
Dendritic cells	Part of the immune system; cells that 'capture' antigens and then 'present' them on their cell surface in order to activate T lymphocytes.
Dermatology, dermatological	The branch of medicine concerned with conditions or diseases of the skin.
Disseminated intravascular coagulation (DIC)	An often fatal and inappropriate activation of the coagulation pathway, often manifesting as large bruises and bleeding at venepuncture sites.
Diverticuli, diverticulitis	Small 'out pouches' or herniations of the muscle of the bowel wall; they can be inflamed, giving rise to abdominal pain and diarrhoea.
Dyspnoea	Shortness of breath, or difficulty breathing; sometimes referred to as 'air hunger'.
Electrocardiogram (ECG)	Assessment of the electrical activity of the heart; used to detect abnormal heart rhythms (arrhythmias) and myocardial infarction ('heart attack').

Electrolytes	Electrically charged molecules (ions) found within cells and extracellular fluids (e.g. sodium, potassium, magnesium and calcium).
Encephalitis	Acute inflammation of the brain caused by bacterial, viral or fungal infections.
Endocarditis	Bacterial infection of the heart valves, giving rise to 'vegetative growths' on the valves.
Endoscope, endoscopy	A flexible or rigid tube with a light source, and sometimes instrument channels, used to examine body cavities.
Epidemic	Occurrence of new cases of a disease in a population.
Epstein–Barr virus	Viral cause of glandular fever (infectious mononucleosis); characterised by lymphadenopathy, fever and extreme tiredness.
Extravasation	The leakage of intravenous fluids, including medication, from the vein into the surrounding tissues.
Factor VIII	An essential blood-clotting protein (known as anti-haemophilliac factor, of AHF).
Fibrosis	Formation of excess fibrous connective tissue.
Gastrectomy	Partial or full surgical removal of the stomach.
Germinate, germination	Begin growth.
Haemodialysis	The removal of waste and excess fluid from the bloodstream. Blood is filtered, 'cleansed' and returned to the body via a haemodialysis ('artificial kidney') machine.
Haemoptysis	The coughing up (expectoration) of blood or blood-stained sputum from the respiratory tract.
Hepatosplenomegaly	Enlargement of the liver and the spleen.
Hyperglycaemia	Elevated blood glucose.
Hypoxia	Oxygen deprivation.
Immunosuppression, immunocompromised	Suppression of the immune system through illness or disease.
Impetigo	A highly infectious skin infection, transmitted via touch/direct contact.
Incubation, incubation period	The time interval between being exposed to an infection and developing symptoms.
Jejunoileal bypass	Surgical anastomosis (joining together) of the jejunum to the ileum (small bowel), bypassing the stomach and the duodenum.
Laminar flow	A continuous flow of 'clean', bacteria-free air that is recirculated under positive pressure into the operating field; also called 'ultraclean ventilation'.
Latent, latency	Dormant, inactive or hidden.
Listeria	Bacteria found in soil, water and animals; causes food poisoning, septicaemia and meningitis and potentially life-threatening infection in pregnancy or if immunocompromised.

Lymphadenopathy	Swollen and/or enlarged lymph glands.
Lyse, lysis	Rupture of the cell membrane resulting in cell death.
Mortality rate	The number of deaths in a population over a period of time. Deaths can be general or due to a specific cause such as infection or disease, or following surgery.
Myasthenia gravis	An autoimmune neuromuscular disorder, affecting voluntary muscle control.
Nanotechnology	The manipulation of atomic and molecular 'matter'.
Oncology	The branch of medicine concerned with the treatment and care of patients with cancer.
Ophthalmology	The branch of medicine concerned with the study and treatment of diseases affecting the eyes.
Opportunistic	Refers to infections and pathogens that take advantage of weakened host immune defences.
Orchitis	Swelling and/or inflammation of one or both testicles.
Osteomyelitis	Bacterial infection of the bone.
Oxygen saturation	Measures the percentage of haemoglobin that is oxygen saturated.
Pandemic	A global outbreak of infection or disease.
Paralytic ileus	Lack or absence of bowel motility and peristalsis.
Pathogenic	Capable of causing disease.
Percutaneous endoscopic gastrostomy (PEG)	An endoscopic procedure whereby an incision is made in the abdominal wall and a feeding tube is inserted.
Pericarditis	Inflammation of the pericardial sac surrounding the heart.
Peripheral neuropathy	Damage through trauma or illness/disease to the nerves outside of the brain and spinal cord.
Peristalsis	Rhythmic, wave-like and involuntary muscular contractions of the bowel wall.
Pleurisy	Inflammation of the lining of the pleural cavity surrounding the lungs.
Prodromal illness	Early symptoms of an impending illness or infection; often non-specific.
Prophylaxis	Protection against illness or disease.
Psoas	A large muscle extending from the bottom of the thoracic spine, along the lumbar spine, through the pelvis and then over the hip joint, attaching to the femur (thigh bone).
Purulent	Discharging, or causing the production of, pus.
Sarcoidosis	A chronic inflammatory condition in which granulomas (lumps) appear at various body sites, most commonly the lungs and thoracic cavity.
Scarlet fever	A highly infectious childhood disease caused by *Streptococcus pyogenes* and characterised by a rash and sore throat.
Seropositive	High levels of specific antibiotic detected in blood serum.
Serotypes	Variations amongst species.

Sigmoidoscopy	Examination of the rectum and sigmoid colon using a sigmoidoscope (a flexible tube with a light source).
Silicosis	An occupational lung disease caused by inhaling silica dust (found in sand, rocks, quarries and mines).
Sterilise, sterilisation	The complete destruction of all microorganisms, inactivating viruses, vegetative bacteria and bacterial spores (but not prions).
Stevens–Johnson syndrome	An immune complex–mediated hypersensitivity reaction involving the skin and mucous membranes.
Stoma	A surgically created artificial opening connecting part of the small bowel, the large bowel or the ureters to the skin for the passage of faeces or urine.
Synovial (fluid)	Lubricating fluid that is naturally secreted into joint cavities to prevent friction.
Systemic	System-wide.
Tachypnoea	Rapid breathing; one of the first signs seen in a deteriorating patient.
Typhus	A bacterial disease spread by lice and fleas.
Urea	A product of protein metabolism that is formed in the liver, filtered by the kidneys and excreted in the urine. Blood urea levels are used as a marker of kidney function.
Vasoconstriction	Narrowing of the blood vessels due to contraction of the blood vessel walls.
Viral hepatitis	Inflammation of the liver caused by hepatitis A.
Viriods	Small infectious agents that are smaller than viruses and cause diseases in plants.
Virulent	Extremely infectious. Used to describe a disease caused by a pathogenic organism which commonly overwhelms the immune defences of the host or spreads rapidly among individuals.
Zoonosis, zoonoses	Disease(s) spread from animals to humans (or humans to animals).

Index

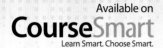
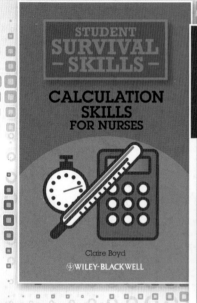
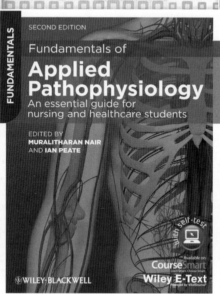
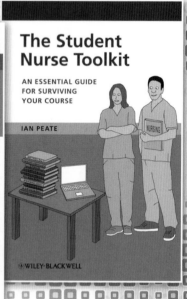